Traumatic Brain Injury

Traumatic Brain Injury

EDITED BY

Pieter E. Vos, MD, PhD

Department of Neurology
Slingeland Hospital
Doetinchem, the Netherlands

Ramon Diaz-Arrastia, MD, PhD

Center for Neuroscience and Regenerative Medicine
Uniformed Services University of the Health Sciences
Bethesda, MD, USA

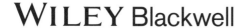

This edition first published 2015 © 2015 by John Wiley & Sons, Ltd.

Registered Office
John Wiley & Sons, Ltd, The Atrium, Southern Gate, Chichester, West Sussex, PO19 8SQ, UK

Editorial Offices
9600 Garsington Road, Oxford, OX4 2DQ, UK
The Atrium, Southern Gate, Chichester, West Sussex, PO19 8SQ, UK
111 River Street, Hoboken, NJ 07030-5774, USA

For details of our global editorial offices, for customer services and for information about how to apply for permission to reuse the copyright material in this book please see our website at www.wiley.com/wiley-blackwell

The right of the author to be identified as the author of this work has been asserted in accordance with the UK Copyright, Designs and Patents Act 1988.

Designations used by companies to distinguish their products are often claimed as trademarks. All brand names and product names used in this book are trade names, service marks, trademarks or registered trademarks of their respective owners. The publisher is not associated with any product or vendor mentioned in this book. It is sold on the understanding that the publisher is not engaged in rendering professional services. If professional advice or other expert assistance is required, the services of a competent professional should be sought.

The contents of this work are intended to further general scientific research, understanding, and discussion only and are not intended and should not be relied upon as recommending or promoting a specific method, diagnosis, or treatment by health science practitioners for any particular patient. The publisher and the author make no representations or warranties with respect to the accuracy or completeness of the contents of this work and specifically disclaim all warranties, including without limitation any implied warranties of fitness for a particular purpose. In view of ongoing research, equipment modifications, changes in governmental regulations, and the constant flow of information relating to the use of medicines, equipment, and devices, the reader is urged to review and evaluate the information provided in the package insert or instructions for each medicine, equipment, or device for, among other things, any changes in the instructions or indication of usage and for added warnings and precautions. Readers should consult with a specialist where appropriate. The fact that an organization or Website is referred to in this work as a citation and/or a potential source of further information does not mean that the author or the publisher endorses the information the organization or Website may provide or recommendations it may make. Further, readers should be aware that Internet Websites listed in this work may have changed or disappeared between when this work was written and when it is read. No warranty may be created or extended by any promotional statements for this work. Neither the publisher nor the author shall be liable for any damages arising herefrom.

Library of Congress Cataloging-in-Publication Data

Traumatic brain injury (Vos)
    Traumatic brain injury / edited by Pieter E. Vos, Ramon Diaz-Arrastia.
      p. ; cm.
    Includes bibliographical references and index.
    ISBN 978-1-4443-3770-9 (cloth)
    I. Vos, Pieter E., editor.   II. Diaz-Arrastia, Ramon, editor.   III. Title.
    [DNLM: 1. Brain Injuries–diagnosis.   2. Brain Injuries–therapy.   WL 354]
    RC387.5
    617.4′81044–dc23
                                        2014028958

A catalogue record for this book is available from the British Library.

Cover image: Drs. Carlos Marquez de la Plata and Ramon Diaz-Arrastia
Cover design by Rob Sawkins

Wiley also publishes its books in a variety of electronic formats. Some content that appears in print may not be available in electronic books.

Set in 9.5/13pt Meridien by SPi Publisher Services, Pondicherry, India
Printed and bound in Malaysia by Vivar Printing Sdn Bhd

1   2015

Contents

List of contributors

Peter S. Amenta
Department of Neurosurgery, Thomas Jefferson University Hospital,
Philadelphia, PA, USA

Philippe Azouvi
AP-HP, Department of Physical Medicine and Rehabilitation, Raymond
Poincaré Hospital, Garches, France
EA HANDIREsP Université de Versailles, Saint Quentin, France
ER 6, Université Pierre et Marie Curie, Paris, France

Rachel P. Berger
Division of Child Advocacy, Department of Pediatrics, Children's Hospital of
Pittsburgh of UPMC, University of Pittsburgh School of Medicine, Pittsburgh,
PA, USA

Peter R.G. Brink
Trauma Center, Maastricht University Medical Center, Maastricht, the
Netherlands

Ramon Diaz-Arrastia
Center for Neuroscience and Regenerative Medicine, Uniformed Services
University of the Health Sciences, Bethesda, MD, USA

Jesse R. Fann
Departments of Psychiatry and Behavioral Sciences, University of Washington,
Seattle, WA, USA
Departments of Rehabilitation Medicine, University of Washington, Seattle,
WA, USA
Departments of Epidemiology, University of Washington, Seattle, WA, USA

Jack Jallo
Department of Neurosurgery, Thomas Jefferson University Hospital,
Philadelphia, PA, USA

Kimbra Kenney
Center for Neuroscience and Regenerative Medicine, Uniformed Services
University of the Health Sciences, Bethesda, MD, USA

C. Christopher King
Department of Emergency Medicine, Albany Medical Center, Albany, NY, USA

Carlos Marquez de la Plata
Department of Behavioral and Brain Sciences, University of Texas at Dallas,
Dallas, TX, USA

Dafin F. Muresanu
Department of Neurology, University CFR Hospital, University of Medicine and
Pharmacy "Iuliu Hatieganu," Cluj-Napoca, Romania

Kathleen F. Pagulayan
VA Puget Sound Health Care System, University of Washington, Seattle, WA,
USA
Departments of Psychiatry and Behavioral Sciences, University of Washington,
Seattle, WA, USA

Lori Shutter
Departments of Neurology and Neurosurgery, University of Pittsburgh
Medical Center, Pittsburgh, PA, USA

Joke M. Spikman
Department of Neuropsychology, University Medical Center Groningen,
Groningen, the Netherlands

Luzius A. Steiner
Department of Anesthesiology, University Hospital of Basel, Switzerland

Claire Vallat-Azouvi
ER 6, Université Pierre et Marie Curie, Paris, France
Antenne UEROS and SAMSAH 92, UGECAM Ile-de-France, France

Joukje van der Naalt
Department of Neurology, University Medical Center Groningen, Groningen,
the Netherlands

Pieter E. Vos
Department of Neurology, Slingeland Hospital, Doetinchem, the Netherlands

Noel S. Zuckerbraun
Division of Pediatric Emergency Medicine, Department of Pediatrics, Children's
Hospital of Pittsburgh of UPMC, University of Pittsburgh School of Medicine,
Pittsburgh, PA, USA

Preface

The idea for this book started 10 years ago. As neurologists who had ventured beyond the traditional path in our specialty by developing an interest in traumatic head injury, we immediately developed a kinship when we met at the annual conference of Neurotrauma Society in California. Noting the progress made in emergency medicine, neurocritical care, and rehabilitation during the last decades of the 20th century, we realized that as a consequence of the increased survival of severely injured patients, traumatic brain injury (TBI) had been transformed from an acute to a much more chronic disease. We also noted that this realization had not yet permeated into the consciousness of the multiple medical specialties caring for patients with TBI. Each discipline was looking at its own part of the elephant, but not fully appreciating the whole picture. We further discussed the fact that the field was poised for further advances in emergency care, diagnostics, and therapeutics and that a multidisciplinary approach would be required for these advances to translate into improved outcomes for our patients.

Injury to the head has been ubiquitous in humans since prehistoric times and remains a common and frequently disabling feature of modern life in all societies. Partly because brain injury is so common, several concepts regarding the injury have remained hidden in plain view until recently. First, the most common causes of disability after brain injury are cognitive and neuropsychiatric. Professionals and lay persons often fail to establish a relationship between the injury and subsequent deficits and alterations in personality. Second, while most patients recover fully after a concussion, a minority does not, making mild TBI and concussion a significant public health burden, particularly individuals who sustain multiple injuries. Third, even patients who make seemingly full or very gratifying recoveries are at risk of developing delayed complications, such as epilepsy or dementia, many years later, placing substantial burdens on their families and society.

These and other reflections led to the foundation cornerstone for the book. Our aim was to explicitly discuss the many phases that the TBI patient undergoes from the time of the accident until reintegration in the society, highlighting aspects of the acute, subacute, and chronic stages. We invited physicians and investigators recognized in diverse disciplines who are involved in treating patients with head injury. We are proud and grateful that so many clinicians in spite of their busy schedule accepted our invitation and were able to both encompass discussion of the clinical aspects of the brain trauma medicine as well as the usefulness and limitations of ancillary investigations and treatment options, helping us move closer to our goal of integrating all of this expertise into a complete picture of TBI medicine.

We hope that this book attracts the attention of physicians and other professionals from all spheres of medicine with an interest in brain trauma. The book may be of interest in critical to those who have a critical role in caring for TBI victims with specialty training in neurology, neurosurgery, emergency medicine, anesthesiology, surgery, critical care medicine, physical medicine and rehabilitation, psychology, and psychiatry. The reader may read this book cover to cover. However, the book is organized in logical episodes from the accident scene, pre-hospital resuscitation, emergency department, in-hospital treatment with emphasis on intensive care, rehabilitation, and finally community reintegration. It is hoped that this approach will introduce physicians and other medical professionals involved at each level also in the challenges that face their colleagues at other stages, and facilitate the development of integrated systems of care that will optimize recovery from one of the most common human diseases.

Pieter E. Vos
Ramon Diaz-Arrastia

Acknowledgments

We would like to thank the authors who contributed chapters and discussions for this book. We are indebted to many colleagues in Europe and the USA for the many insights they have provided during clinical and scientific collaborations, which we have strived to include. We also thank our families who have been unwaveringly supportive through the peaks and valleys of careers in academic neurology. We are finally grateful to our patients for their selflessness, for their participation in scientific studies, and for allowing us to be their doctors.

PART I
Introduction and imaging

CHAPTER 1

The clinical problem of traumatic head injury

Ramon Diaz-Arrastia[1] and Pieter E. Vos[2]

[1]*Center for Neuroscience and Regenerative Medicine, Uniformed Services University of the Health Sciences, Bethesda, MD, USA*
[2]*Department of Neurology, Slingeland Hospital, Doetinchem, the Netherlands*

Introduction

Traumatic brain injury (TBI) is among the oldest and most common medical afflictions affecting humankind. A South African australopithecine skull estimated to be 3 million years old shows evidence of a lethal skull fracture administered by another early hominid [1], and injuries to the cranium are commonly found in skeletal remains of prehistoric humans. Between 10 and 50% of skulls of prehistoric humans show evidence of cranial trauma [2, 3]. Most of these injuries were a consequence of warfare, but it is also likely that many of these TBIs were accidental and occurred during hunting or otherwise interacting with a harsh environment. The advance of civilization has resulted in a dramatic decrease in interpersonal violence, as recently pointed out in an influential book by Steven Pinker of Harvard University [4], but TBI remains a common and frequently disabling feature of modern life in industrialized as well as industrializing societies.

This book is organized so that the information is maximally useful to practicing clinicians as they encounter patients with TBIs. This often starts at the site of injury, where the decision of regarding transport to an emergency department (ED) for higher-level evaluation and management is made. In cases of severe TBI, some interventions must be started in the field in order to minimize secondary injury. In the ED, the diagnostic and management algorithm is determined by the patient's level of consciousness, the extent of cranial and extracranial injuries, and findings on neuroimaging studies, usually cranial computerized tomography (CT). A subset of patients require emergent surgical treatment, and care by a neurosurgeon is often lifesaving at this stage. Subsequent to the ED (or operating theater), patients are usually cared for in the intensive care unit, where careful monitoring and interventions are aimed at lowering intracranial pressure and maximizing cerebral perfusion pressure

---

Traumatic Brain Injury, First Edition. Edited by Pieter E. Vos and Ramon Diaz-Arrastia.
© 2015 John Wiley & Sons, Ltd. Published 2015 by John Wiley & Sons, Ltd.

to minimize secondary brain injury. Neurocritical care medicine is a new and rapidly growing subspecialty of neurology and represents a fertile area of research in neurotrauma. Some patients with milder injuries are discharged from the ED with instructions to seek follow-up care in the community, while others with moderate injuries may be admitted to the general hospital ward for close observation. Upon discharge from the hospital, many patients, particularly those with moderate and severe injuries, require inpatient rehabilitation therapy, while others are sent home for outpatient rehabilitation services. The availability of rehabilitation services and specialists varies widely even in wealthy countries, and while it is generally accepted that rehabilitation treatments are valuable, research to identify optimal rehabilitative strategies is still in its infancy. Ultimately, most TBI patients attempt to reintegrate into their communities and resume their normal lives. While many can do so successfully, a substantial fraction experience disabilities that limit their ability to resume their preinjury lifestyle. During the chronic stage after injury, many patients experience long-term and sometimes delayed complications that require continued medical attention.

TBI patients encounter different physicians at each stage of the continuum of care, and while specialists from different disciplines (including emergency medicine, neurosurgery, neurology, neuroradiology, critical care medicine, rehabilitation medicine, psychiatry, and psychology) are involved at each stage, the best care is provided by medical systems that integrate and coordinate care at each stage along the continuum. Unfortunately, such integrated systems of care are rare, even in wealthy countries. This book is a small attempt to bridge that gap by introducing physicians involved at each level with the challenges that face their colleagues at other stages and to point out the needs to those involved in developing integrated systems of care for one of the most common human maladies.

Social burden of TBI
US estimates

TBI is a major cause of death and disability. In the USA alone, approximately 1.7 million sustain a TBI each year, of which 52 000 people die, and another 275 000 are hospitalized and survive [5]. High-risk age groups are those under 4, 15–19, and greater than 65. These figures do not include injury data from military, federal, and Veterans Administration hospitals. As has been the case since prehistory, military personnel are at particular risk of TBI, which reportedly occurs in approximately 15% of those involved in combat operations [6, 7]. TBI is also a common cause of long-term disability. It is estimated that in the USA, 80 000–90 000 people annually experience permanent disability associated with TBI. Currently, more that 3.2 million Americans (or 1% of the population) live with TBI-related disabilities [8]. This results in an enormous burden on patients, their families, and society. Similar data are available from other developed countries. The social burden in mid- and lower-income countries is likely even higher.

European estimates

In Europe, TBI figures are in general comparable to those in the USA. In a recent survey on the costs of brain disorders in Europe, the best available estimates of the prevalence and cost per person for 19 groups of disorders of the brain were identified via a systematic review of the published literature. An economic model was developed to estimate the mean annual costs of persons sustaining a TBI [9]. Most brain disorders have an insidious onset followed by worsening and often chronic symptoms, and for such conditions, the most reliable epidemiologic data constitute prevalence estimates derived from community-based samples. However, TBI differs from other disorders in that their onset is sudden and followed by an intensive period of care followed by rehabilitation and potentially cure. For TBI, incidence rates are mainly available and the cost of patients during a period following disease onset. In the European study, also estimates on the cost of patients suffering from the long-term consequences of TBI were included as an approximation of the costs for patients with a previous onset of disease. The identified cost of TBI studies presented the mean indirect cost of the whole population, including also the zero estimates of patients not working because of other causes than the disorder (e.g., being underage or retired). The economic model was designed to estimate the number and costs of persons in acute trauma care, in rehabilitation, or suffering from the long-term consequences of a previous TBI. We assumed a time horizon of 20 years divided into three phases: acute (first 6 months following the injury), rehabilitation (the following 18 months), and finally a long-term phase. The cost estimate of TBI based on separate estimates for each severity (mild, moderate, and severe TBI) for 2010 was 33.0 billion €PPP [9].

The problem of mild TBI

TBI is usually classified as mild, moderate, and severe, based on the initial Glasgow Coma Score (GCS) recorded in the ED. Severe TBI is defined by a score between 3 and 8, moderate TBI by GCS between 9 and 12, and mild TBI (mTBI) by GCS 13 and 15 [10]. Although it is recognized that this classification scheme has a lot of limitations [11], it has been universally utilized in clinical practice as well as in clinical research. Although severe TBI has been the primary focus of investigation over the past 30 years [12], mTBI is at least 10-fold more prevalent [13, 14]. While the likelihood of favorable recovery is higher in mTBI compared to moderate and severe TBI, many patients with mTBI are left with disabilities that impair their ability to fulfill their work, school, or family responsibilities. It is likely that the social burden resulting from mTBI is at least equivalent to that resulting from severe TBI, given its much higher prevalence [13]. Using incidence and cost data from 1985, Max *et al.* [15] concluded that 44% of the total lifetime costs associated with TBI were due to mTBI. Since this study did not consider the costs of lost productivity and reduced quality of life, as well as indirect costs borne by family and others, it is likely to be an underestimate of the true societal burden of mTBI.

Mild TBI has been relatively understudied for several reasons. First, most mTBI patients make a seemingly complete recovery, and early identification of mTBI patients who are most likely to suffer persistent symptoms and develop cognitive and neuropsychological deficits is difficult. Second, since mortality and functional dependence on others are relatively rare in mTBI, the outcome assessments that are traditionally used for severe TBI are insufficiently sensitive for the type of cognitive and behavioral disabilities that most commonly result from mTBI [12]. The cognitive and psychiatric consequences of TBI are often nonspecific and overlap with conditions such as developmental, behavioral, mood and thought disorders, and dementia. Further, many of the long-term consequences of TBI manifest years after the trauma and may not be ascribed to the brain injury from which there was an apparently initial complete recovery. For example, TBI early in the preschool years may alter the developmental potential of the young brain and result in problems that only manifest during adolescence and young adulthood, such as substance abuse disorders, mood disorders, and conduct disorders [16]. Similarly, there is an increased risk of late-life dementia in individuals who suffered a TBI in early to midlife, even after an apparent initial complete recovery [17].

TBI as a chronic, lifelong condition

TBI has traditionally been conceptualized as an event, from which there is either complete or incomplete recovery, and that once recovery has plateaued, whatever residual deficits remain have been assumed to be stable. Recently, it has been recognized that TBI is best conceptualized as a lifelong chronic health condition, which begins at the time of the injury but has chronic effects that persist for life and, in many cases, manifest only after a latency of several to many years [18, 19]. These chronic health effects merit careful monitoring and continued therapeutic interventions.

It has long been recognized that neurological disorders such as posttraumatic epilepsy are a consequence of TBI, which may manifest years after the injury [20, 21]. This is a direct evidence for the fact that traumatic insults trigger synaptic plasticity and circuit rewiring that persists for months and years and is likely lifelong. This plasticity is usually beneficial and allows for repair and recovery but, in some cases, results in a maladaptive neural circuit. Other neurological disorders such as Alzheimer's disease, Parkinson's disease, and chronic traumatic encephalopathy are also well-recognized long-term sequelae of neurotrauma [22]. Disorders of the hypothalamic–pituitary axis are noted in up to 30% of survivors of moderate and severe TBI [23] and can have protean long-term consequences, including sleep disorders [24]. As a consequence of these and perhaps other chronic health conditions, individuals who experience moderate-to-severe TBIs have a reduction in life expectancy of approximately 4–7 years [25, 26].

Patients who survive more than 1 year after moderate-to-severe TBI are 37 times more likely to die from seizures, 12 times more likely to die from septicemia, and 4 times more likely to die from pneumonia than a matched control group from the general population [27].

Paucity of specific therapies for TBI

The high social burden resulting from TBI has led to extensive preclinical studies and numerous clinical trials aimed at developing therapies to improve functional outcome [12]. In animal models, therapeutic interventions aimed at modulating molecular pathways identified to be induced after TBI have been successful in limiting the extent of injury and improving neurologic recovery [28–30]. These experimental observations constitute a convincing proof of the principle that opportunity exists for therapeutic interventions. However, phase III clinical trials of several of these therapies in patients with severe brain injuries have failed to demonstrate efficacy [31]. It is likely that one of the main reasons for this failure to translate therapies from the lab to the bedside is the heterogeneity of TBI [32]. Not all is bleak, however. A retrospective review of neurosurgical databases in the USA found that mortality from severe TBI declined from 39 to 27% from 1984 to 1996 [33]. Most of this remarkable improvement is due to advances in supportive care and the development of specialized neurocritical care units.

Pharmacologic interventions targeting repair, regeneration, and protection after TBI are particularly lacking. Drug development for TBI has traditionally focused on limiting secondary brain injury after the initial traumatic event, based on the belief that the capacity of the central nervous system for repair and regeneration was limited. New evidence now indicates that the adult brain has substantial regenerative capacity, and repair and regeneration processes can be activated or enhanced by pharmacologic and nonpharmacologic treatment. Brain repair mechanisms that are potential therapeutic targets include angiogenesis, axon guidance and remodeling, remyelination, neurogenesis, and synaptogenesis. Pharmacologic interventions supporting regeneration and repair may have a longer therapeutic window than pharmacologic interventions designed to limit injury, and they are also potentially effective in the acute, subacute, postacute, and chronic phases after TBI. Thus, repair and regeneration therapies have the potential advantage of being effective over a prolonged period of time following TBI.

Pharmacologic interventions designed to treat the persistent symptoms associated with the chronic stage of TBI (e.g., memory disturbances, depression, headache) are widely used off-label by clinicians. These usually include pharmacotherapies aimed at modulating the dopaminergic, noradrenergic, serotonergic, glutamatergic, and cholinergic systems. However, strong evidence for their efficacy and safety is lacking. As a result, the selection of drug for individual patients, or drug dose and duration, is empirical and highly variable among health systems. Clinical trials are needed to assess the efficacy and toxicity of these pharmacologic interventions.

Finally, it is likely that combination therapy will ultimately be required to promote maximal recovery and optimize outcome after TBI. Because TBI damages the brain by multiple mechanisms, combination therapy designed to simultaneously target multiple mechanisms of injury will likely be required. Pharmacotherapy that blocks downstream cellular and molecular mechanisms in the brain combined with pharmacotherapy that targets symptoms resulting from TBI may provide one reasonable strategy. Thus, drug combinations have the potential of having a larger therapeutic efficacy than that of individual drugs. Additionally, nonpharmacologic therapies such as exercise and physical and occupational therapies may also facilitate repair and regeneration. It is likely that the combination of pharmacologic and nonpharmacologic therapies may ultimately prove most successful.

Classifying a multidimensional process

Multiple paradigms exist for classifying TBI, including classification by injury severity, mechanism, pathoanatomy, and pathophysiology. The most widely used classification is by injury severity and is based on factors such as the neurological exam (usually operationalized through the Glasgow Coma Scale) and the duration of loss of consciousness and posttraumatic amnesia [34]. However, it is well recognized that such measures provide only a one-dimensional view and are of limited utility for guiding therapy and prognostic counseling.

A pathoanatomic classification, guided by neuroimaging findings, provides additional valuable information. TBI can result from either focal or diffuse insults, though both patterns may exist in a given patient to varying degrees. Focal injuries result from force directly transmitted to the head upon contact and include skull fractures, extra-axial hemorrhage (epidural or subdural), contusions, lacerations, and focal vascular injuries that produce strokes. Diffuse injuries result from acceleration/deceleration of the head and are characterized by diffuse axonal injury, traumatic subarachnoid hemorrhage, traumatic vascular injury, inflammation, and neuroendocrine dysfunction. Neuroimaging with cranial CT scanning is excellent at detecting focal injuries, but poor at detecting diffuse injuries. Magnetic resonance imaging (MRI) is superior to CT, particularly for identifying diffuse injuries. A single patient, particularly one with injury in the severe end of the spectrum, may manifest both focal and diffuse injuries and multiple pathoanatomic types of each. Recent emphasis has been placed on multidimensional classification, encompassing severity as well as pathoanatomic characteristics that likely have pathophysiologic mechanisms in common. Such schemes, based heavily on patterns seen on neuroimaging studies, hold promise that such an understanding will lead to the development of targeted and more effective therapies [35].

It is also clear that demographic factors such as age, gender, and possibly genetic background play an important role in the response of neural tissue to traumatic injury and will have to be considered when selecting therapeutic strategies. An equivalent mechanical force is likely to result in a more severe and pathoanatomically complex injury in an infant or older person than in an adolescent or young adult, and the long-term consequences of such an injury will also likely differ.

Understanding the endophenotypes of TBI

The term endophenotype, initially coined in the field of psychiatric genetics [36, 37], refers to internal phenotypes discoverable by biochemical, physiological, radiological, pathological, or other techniques, which are intermediate between a complex phenotype and the presumptive genetic or environmental contribution to the complex disease. Discovering the genetic and environmental factors contributing to complex human diseases, as well as developing effective therapies for them, often requires understanding the endophenotypes of the disease. For example, the discovery of genetic factors contributing to coronary artery disease [38] and the eventual development of effective therapies based on HMG-CoA reductase inhibition was made possible by understanding the endophenotype of hypercholesterolemia, which is measurable through a simple blood test. It is likely that the development of effective therapies for TBI will require a thorough understanding of endophenotypes discoverable through methods such as MRI, biochemical assays of biomarkers in blood or cerebrospinal fluid, electroencephalography or other physiologic techniques, and neuropathology. Although this work is in its infancy, preliminary observations are starting to point out the broad outlines of the endophenotypes of TBI.

Such TBI endophenotypes may be represented by a vector-based scheme (see Figure 1.1, modified from Saatman *et al.* [35]). Each measured endophenotype can be represented by a single vector, with the magnitude of the vector representing deviation from normal. Vectors can be arranged radially about a central point representing normal, and the angle between each vector represents the correlation between each measure. For example, endophenotypes that are highly correlated with each other are represented by vectors at small (acute) angles, while those that are not correlated are represented by vectors orthogonal to each other. The surface area mapped out by the vectors represents injury severity, and the shape reflects heterogeneity. Additionally, multivariate statistical analysis can facilitate transformation of univariate statistical relations to multivariate representations, such as path diagrams that convey cause and effect. Improved characterization of data sets via multivariate statistical analysis could also guide the design of testing parameters, thereby enhancing applicability of results and increasing efficiency of bench-to-bedside translation.

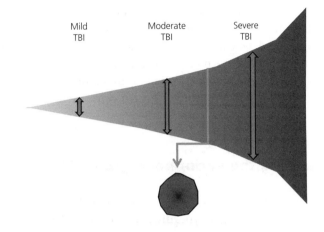

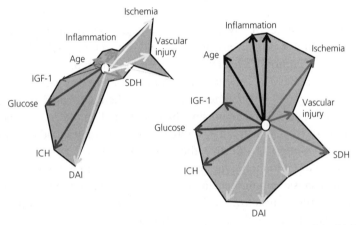

Figure 1.1 Multiple vector-based analytical scheme. Tensor representations of the high-dimensional data associated with TBI may improve classification and guide therapeutic interventions, as has been demonstrated in other field such as oncology. Patient B is shown to have greater injury severity than Patient A, reflected by the greater area of the shape determined by the degree to which vector components deviate from normal (the central point) (Adapted from Saatman *et al.* [32]).

Conclusion

TBI is one of the most common medical afflictions affecting mankind, and since it often affects children and young adults and interrupts their education, social, and professional development, its impact on society is disproportionate. Despite much progress over the past decades, much remains to be done. Recent advances in neuroimaging and in understanding the biochemistry and physiology of neurotrauma hold much promise for improved diagnosis, better understanding of endophenotypes, and identification of the most therapies. Success will ultimately require collaborations between medical and nonmedical specialists from various disciplines and the development of integrated systems of care.

References

1 Dart, R.A. (1949) The predatory implemental technique of Australopithecus. *Journal of Physical Anthropology*, **7**, 1–38.

2 Tung, T.A. (2007) Trauma and violence in the Wari empire of the Peruvian Andes: warfare, raids, and ritual fights. *American Journal of Physical Anthropology*, **133**, 941–956.

3 Torres-Rouff, C. & Costa Junqueira, M.A. (2006) Interpersonal violence in prehistoric San Pedro de Atacama, Chile: behavioral implications of environmental stress. *American Journal of Physical Anthropology*, **130**, 60–70.

4 Pinker, S. (2011) *The Better Angels of Our Nature: Why Violence Has Declined*. Viking Books, New York.

5 Faul M., Xu, L., Wald, M.W., & Coronado, V.G. (2010) *Traumatic Brain Injury in the United States: Emergency Department Visits, Hospitalizations, and Deaths 2002–2006*. Centers for Disease Control and Prevention, National Center for Injury Prevention and Control, Atlanta, GA, pp. 1–71.

6 Hoge, C.W., McGurk, D., Thomas, J.L., Cox, A.L., Engel, C.C., & Castro, C.A. (2008) Mild traumatic brain injury in U.S. Soldiers returning from Iraq. *New England Journal of Medicine*, **358**, 453–463.

7 Schneiderman, A.I., Braver, E.R., & Kang, H.K. (2008) Understanding sequelae of injury mechanisms and mild traumatic brain injury incurred during the conflicts in Iraq and Afghanistan: persistent postconcussive symptoms and posttraumatic stress disorder. *American Journal of Epidemiology*, **167**, 1446–1452.

8 Zaloshnja, E., Miller, T., Langlois, J.A., & Selassie, A.W. (2008) Prevalence of long-term disability from traumatic brain injury in the civilian population of the United States, 2005. *The Journal of Head Trauma Rehabilitation*, **23**, 394–400.

9 Gustavsson, A., Svensson, M., Jacobi, F., *et al.* (2011) Cost of disorders of the brain in Europe 2010. *European Neuropsychopharmacology*, **21**, 718–779.

10 Stein, S.C. (1996) Classification of head injury. In: R. K. Narayan, J. T. Povlishock, & J. E. Wilberger (eds), *Neurotrauma*, pp. 31–42. McGraw Hill, New York.

11 Thurman, D.J., Coronado, V., & Selassie, A. (2007) The epidemiology of TBI: implications for public health. In: N. D. Zasler, D. I. Katz, & R. D. Zafonte (eds), *Brain Injury Medicine: Principles and Practice*, pp. 45–55. Demos, New York.

12 Narayan, R.K. & Michel, M.E.; The Clinical Trials in Head Injury Study Group (2002) Clinical trials in head injury. *Journal of Neurotrauma*, **19**, 503–557.

13 National Center for Injury Prevention (2003). *Report to Congress on Mild Traumatic Brain Injury in the United States: Steps to Prevent a Serious Public Health Problem*. Centers for Disease Control and Prevention, Atlanta, GA.

14 Bazarian, J.J., McClung, J., Shah, M.N., Cheng, Y.T., Flesher, W., & Kraus, J. (2005) Mild traumatic brain injury in the United States, 1998–2000. *Brain Injury*, **19**, 85–91.

15 Max, W., MacKenzie, E.J., & Rice, D.P. (1991) Head injuries: costs and consequences. *The Journal of Head Trauma Rehabilitation*, **6**, 76–91.

16 McKinlay, A., Grace, R., Horwood, J., Fergusson, D., & MacFarlane, M. (2009) Adolescent psychiatric symptoms following preschool childhood mild traumatic brain injury: evidence from a birth cohort. *The Journal of Head Trauma Rehabilitation*, **24**, 221–227.

17 Shively, S., Scher, A.I., Perl, D.P., & Diaz-Arrastia, R. (2012) dementia resulting from traumatic brain injury: what is the pathology? *Archives of Neurology*, **69**, 1245–1251.

18 Masel, B.E. & Dewitt, D.S. (2010). Traumatic brain injury: a disease process, not an event. *Journal of Neurotrauma*, **27**, 1529–1540.

19 Corrigan, J.D. & Hammond, F.M. (2013). Traumatic brain injury as a chronic health condition. *Archives of Physical Medicine and Rehabilitation*, **94**, 1199–1201.

20 Diaz-Arrastia, R., Agostini, M.A., Madden, C.J., & Van Ness, P.C. (2009) Posttraumatic epilepsy: the endophenotypes of a human model of epileptogenesis. *Epilepsia*, **50** (Suppl 2), 14–20.

21 Annegers, J.F., Hauser, W.A., Coan, S.P., & Rocca, W.A. (1998) A population-based study of seizures after traumatic brain injuries. *The New England Journal of Medicine*, **338**, 20–24.

22 Institute of Medicine Committee on Gulf War and Health (2009) Neurologic outcomes. In: Institute of Medicine (ed), *Gulf War and Health. Volume 7. Long-Term Consequences of Traumatic Brain Injury*, pp. 197–264. National Academies Press, Washington, DC.

23 Schneider, H.J., Kreitschmann-Andermahr, I., Ghigo, E., Stalla, G.K., & Agha, A. (2007) Hypothalamopituitary dysfunction following traumatic brain injury and aneurysmal sub-arachnoid hemorrhage: a systematic review. *The Journal of the Medical Association*, **298**, 1429–1438.

24 Masel, B.E., Scheibel, R.S., Kimbark, T., & Kuna, S.T. (2001) Excessive daytime sleepiness in adults with brain injuries. *Archives of Physical Medicine Rehabilitation*, **82**, 1526–1532.

25 Harrison-Felix, C., Whiteneck, G., Devivo, M., Hammond, F.M., & Jha, A. (2004) Mortality following rehabilitation in the Traumatic Brain Injury Model Systems of Care. *NeuroRehabilitation*, **19**, 45–54.

26 Harrison-Felix, C.L., Whiteneck, G.G., Jha, A., DeVivo, M.J., Hammond, F.M., & Hart, D.M. (2009) Mortality over four decades after traumatic brain injury rehabilitation: a retrospective cohort study. *Archives of Physical Medicine Rehabilitation*, **90**, 1506–1513.

27 Harrison-Felix, C., Whiteneck, G., DeVivo, M.J., Hammond, F.M., & Jha, A. (2006) Causes of death following 1 year postinjury among individuals with traumatic brain injury. *The Journal of Head Trauma Rehabilitation*, **21**, 22–33.

28 McIntosh, T.K. (1993) Novel pharmacologic therapies in the treatment of experimental brain injury: a review. *Journal of Neurotrauma*, **10**, 215–261.

29 McIntosh, T.K., Juhler, M., & Wieloch, T. (1998) Novel pharmacologic strategies in the treatment of experimental brain injury: 1998. *Journal of Neurotrauma*, **15**, 731–769.

30 Marklund, N., Bakshi, A., Castelbuono, D.J., Conte, V., & McIntosh, T.K. (2006) Evaluation of pharmacological treatment strategies in traumatic brain injury. *Current Pharmaceutical Design*, **12**, 1645–1680.

31 Doppenberg, E.M.R. & Bullock, R. (1997). Clinical neuroprotective trials in severe traumatic brain injury: lessons from previous studies. *Journal of Neurotrauma*, **14**, 71–80.

32 Saatman, K.E., Duhaime, A.C., Bullock, R., Maas, A.I., Valadka, A., & Manley, G.T. (2008) Classification of traumatic brain injury for targeted therapies. *Journal of Neurotrauma*, **25**, 719–738.

33 Lu, J., Marmarou, A., Choi, S., Maas, A., Murray, G., & Steyerberg, E.W. (2005) Mortality from traumatic brain injury. *Acta Neurochirurgica*, **95** (Suppl), 281–285.

34 Menon, D.K., Schwab, K., Wright, D.W., & Maas, A.I. (2010) Position statement: definition of traumatic brain injury. *Archives of Physical Medicine and Rehabilitation*, **91**, 1637–1640.

35 Stahl, R., Dietrich, O., Teipel, S.J., Hampel, H., Reiser, M.F., & Schoenberg, S.O. (2007) White matter damage in Alzheimer disease and mild cognitive impairment: assessment with diffusion-tensor MR imaging and parallel imaging techniques. *Radiology*, **243**, 483–492.

36 Gottesman, I.I. & Shields, J. (1973) Genetic theorizing and schizophrenia. *The British Journal of Psychiatry*, **122**, 15–30.

37 Gottesman, I.I. & Gould, T.D. (2003) The endophenotype concept in psychiatry: etymology and strategic intentions. *The American Journal Psychiatry*, **160**, 636–645.

38 Brown, M.S. & Goldstein, J.L. (1986) A receptor-mediated pathway for cholesterol homeostasis. *Science*, **232**, 34–47.

CHAPTER 2

Neuroimaging in traumatic brain injury

Pieter E. Vos[1], Carlos Marquez de la Plata[2], and Ramon Diaz-Arrastia[3]

[1]Department of Neurology, Slingeland Hospital, Doetinchem, the Netherlands
[2]Department of Behavioral and Brain Sciences, University of Texas at Dallas, Dallas, TX, USA
[3]Center for Neuroscience and Regenerative Medicine, Uniformed Services University of the Health Sciences, Bethesda, MD, USA

Cranial computed tomography

Computed tomography (CT) scanning of the head is the principal diagnostic tool to demonstrate brain damage in TBI [1]. Since its introduction in the 1970s, it has revolutionized the management of TBI and has doubtlessly saved many lives. The primary use of cranial CT scanning is to detect life-threatening traumatic intracranial abnormalities that require immediate neurosurgical intervention or admission to an intensive care unit for careful monitoring of neurologic status. CT is sensitive and specific in detecting skull fractures, intracranial hemorrhages (subdural hematomas, epidural hematomas, traumatic subarachnoid or intraventricular hemorrhages, and parenchymal contusions) (see Table 2.1, Figure 2.1). CT is also able to detect local or diffuse brain edema, which can be identified as areas of hypodensity or indirectly by findings such as effacement of cortical sulci, disappearance of the normal gray–white matter demarcation, midline shift, or effacement of basal cisterns (see Figure 2.1). Approximately 10% of patients with severe TBI require a craniectomy based on the findings from an initial CT scan. According to the Brain Trauma Foundation guidelines, these findings include extra-axial hematomas larger than 30 mL in size or associated with greater than 5 mm of midline shift and parenchymal hematomas in a noneloquent cortex greater than 20 mL in size [1]. Patients in whom the original CT scan shows small- or moderate-sized parenchymal hematomas, traumatic subarachnoid hemorrhage, or extra-axial hemorrhages (subdural or epidural hematomas) are admitted to the hospital and usually rescanned within 24 h or sooner if there is a deterioration of neurologic status, as clinically significant expansion of intracranial hematomas is common [1].

In mild-to-moderate brain injury, CT is useful in identifying traumatic lesions that may affect clinical management such as small hematomas that may

Traumatic Brain Injury, First Edition. Edited by Pieter E. Vos and Ramon Diaz-Arrastia.
© 2015 John Wiley & Sons, Ltd. Published 2015 by John Wiley & Sons, Ltd.

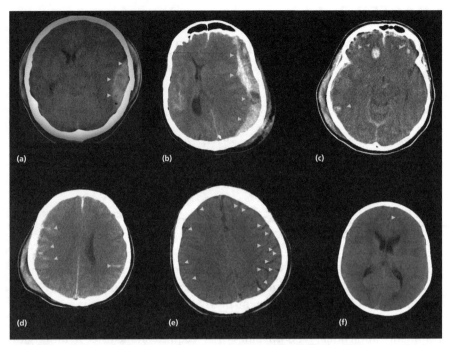

Figure 2.1 Intracranial traumatic lesions. (a) Left epidural hematoma and skull fracture. (b) Left subdural hematoma. (c) Bifrontal intraparenchymal contusions. Right intraparenchymal temporal contusion. (d) Bilateral traumatic cortical subarachnoid hemorrhage. (e) Right-sided edema. Effacement of cortical sulci on the right side as compared to the left. (f) Punctate hemorrhage at frontal gray–white matter interface (may indicate DAI).

subsequently expand or traumatic subarachnoid or intraventricular hemorrhages that may result in posttraumatic hydrocephalus [2–4, 7]. However, CT findings relate poorly to long-term outcome in mild TBI (mTBI). In mTBI, the abnormalities identified by acute CT are not associated with long-term functional outcome [8]. Approximately 10% of patients who sustain mTBI with no significant abnormalities on the acute CT have significant problems returning to work [9]. An explanation for this inability to predict outcome may be the insensitivity of CT to detect the diffuse microstructural white matter damage that is characteristic of diffuse axonal injury (DAI) or its failure to identify deficits in cerebral perfusion or cerebrovascular reactivity [9].

This chapter will introduce a systematic approach in the reading of CT, to assist the clinician in recognizing parameters that adversely affect outcome, ascertaining optimal treatment, making clinical decisions, and estimating prognosis. In addition, validated scales for rating CT scans like the Trauma Coma Data Bank (TCDB) classification or Rotterdam CT score, which are helpful in clinical research as well as for stratifying participants by injury severity, will be introduced [2–4]. Although positron emission tomography and technetium-99m-hexa-methyl propylene amine oxime single-photon emission computed tomography (SPECT) may sometimes show abnormalities in the acute and

Table 2.1 Systematic approach to describe CT findings after TBI.

Extracranial	Look for	Describe anatomical position
Skin	Laceration	Frontal
	Contusion	Temporal
		Parietal
		Occipital
Cranium		
Bone (in bone setting)	Skull fracture	Frontal
	Depressed skull fracture	Temporal
	Basal skull fracture	Parietal
		Occipital
Facial	Frontal bone, nasal, orbital, maxilla, zygoma, mandibula	
Sinuses	Frontal, maxillaris, sphenoidalis	
Intracranial		
Extracerebral	Epidural	Side and site
	Subdural	
	Subarachnoid	
	Intraventricular	
Intracerebral		
Gray matter	Cortical Contusion	Coup
		Contre coup
	Cortical edema	Efficacement of sulci
		Fading of gray–white matter difference
	Subcortical contusion	
White matter	Frontal, CC	
	DAI (punctate hemorrhage <15 mm in diameter)	Gray–white matter interface
		Internal capsule/CC
		Mesencephalon
		Pons
Ventricles	Lateral	Present
	Third	Compressed
	Fourth	Absent
		Blood
Cisterns	Sylvii	Present
	Suprasellar	Compressed
	Ambient/quadrigemina	Absent
	Prepontine	
Shift	At the level of septum pellucidum	Left–right
Herniation pneumocephalus	Falx	
	Diencephalic	
	Temporal/uncal tonsillar	

chronic stages when CT or magnetic resonance imaging (MRI) and neurological examination do not show damage, we will consider these and other imaging modalities like magnetic resonance spectroscopy beyond the scope of this book.

How to read the CT?

Because immediate and accurate recognition of intracranial emergencies on head CT is vital to initiate proper treatment, a formalized systematic approach to interpretation of head CTs is useful. In 1998, *Perron et al.* proposed a mnemonic "*Blood Can Be Very Bad*" [10]. The use of this mnemonic resulted in a significant improvement in the accuracy rate of CT interpretation by emergency residents. *B* stands for *blood* to remind examiners to search for intracranial hematomas, *C* stands for the appearance of the four key *cisterns*, *B* stands for *brain* to check sulcal patterns and evidence of midline shift, *V* prompts reviewing the four *ventricles*, and finally, *B* is a reminder to assess the bones of the cranium (see Figures 2.1–2.4). As a general

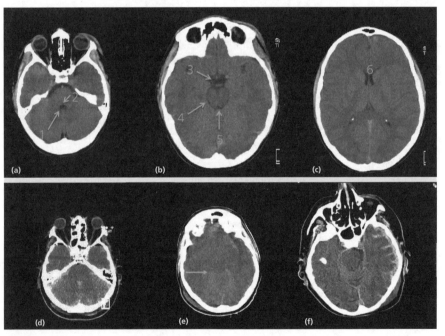

Figure 2.2 (a) Normal CT scan of the head in a 46-year-old patient suffering from a mild TBI. 1. Fourth ventricle, 2. prepontine cistern; (b) normal CT, 3. pentagon (suprasellar) cistern, 4. right ambient cistern, 5. quadrigeminal cistern (lower part); (c) normal CT, 6. at the level of the lateral ventricles and septum pellucidum; (d) subtentorial brain swelling and herniation. Fourth ventricle and prepontine cistern compressed. (e) Diffuse brain swelling and shift. Basal cisterns not visible. (f) Left-sided subdural hematoma, subarachnoid hemorrhage, and right-sided shift of the brainstem due to herniation. Contralateral compression and ipsilateral (left side) widening of cisterna ambiens.

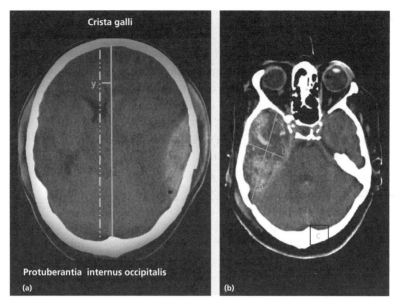

Figure 2.3 (a) Shift is measured at the level of the septum pellucidum. Right line is the middle line between the crista galli and the protuberantia internus occipitalis. y is the shift measured as the distance between the line through the septum pellucidum and the interhemispheric line. (b) Volume measurement of traumatic intracranial lesions. Right temporal contusion. Volume can be assessed with the formula: **volume = 4/3 π × 0.5 a × 0.5 b × 0.5 c = 0.52 × a × b × c.** a = largest diameter of the contusion zone (in cm), b = largest diameter perpendicular to a (in cm), c = number of slices of the contusion zone times slice thickness (in cm).

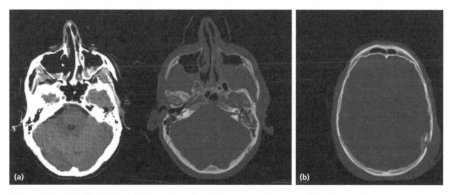

Figure 2.4 (a) Left-sided skull base fracture: left, normal setting; right, bone CT setting. (b) Bone setting left temporoparietal depressed skull fracture.

guide, use of the mnemonic can be useful to systematically approach the CT. Nevertheless, other specific issues must be taken into account in relation to traumatic lesions.

Blood: Lesion volume

A wide variety of threshold values for hematoma volume, ranging from 5 to 150 mL, have been proposed to ascertain the relationship between hematoma size and outcome [11, 13–15]. Internationally acknowledged injury severity models use different cutoff values to classify trauma victims with multiple (systemic) injuries or isolated head injuries (see Figure 2.3). The Abbreviated Injury Scale (AIS) and the Injury Severity Score both use threshold values of 15, 30, and 50 mL to estimate decreasing probabilities of survival after TBI (Table 2.1) [11, 16]. Reevaluation of 13 962 patients in a large European trauma registry between 2001 and 2008 with a GCS less than 15 at presentation or any head injury with AIS severity code 3 and above demonstrated that large compared to small epidural, subdural, and intraparenchymal hematomas are associated with a substantially higher probability of hospital mortality (Table 2.1) [17]. Although the use of threshold values can support clinical decisions, using lesion volume as continuous variable in prognostic models has been recommended recently [15].

Brain: Shift

A linear relationship between midline shift, measured at the level of the septum pellucidum, and outcome exists in patients with severe TBI [5, 18] (see Figure 2.3). Cutoffs ranging from 3.0 to 20.0 mm have been tested for their association with outcome. Prognosis is worse in the presence of shift above various cutoff values (reviewed in reference [15]). The TCDB CT classification uses a shift cutoff value of 5 mm (Table 2.1) [3].

Basal cisterns

One of the most prominent CT characteristics and a powerful predictor of outcome is the status of the basal cisterns. The term *perimesencephalic cisterns* is frequently used to denote the basal cisterns (see Figure 2.1). However, no clear definition exists to anatomically delineate the basal cisterns [11]. Complete and partially obliterated basal cisterns are a sign of raised intracranial pressure [12] (see Figure 2.2). Basal cisterns' compression results in a two- to fourfold increase in mortality or unfavorable outcome compared to normal visibility of the basal cisterns [12–14]. Regarding the aspect of the distinct compartments of the basal cisterns, systematic evaluation of the predictive value of the individual cisterns has been performed by our group, demonstrating that absence (complete obliteration) or compression of both the ambient cisterns and the fourth ventricle is independently related to unfavorable outcome and death [20]. The assessment of the ambient cisterns and the fourth ventricle has satisfactory inter- and intrarater reliabilities (kappa coefficients: 0.80–0.95).

Ventricles

The predictive value of compression of the cerebral ventricles (lateral, third, fourth) in TBI has not been as extensively studied as effacement of basal or perimesencephalic cisterns. Obliteration of the third ventricle is associated with raised ICP and adverse outcome after severe TBI [21, 22] and an independent prognostic variable in a multivariate predictive model of TBI [23]. Small or asymmetrical lateral ventricles are probably not related to outcome [13]. Determining the presence or absence of the status of ventricles on CT by visual inspection is susceptible to interobserver variation. Inter- and intrarater variability for the lateral and third ventricles have not been studied. We found a satisfactory inter- and intrarater reliability of the fourth ventricle. The interrater kappa coefficients of the status of the fourth ventricle were 0.93 (normal vs. abnormal) and 0.95 (normal, compressed, or absent) [20]. The intrarater kappa coefficients of the fourth ventricle score (normal vs. abnormal) were 0.89 and for the three-point scale (normal, compressed, or absent) 0.80. Obliteration of the fourth ventricle and foramen magnum indicates a bad prognosis from the presence of infratentorial brain swelling, a cerebellar mass lesion, or an end stage of progressive vertical brain herniation.

Bone

X-skull radiography and echo were the primary diagnostic tools in the detection of intracranial abnormalities before the introduction of the CT in 1972. X-skull is in particular sensitive to detect fractures. Fractures were then noted as indicators of an increased chance for the presence of intracranial hematoma. The diagnostic value of plain skull radiography as an indirect indicator of the presence of hematoma decreased since the introduction of the CT. Compared with X-skull radiography, CT is also excellent at demonstrating depressed or comminuted skull fractures. Only fractures parallel to the plane of the scan slice such as those involving the vertex of the skull are sometimes missed. CT is also sensitive in visualizing facial fractures and skull base fractures. The importance of detecting skull fractures in TBI is related to (i) an increased risk of cerebrospinal fluid (CSF) leakage and CSF fistula formation after a skull base or temporal bone fracture or open fracture [23], (ii) increased odds for developing meningitis in the presence of a skull base fracture, and (iii) a growing skull fracture in children. Of note, to evaluate the presence of a fracture (skull, facial, skull base), a different *window* setting is used from the settings to highlight soft tissue or blood or brain parenchyma (see Figure 2.4).

Trauma Coma Data Bank classification

In 1991, a CT scan classification of head injury including four categories of diffuse injury and two surgical mass lesion categories was developed by the TCDB study [3]. This CT classification was the first official system to categorize intracranial injury after moderate and severe TBI in a systematic way and to discriminate between diffuse injury and mass lesions. Four categories indicate diffuse injury of increasing severity, whereas two categories indicate the presence of a mass lesion [3]. The TCDB CT classification categorizes TBI patients into six groups. The primary distinction is made between diffuse injury (categories I–IV) and the presence of mass lesions (evacuated or nonevacuated) (Table 2.2).

A strong association exists between outcome and the initial CT scan diagnosis according to the TCDB CT classification. The TCDB classification (also known as the Marshall classification, after its first author) is widely used in research trials and prognostic studies of moderate and severe TBI to characterize and categorize patients.

The TCDB classification is a composite score of certain individual aspects of the CT evaluation: the mesencephalic cisterns, the degree of midline shift in millimeters, and the volume of intracerebral or extracerebral hematoma [3]. Recent prognostic models based on large international patient cohorts confirmed that the type of intracranial lesion and intracranial hematoma size, effacement of cisterns, and shift of the cerebral midline structures are strong outcome predictors [6, 19, 23]. Controversy remains about how best to combine these parameters into a prognostic scheme, and whether to use threshold values or continuous variables.

Table 2.2 Traumatic Coma Data Bank CT (Marshall) classification for traumatic brain injury.

Category	Definition
Diffuse injury I	No visible intracranial pathology
Diffuse injury II	Cisterns are present with midline shift 0–5 mm and/or lesion densities present, no high- or mixed-density lesions ≥ 25 mL
Diffuse injury III	Cisterns compressed or absent, with midline shift 0–5 mm, no high- or mixed-density lesions ≥ 25 mL
Diffuse injury IV	Midline shift > 5 mm, no high- or mixed-density lesion ≥ 25 mL
Evacuated mass lesion (V)	Any lesion surgically evacuated
Nonevacuated mass lesion (VI)	High- or mixed-density lesion ≥ 25 mL, not surgically evacuated

While the predictive value of the TCDB CT classification has been confirmed in several studies, there are several limitations that have led to efforts to develop new classification schemes. The TCDB classification does not take into account the presence of traumatic subarachnoid hemorrhage, which is found in 23–63% of patients with severe TBI [24]. Proposals for adding subarachnoid hemorrhage in CT classification systems to enhance the predictive power on outcome appeared in the 1990s [24, 25]. Moreover, the TCDB classification does not recognize the difference between subdural and epidural hematomas. This forms a significant limitation given the more favorable prognosis associated with epidural hematomas. Finally, the TCDB classification can be improved by combining categories V and VI that assess the volume of any mass lesion [26].

The Rotterdam CT score

The Rotterdam CT score demonstrated that discrimination can be further improved by adding intraventricular and traumatic subarachnoid hemorrhage and by a more detailed differentiation of mass lesions and basal cisterns and taking into account the presence of epidural hematoma (Table 2.3) [5]. Several prognostic models have now demonstrated superior prediction of the Rotterdam CT score over the TCDB classification (REF).

Table 2.3 The Rotterdam CT score.

Predictor value	Score
Basal cisterns	
Normal	0
Compressed	1
Absent	2
Midline shift	
No shift or shift ≤ 5 mm	0
Shift >5 mm	1
Epidural mass lesion	
Present	0
Absent	1
Intraventricular blood or tSAH	
Absent	0
Present	1
Sum score	1

The Rotterdam CT score chart for the probability of mortality in patients with severe or moderate TBI.
Abbreviation: tSAH, traumatic subarachnoid hemorrhage.
The sum score adds plus 1 to make the grading numerically consistent with the grading of the motor score of the GCS and with the Marshall CT classification.

Table 2.4 Utility of MRI sequences for TBI-related pathology.

Sequence density (high or low)	Principles and lesion appearance	Strengths and weaknesses
T1	Sensitive to hematomas and parenchymal lesions	+ Excellent gray–white matter differentiation – Unspecific, low diagnostic specificity
T2WI	Conventional MRI with long TR and TE	+ Sensitive to edema, contusions, lesions near the skull base, and orbitofrontal and lower temporal areas
High	↑ Hemorrhage°, edema, gliosis, nonhemorrhagic axonal injury, ischemia	+ Allows for the estimation of oldness of hemorrhage
Low	↓ Hemorrhage°	– Relatively low sensitivity for intraparenchymal hemorrhage
FLAIR	T2WI with the suppression of the CSF signal	+ Increased differentiation between CSF and parenchymal tissue with better detection of periventricular and superficial cortical lesions
High	↑ Hemorrhage°, edema, gliosis, nonhemorrhagic axonal injury, ischemia	+ Equal or more sensitive in detecting brain lesions (including DAI) than T2WI
Low	↓ Hemorrhage°	– Relatively long acquisition time
T2*-GRE	Magnetic susceptibility differences resulting from the paramagnetic effects of blood breakdown products lead to local field inhomogeneities	+ Highly sensitive in the detection of DAI-related punctate hemorrhages
High	↑ Nonhemorrhagic axonal injury	– Large artifacts at the air/tissue interfaces (e.g., orbitofrontal bone, sinuses, mastoid)
Low	↓ Hemorrhage	
SWI	Combination of magnitude and phase† images with a three-dimensional, velocity-compensated gradient echo sequence	+ Highly sensitive in the detection of small DAI-related punctate hemorrhages
Low	Hemorrhage (can be accompanied by ↑ within the lesion)	+ Less unwanted magnetic field inhomogeneities artifacts than T2*-GRE + Good visualization of venous structures – Relatively long acquisition time – Sensitive to motion artifacts

MRI

MRI uses a combination of static and dynamic magnetic fields in conjunction with radiofrequency pulses to generate a signal from water protons within tissues. For example, T1- or T2-weighted images measure differences in the longitudinal recovery or transverse decay of excited protons, which permits characterization of subtle differences between normal and injured tissues. In addition, numerous more specialized MR techniques, including sequences that are highly sensitive for microhemorrhages (e.g., susceptibility-weighted imaging [SWI]), techniques that may depict the microstructure of the brain and produce a map of the axon cell processes (diffusion tensor imaging [DTI]), and methods to probe brain physiology directly (e.g., functional MRI [fMRI]), have been introduced during the last 20 years enabling the detection of subtle but functionally important consequences of TBI.

Conventional MRI

Conventional MRI sequences include T1- and T2-weighted, T2* gradient-recalled echo (T2*-GRE), fluid-attenuated inversion recovery (FLAIR), and diffusion-weighted imaging (DWI) (Table 2.4).

T1-weighted sequences are susceptible to the presence of blood or fat in brain tissue depicted by high signal intensities. However, T1 offers minimal diagnostic specificity as abnormal attenuation on T1 sequences is unspecific and may indicate multiple etiologies such as hematomas, parenchymal lesions, or vascular tumors. T2*-weighted gradient echo MR imaging detects brain hemorrhage better than T1 images, but high signal intensities from the CSF in these images complicate the identification of DAI/TAI lesions. FLAIR MRI imaging detects cerebral edema and allows for easier identification of injured tissue, as it nullifies CSF signal and greatly increases the contrast between normal and abnormal brain matter [27, 28]. In addition, FLAIR-weighted MRI can be used to quantify the degree of white matter damage after trauma [29, 30, 38].

Conventional MRI is more sensitive than CT for detecting TBI-related lesions. In particular, it is much better than CT in detecting nonhemorrhagic contusions, edema, punctuate hemorrhages, and DAI [31]. In addition, MRI provides higher spatial and contrast resolution than CT and higher sensitivity to detect indirect brain damage from systemic injuries including hypoxic–ischemic injury and fat embolism [28, 31–34]. In a prospective study directly comparing CT with conventional MRI in level I trauma centers, 27% of mTBI patients with normal admission head CT had trauma-related abnormalities on MRIs done approximately 2 weeks after injury [101]. The most common MRI abnormalities were subcortical microhemorrhages, indicative of traumatic axonal injury, noted on T2*-weighted gradient echo sequences.

MRI is primarily used in the subacute and chronic phases of TBI, when patient safety issues related to transport and prolonged time in the imaging suite play a less important role. In moderate and severe TBI, MRI is often done to explain a neurologic status worse than predicted by a normal or near-normal CT scan, raising suspicion of a more serious injury. Such information can be useful prognostically as well as for guiding rehabilitation strategies. In mTBI with persistent postconcussive syndrome and cognitive deficits, MRI can be useful for counseling and forensic indications.

For clinical usefulness, the ease and reliability of traumatic lesion detection are important. Lesion number, volume, and lesion location may all affect clinical status and outcome. Brainstem injury is a predictor of mortality and poor functional outcome [35, 36]. Lesions at the temporal and frontal lobes may explain memory and executive functioning disorders [37]. The number of white matter hyperintensities by FLAIR MRI is significantly associated with long-term outcome after TBI [30, 38]. In 18 patients with severe TBI, the number of hyper-intensities seen on FLAIR was positively associated with functional outcome [30]. In 37 patients with severe TBI, FLAIR lesion volumes in the corpus callosum (CC) correlated with disability and cognition in the first months following injury. FLAIR lesion volume in the frontal lobes correlated significantly with clinical scores at 1 year [38].

Quantification of the volume of white matter FLAIR hyperintensities among patients with moderate-to-severe DAI demonstrated poorer outcomes among patients with greater lesion volumes [29]. FLAIR imaging results are also associated with chronic alterations in brain structure, as FLAIR hyperintensities identified acutely after injury are strongly predictive of posttraumatic tissue atrophy 6 months after injury [39].

FLAIR imaging can also be used longitudinally to quantify changes in lesion volume over time and detect the appearance of new lesions [38, 39, 57]. However, in patients with mild-to-moderate brain injury, MRI is at best a modest predictor of long-term recovery and return to work status. Emerging advances in MRI technology, as discussed in the following section, have resulted in enhanced sensitivity for microstructural axonal damage and improved the prognostic value.

DWI is an MRI modality that has revolutionized the field of stroke neurology. DWI allows for early spatial identification and quantification of cytotoxic and vasogenic edema that accompanies brain injuries, including after TBI. DWI relies on differences in the random thermal or self-diffusion of protons in water throughout the brain and quantifies these differences using the apparent diffusion coefficient (ADC). Areas with restricted proton diffusion appear hyperintense on DWI images and have low ADC values, while the reverse is true in regions with increased diffusion. DWI can detect diffusion abnormalities within days or even hours after TBI in patients with mild and severe head injuries [40–44]. DWI has a higher sensitivity for edematous lesions than FLAIR and T2-weighted MRI, although it is less sensitive for detecting hemorrhagic DAI/TAI than T2 sequences [40]. With regard to prognosis, the volume of lesions identified acutely by

DWI is more strongly correlated with clinical outcome than the aforementioned MRI sequences, supporting the use of acute DWI as a biomarker for outcome after TAI [45].

DWI also has the potential to distinguish between vasogenic and cytotoxic edema. Vasogenic edema, resulting from fluid leakage from the local vasculature into the extracellular space, results in areas of increased water diffusion and higher ADC values, while cytotoxic edema is characterized by a shift of water from extracellular to intracellular compartments and results in restricted diffusion, hyperintense DWI-weighted MRI signal, and lower ADC values [40, 46]. In theory, vasogenic edema represents lesions that may potentially be reversed with appropriate medical management, while cytotoxic edema likely identifies areas of largely irreversible axonal damage, although this remains to be proven. Both cytotoxic and vasogenic edema may contribute to long-term functional outcome after TBI.

Emerging MRI modalities for TBI

SWI

SWI is an MRI technique originally developed for improved visualization of the venous system but that proved very suitable in demonstrating small hemorrhagic lesions associated with TBI and provides increased sensitivity over conventional gradient echo MRI. SWI utilizes the differing magnetic susceptibility properties of brain tissue and blood (or blood products such as hemosiderin) in order to identify microscopic areas of extravasated blood early after trauma [47]. SWI substantially increases the sensitivity for detection and quantification of hemorrhagic lesions over T2-weighted MRI [48–51]. Moreover, while conventional MRI sequences and even CT may be useful in identifying large hemorrhagic lesions after closed head injury, many small hemorrhages associated with the shearing forces of DAI/TAI may only be detected by SWI [47, 48].

In pediatric TBI, the number and volume of lesions identified by SWI are associated with poor neuropsychological outcomes and decreased intelligence quotient (IQ) scores several years after injury [50]. Moreover, children with moderate or severe disability between 6 and 12 months after TBI have a greater number and volume of SWI-identified lesions than those with mild disability or normal outcome [49].

DTI

DTI has received increasing attention over the last 10 years as a marker for white matter injury in several neurologic conditions, including TBI.

DTI utilizes the magnetic properties of water, to measure the thermally induced molecular self-diffusion occurring within the tissue compartments of the brain (i.e., the intra- and extracellular spaces). The amounts and spatial distribution of diffusion can be measured in one given direction at a time; by successive manipulation of the MRI system, the average amount of water diffusion occurring across all directions measured can be obtained and is termed mean diffusivity (MD), and the relative directionality of water diffusion can be computed as the normalized standard deviation of these measurements and is referred to as its fractional anisotropy (FA). FA is calculated by measuring the amount of diffusion in multiple (six or more) directions and computing the composite 3D tensor value for each voxel in the brain: from a diagonalization of this tensor, three eigenvalues are obtained and used to compute MD, FA, and other scalar mappings. Diffusion is said to be isotropic if water diffuses in a nonrestricted and random manner (in this case, all three eigenvalues are equal) and anisotropic if water molecules diffuse in a relatively directional or restricted manner, as is the case when water diffuses along the length of a bundle of axons but not in a perpendicular fashion (in this case, one eigenvalue is much larger than the other two).

DTI is able to demonstrate clear differences in MD and FA within several clinical populations including TBI. The distribution of DTI-derived metrics for voxels throughout the brain may identify gross structural integrity differences between patients with TBI and normal controls [52–54]. For example, in patients with chronic TBI the shape of FA histograms is more peaked (kurtotic) and skewed, as compared to histograms of controls [53]. The FA distributions are significantly shifted toward lower values compared to normal controls indicating more isotropic diffusion [52]. Furthermore, these measures of microstructural integrity correlate with postconcussive symptoms 1 month after injury. Interestingly, a longitudinal study found both increases and decreases in FA over time during 6 months postinjury in patients with mTBI [55].

DTI has also demonstrated microstructural compromise in centroaxial white matter regions commonly impacted in DAI using a whole-brain analysis technique called voxel-based analysis [18, 53, 56, 59]. In a study of 9 severe TBI patients scanned 4 years after TBI and 11 controls using VBA, patients had lower FA within major white matter structures than controls [44]. Specifically, compromise to the integrity of the CC, internal capsule, superior and inferior longitudinal fasciculi, and the fornix occurs in severe TBI. Two other studies found similar results in patients whose brains were imaged earlier after TBI (i.e., approximately 1 year postinjury) [58, 59]. Our group has examined DTI data from moderately to severely injured patients with TAI scanned approximately 8 months after injury and revealed compromise to various white matter regions, as compared to controls, and their degree of white matter compromise correlates well with functional and neurocognitive outcomes [100].

Interestingly, Bendlin *et al.* examined the same cohort of patients on two occasions: once at approximately 2 months postinjury and again within 1 year of injury [58]. Using VBA analysis on DTI-derived data in this longitudinal fashion, they observed significant white matter volume loss within the CC, cingulum, longitudinal fasciculi, uncinate fasciculus, and brainstem fiber tracts over time. Figures 2.6 and 2.7 illustrate data from one of our injured participants and shows the evolution of white matter compromise as measured FA over a

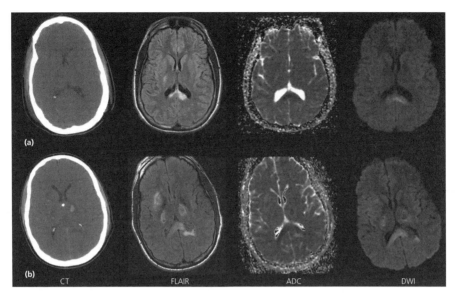

Figure 2.5 (a) Cytotoxic edema in deep white matter structures. (b) Mixed cytotoxic and vasogenic edema in deep white matter structures.

6-month period and demonstrates relatively greater sensitivity for white matter lesions in using DTI compared to FLAIR.

Nakayama and colleagues carefully selected participants who had experienced a nonmissile TBI and demonstrated significant injury-related cognitive impairment without detectable lesions on conventional neuroimaging [59]. Using VBA on DTI scans acquired an average of 14 months postinjury, they observed significant decreases in FA of the CC. Given the stringent inclusion criteria in their study, the results strongly suggest that a voxel-based approach to analyzing white matter integrity can detect areas of damage that may be associated with clinical outcome after TAI. Additionally, diffusion tensor tractography demonstrated qualitative differences in length and volume of the CC and fornix between patients and controls

Diffusion tensor tractography is a technique used to three-dimensionally reconstruct white matter structures based on the directionality of water diffusion within each voxel. White matter tracts are reconstructed using either deterministic or probabilistic methods [103]. Because water diffuses more anisotropically along axons than perpendicular to them, adjacent voxels within subcortical regions with similar FA values, and similar directions of maximal or preferred diffusion, can be tracked and are said to be structurally connected. Diffusion tensor tractography has shown sensitivity to compromised white matter in TAI [56, 59–62]. Wilde *et al.* examined 16 children for an average of 3 years post-severe TBI and found that the reconstructed CC in this group had lower average FA values than age-matched uninjured counterparts [60]. Additionally, they found that higher FA in the CC is associated with better functional outcomes among patients. Nakayama et al. and Xu *et al.* used tractography and voxel-based approaches to examine the integrity of the CC and fornix post-TBI [56, 59]. Their studies allowed for comparison between approaches, concluding that compromise to the CC can be observed using either approach. Interestingly, Nakayama and colleagues found that tractography was sensitive to compromise within the fornix, while FA within this structure measured using VBA was not different from controls. Their results suggest that TAI-related white matter compromise in certain structures may be best detected by different DTI techniques, such as trading in-plane resolution with slice thickness to maintain signal but increase structural resolution.

Wang *et al.* reconstructed several white matter tracts among moderately to severely injured patients with TAI, in acute and chronic phases, and age- and gender-matched controls [61]. They demonstrated significantly lower FA within the CC (genu, posterior body, splenium), fornix, and peduncular projections to occipital and parietal cortices of patients. Additionally, they found that the integrity of the splenium of the CC was strongly associated with the Glasgow Outcome Score—Extended. Data from our group was used to examine the integrity of several white matter structures, finding that FA within the CC, fornix, right inferior longitudinal fasciculus, and bilateral inferior fronto-occipital fasciculi is strongly correlated to neurocognitive performance approximately 8 months postinjury [65] (Figure 2.6).

Quantitative volumetric techniques

Cerebral atrophy, progressing for months and possibly years after injury, is a common consequence of TBI and is associated with poor patient outcomes [63–65, 104]. While the predominant view is that loss of structural volume results from direct insult to neuron bodies, it is possible that atrophy, in the absence of focal trauma, may originate primarily from axonal damage with subsequent Wallerian degeneration and neuronal cell death [39]. With regard to TAI, recent evidence indicates that posttraumatic atrophy is not globally diffuse, but rather, some brain regions are highly susceptible to volume loss, while others show marked resilience [65]. Moreover, atrophy in particular brain regions may hold prognostic value for disability or functional recovery, and accurate measurement of *in vivo* structural changes utilizing 3D structural MRI may serve as a potential biomarker for outcome after TBI.

Numerous neuroimaging techniques have been proposed for the measurement of atrophy rates after TBI. Cross-sectional methods compare the volume of brain tissue (typically gray and white matter with exclusion of CSF) against a common normalization volume such as total intracranial volume for patient–control group comparisons, while longitudinal studies utilize repeated MRI scans for between-scan comparisons and tend to incur lower absolute measurement error than cross-sectional studies [66]. There are relatively few longitudinal studies of atrophy after TBI [58, 63, 65, 67–69]. Of these, the majority assessed volume loss

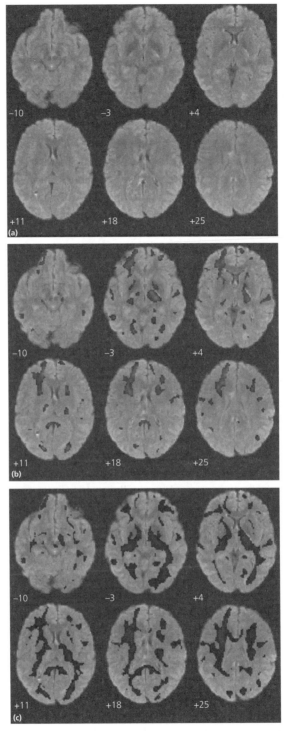

Figure 2.6 Acute and chronic white matter compromise for a 23-year-old male with a severe TBI (GCS = 3) consistent with TAI. (a) Acute FLAIR image showing subtle hyperintensities on the right posterior limb of the internal capsule and fornix. (b) Acute and (c) chronic subnormal FA lesions superimposed on the patient's acute FLAIR image. Note reduced FA in midbrain and other subcortical white matter regions during the acute phase (hot colors) that were not hyperintense in the acute FLAIR. Also, notice even more areas of decreased FA at the chronic phase (winter colors), some of which, but not all, were areas of subnormal FA at the acute phase.

occurring between the subacute and chronic time periods, finding volume loss between 1 and 4% [13, 58, 67, 68]. Two recent studies assessed atrophy beginning acute after injury (within 1 week), finding global atrophy rates of 5 and 8% within 6–8 months of injury [65, 70]. The clearance of acute brain edema did not account for the observed decreases. For the sake of comparison, global atrophy rates in Alzheimer's disease are on the order of 1–2% per year [71, 72]. This suggests that atrophy after TBI begins very early and progresses at an astounding pace. In addition, it is probable that the rate of posttraumatic volume loss is dependent on time after injury. In order to determine the best time for intervention in future clinical trials of therapies targeted at preserving brain parenchyma, it will be essential to determine the progression of whole-brain volume loss occurring at shorter time intervals and over a longer study period.

Quantifying regional variations in atrophy rates represents a formidable challenge in patients with TBI. This is due in large part to regional morphometric distortions caused by focal traumatic lesions, leading to complications with image registration, intensity normalization, and tissue segmentation. Nevertheless, several quantitative techniques utilizing 3D structural T1-weighted MRI images have been developed and applied to TBI. One of the earliest approaches is region-of-interest (ROI) analysis, a morphometric procedure that relies heavily on manual tracing of readily identifiable cerebral structures. While ROI studies provide evidence for atrophy in a variety of brain regions (for a review, see reference [73]), methodological limitations greatly undermine their ability to identify areas of marked susceptibility to atrophy after TBI. As ROI analyses rely on manual identification and delineation of cerebral structures, they are limited in their ability to quantify brain regions lacking clear structural boundaries. Moreover, ROI analyses typically focus on only a small set of structures and are unable to provide a complete assessment of changes in brain morphometry.

Recognizing these limitations, several quantitative and automated MRI approaches have been developed for the calculation of tissue volume per brain voxel, thereby achieving a more comprehensive picture of structural changes after trauma. Voxel-based morphometry (VBM) registers structural MRI images to a common 3D reference space; segments tissue based on signal intensities to delineate the gray matter, white matter, and CSF; and smoothes across neighboring voxels for the creation of composite brain tissue maps. Tensor-based morphometry (TBM) allows for improved nonlinear image registration and may be less sensitive to inaccuracies in tissue segmentation than VBM [13, 26]. The FreeSurfer image analysis suite (www.http://freesurfer.net/) permits high-resolution quantification of thickness, surface area, curvature, and volume of numerous atlas-derived brain regions, increasing the sensitivity cortical morphometric changes over other voxel-wise approaches. Employing these techniques, posttraumatic atrophy has been noted in a variety of brain regions including the amygdala, brainstem, CC, hippocampus, thalamus, putamen, precuneus cortex, and several regions of the parietal and frontal cortices among others [58, 63, 65, 74, 76] (Figure 2.8). Interestingly, many of the regions highly susceptible to atrophy after trauma are heavily involved in the default mode network (DMN) and also undergo particularly high rates of volume loss in Alzheimer's disease, perhaps hinting toward a similar neurodegenerative mechanism shared by both diseases [65, 75]. Clearly, future studies are needed to advance our understanding of the implications of regional variations in atrophy rates after TBI.

FreeSurfer remains a research tool, but its developers have created a program designed to be useful in the routine practice of neuroradiology. NeuroQuant® is an FDA-approved software that evaluates the patient's MRI for brain atrophy in several key regions and compares the results to an FDA-approved database of people of the same age that have healthy brains. A pilot study comparing NeuroQuant® volumetric analysis with visual inspection by a neuroradiologist found that NeuroQuant® identified atrophy in 50% of patients with mild and moderate TBI, while the neuroradiologist's traditional approach found atrophy in only 10% [78] (Figures 2.7 and 2.8).

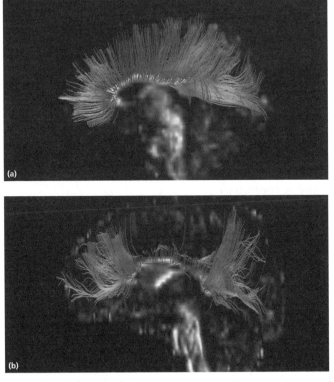

Figure 2.7 Reconstructed CC using diffusion tensor tractography. (a) Reconstructed CC in a healthy, non-brain-injured control participant. (b) CC of an age- and gender-matched individual 6 months posttraumatic axonal injury.

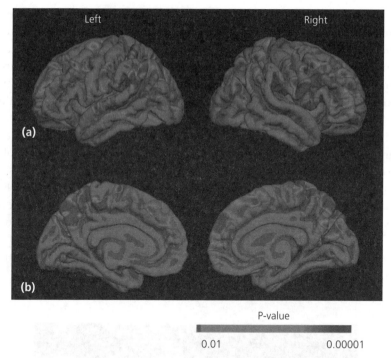

Figure 2.8 Cortical atrophy after traumatic axonal injury in 25 adults. MRI scans were obtained within 1 week of injury and repeated 8 months later. Highlighted regions represent areas of significant brain volume loss between the two-time periods as measured by FreeSurfer morphometry. (a) Lateral and (b) midsagittal views displayed at the pial layer.

Assessment of functional connectivity

Resting state
Interhemispheric connectivity
Resting-state functional connectivity MRI (fcMRI) is an imaging modality used to determine the functional relatedness of selected brain regions while the brain is at rest. It is based on the temporal correlation of blood oxygenation level-dependent (BOLD) signal between various regions [77, 78]. The resting brain shows spontaneous low-frequency neuronal fluctuations that are synchronous over spatially distributed networks. These fluctuations can be measured as the BOLD response during rest with fMRI [114]. The temporal correlation of the time courses between brain regions gives a measure of functional connectivity. It has been proven that the analysis of functional connectivity during rest reveals whole-brain resting-state networks involved in visual, auditory, and sensorimotor processing and in higher cognitive functions like attention, memory, executive functioning [115, 117, 118]. fcMRI may have advantages over task fMRI for studying TBI. Task-based fMRI may present information on the functional

reorganization after injury. However, depending on the activity during a given task, fMRI provides only information on brain regions, participating in a particular task, rather than the whole brain.

A majority (60–80%) of the brain's resources are utilized at rest [120]. fcMRI allows for global analysis of brain activity at rest and may thus help to understand better how brain functions are influenced by TBI. In other words, resting-state fMRI yields unique information about brain functional networks in the absence of direct stimulation.

Functional connectivity patterns among healthy individuals demonstrate a functional link between various regions known to communicate during various tasks and at rest. In contrast, connectivity patterns among clinical populations with compromise to white matter deviate considerably from those observed among healthy brains. fcMRI studies have shown TBI-induced functional changes and changes in functional connectivity during cognitive tasks including working memory, episodic memory, attention, and motor function [105–109, 110, 116]. For example, the relationship between CC integrity and functional connectivity was demonstrated by Quigley and colleagues, who found that patients with agenesis of the CC had significantly reduced interhemispheric connectivity as compared to healthy controls [79]. Likewise, after a complete callosotomy, interhemispheric functional connectivity was significantly reduced while intrahemispheric connectivity was relatively preserved, suggesting the CC plays a significant role in the degree of interhemispheric functional connectivity observed using fcMRI [80].

Given that the CC is the most commonly injured white matter structure after TAI [81–84], and compromise to the integrity of the CC results in compromised interhemispheric functional connectivity among clinical populations, fcMRI may be useful for detecting functional compromise among patients with TAI as well. McDonald and colleagues examined one patient with severe TBI with a GCS of 3 presenting with verbal memory impairment and observed decreased functional connectivity in the left hippocampal network [85]. While these results suggest that functional disconnection may be associated with impairment in neurocognitive function, it was merely a case study. On a group level, a study conducted by our research group found that patients with moderate-to-severe TAI had significantly lower interhemispheric functional connectivity between the hippocampi and the anterior cingulate than controls [99]. Furthermore, interhemispheric functional connectivity for hippocampi was significantly correlated with delayed verbal memory. These findings support the hypothesis that white matter damage due to TAI negatively impacts functional connectivity of certain brain regions. Studies are underway to examine the degree to which compromise in anatomical connectivity influences functional connectivity. Future studies in fcMRI may also benefit from examining the integrity of intrinsic functional networks after TAI, as compromise to the DMN has been demonstrated in other clinical populations including Alzheimer's disease [86–92], major depression [93], and schizophrenia [94–98]. In contrast, mTBI patients exhibited decreased BOLD connectivity within the DMN, hyperconnectivity between the rACC and lateral prefrontal cortical areas, and hyperconnectivity between the right prefrontal cortex and posterior parietal cortex [102].

(m)TBI affects the whole-brain functional networks rather than local sites

As discussed in the previous pages, much has been learned in the past 20 years from structural MRI about what happens in the brain after TBI. However, the use of structural MRI has not translated into clear clinical benefit. For example, approximately 30% of mTBI patients have abnormal structural MRI scans [57], but roughly only 10% of mTBI patients develop cognitive impairments related to attention, executive functions, memory including working memory, episodic memory, visual memory, or prospective memory (see Chapter 9). Structural MRI abnormalities are at best weakly correlated with abnormal neuropsychological test scores. One line of reasoning explains these inconsistencies by the small size and subtle nature of structural lesions caused by mTBI (like microscopic DAI) that remain undetected with conventional imaging techniques [121].

A major challenge in TBI is to sort out the high heterogeneity of brain damage to identify and classify those patients who are most likely to benefit from the treatment [2]. Brain lesions caused by TBI are not restricted to vascular territories of the gray or white matter, but virtually every region in the brain can be damaged as a result of impact to the head. Injury mechanism (traffic accident, fall, sport accident, military injury, etc.) and the biomechanics of impact (angular vs. linear acceleration, duration) are important factors defining injury location and severity of TBI (see [119] for review). Further, interindividual differences in premorbid factors (including age, prior head injury, substance abuse, psychiatric history, genotype, IQ, social circumstances) lead to widely variable TBI outcomes. Finally, functional outcomes after TBI are extremely diverse ranging from full recovery to persistent life-changing clinical sequelae including somatic, cognitive, emotional symptoms and psychiatric diagnoses like depression, substance dependence, anxiety disorder. This heterogeneity makes the analysis of injury-induced consequences difficult.

Mapping of symptoms to focal lesions and focusing on local functions within brain regions, although a successful approach for some neurological diseases, limit progress in understanding TBI pathology. Recent studies suggest that cognitive changes after mild and moderate TBI arise rather from damage to distributed functional networks than from focal lesions [102, 111]. In other words, impaired interaction between regions constituting networks that mediate specific brain functions may underlie TBI-related signs and symptoms [112, 113].

fcMRI in mTBI

Using a group independent component analysis approach, we and others identified patterns of altered whole-brain resting-state functional connectivity in mTBI patients [112, 113]. We found a decrease in functional connectivity within the motor-striatal network in the mTBI patients compared to a control group. At the same time, patients showed deficits in psychomotor speed as well as in speed of information processing. We hypothesize that although disorders in motor function after mTBI are rarely reported, injury still has an effect on motor functioning, which in its turn may also explain the reduction in speed of information processing. Further, we found a cluster of increased functional connectivity in the right frontoparietal network in the mTBI group. Interestingly, this abnormal increased connectivity might reflect increased awareness to external environment and explain excessive cognitive fatigue reported by patients with mTBI. It might also underlie the physical postconcussive symptoms, such as headache and increased sensitivity to noise/light [112].

Resting-state fcMRI and prediction of outcome from TBI

The ultimate goal of fcMRI in TBI is to provide clinicians with prognostic information in individual patients. Even more important, the resting-state fMRI approach provides information on the whole-brain collection of functional networks, which allows for prediction of outcome in all functional domains instead of a single function (as tested in task paradigms). Resting-state functional connectivity can be measured even in comatose patients [122]. Healthy controls, locked-in syndrome patients, minimally conscious and vegetative patients, and coma patients were compared with fcMRI. In noncommunicative brain-damaged patients, connectivity in the DMN areas negatively correlated with the degree of clinical consciousness impairment [122].

Summarizing, resting-state functional connectivity fMRI seems to be a promising tool that can be incorporated into the clinical realm in future. Providing good signal-to-noise ratio, giving the measure of whole-brain functional connectivity, and requiring minimal patient involvement, it can be used for obtaining diagnostic and prognostic information on TBI outcome on individual level.

References

1 Bratton, S.L., Chestnut, R.M., Ghajar, J., *et al.*; Brain Trauma Foundation; American Association of Neurological Surgeons; Congress of Neurological Surgeons; Joint Section on Neurotrauma and Critical Care, AANS/CNS. Guidelines for the management of severe traumatic brain injury. VI. Indications for intracranial pressure monitoring. *Journal of Neurotrauma,* 2007; **24 (Suppl 1)**, S1–S106.

2 Saatman, K.E., Duhaime, A.C., Bullock, R., Maas, A.I., Valadka, A., & Manley, G.T. (2008) Classification of traumatic brain injury for targeted therapies. *Journal of Neurotrauma*, **25** (7), 719–738.

3 Marshall, L.F., Marshall, S.B., Klauber, M.R. *et al.* (1992) The diagnosis of head injury requires a classification based on computed axial tomography. *Journal of Neurotrauma*, **1992;(9 Suppl** 1), S287–S292.

4 Maas, A.I., Hukkelhoven, C.W., Marshall, L.F., & Steyerberg, E.W. (2005) Prediction of outcome in traumatic brain injury with computed tomographic characteristics: a comparison between the computed tomographic classification and combinations of computed tomographic predictors. *Neurosurgery*, **57** (6), 1173–1182.

5 Maas, A.I., Steyerberg, E.W., Butcher, I. *et al.* (2007) Prognostic value of computerized tomography scan characteristics in traumatic brain injury: results from the IMPACT study. *Journal of Neurotrauma*, **24** (2), 303–14.

6 Steyerberg, E.W., Mushkudiani, N., Perel, P. *et al.* (2008) Predicting outcome after traumatic brain injury: development and international validation of prognostic scores based on admission characteristics. *PLoS Med*, **5**(8), e165.

7 Vos, P.E., Alekseenko, Y., Battistin, L. *et al.* (2012). Mild traumatic brain injury. *European Journal of Neurology*, **19** (2), 191–198.

8 Jacobs, B., Beems, T., Stulemeijer, M. *et al.* (2010) Outcome prediction in mild traumatic brain injury: age and clinical variables are stronger predictors than CT abnormalities. *Journal of Neurotrauma*, **27** (4), 655–668.

9 Metting, Z., Rodiger, L.A., Stewart, R.E., Oudkerk, M., De, K.J., & van der, N.J. (2009) Perfusion computed tomography in the acute phase of mild head injury: regional dysfunction and prognostic value. *Annals of Neurology*, **66** (6), 809–816.

10 Perron, A.D., Huff, J.S., Ullrich, C.G., Heafner, M.D., & Kline, J.A. (1998) A multicenter study to improve emergency medicine residents' recognition of intracranial emergencies on computed tomography. *Annals of Emergency Medicine*, **32** (5), 554–562.

11 The American Association of Neurological Surgeons. The Brain Trauma Foundation. The American Association of Neurological Surgeons. The Joint Section on Neurotrauma and Critical Care. (2000) Computed tomography scan features. *Journal of Neurotrauma*, **17** (6–7), 597–627.

12 Toutant, S.M., Klauber, M.R., Marshall, L.F. *et al.* (1984) Absent or compressed basal cisterns on first CT scan: ominous predictors of outcome in severe head injury. *Journal of Neurosurgery*, **61** (4), 691–694.

13 Choksey, M., Crockard, H.A., & Sandilands, M. (1993) Acute traumatic intracerebral haematomas: determinants of outcome in a retrospective series of 202 cases. *British Journal of Neurosurgery*, **7**, 611–622.

14 Lobato, R.D., Rivas, J.J., Cordobes, F. *et al.* (1988) Acute epidural hematoma: an analysis of factors influencing the outcome of patients undergoing surgery in coma. *Journal of Neurosurgery*, **68**, 48–57.

15 Jacobs, B., Beems, T., van der. Vliet T., Diaz-Arrastia, R.R., Borm G.F., & Vos P.E. (2011) Computed tomography and outcome in moderate and severe traumatic brain injury: hematoma volume and midline shift revisited. *Journal of Neurotrauma*, **28** (2), 331–340.

16 Baker, S.P., O'Neill, B., Haddon, W. Jr., & Long, W.B. (1974) The injury severity score: a method for describing patients with multiple injuries and evaluating emergency care. *Journal of Trauma*, **14**, 187–196.

17 Perel, P., Roberts, I., Bouamra, O., Woodford, M., Mooney, J., & Lecky, F. (2009) Intracranial bleeding in patients with traumatic brain injury: a prognostic study. *BMC Emergency Medicine*, **9**, 15.

18 Eisenberg, H.M., Gary, H.E., Jr., Aldrich, E.F. *et al.* (1990) Initial CT findings in 753 patients with severe head injury. A report from the NIH Traumatic Coma Data Bank. *Journal of Neurosurgery*, **73** (5), 688–698.

19 van Dongen, K.J., Braakman, R., & Gelpke, G.J. (1983) The prognostic value of computerized tomography in comatose head- injured patients. *Journal of Neurosurgery*, **59** (6), 951–957.

20 Jacobs, B., Beems, T., van der Vliet, T., Borm, G.F., & Vos, P.E. (2010) The status of the fourth ventricle and ambient cisterns predict outcome in moderate and severe traumatic brain injury. *Journal of Neurotrauma*, **27** (2), 331–340.

21 Colquhoun, I.R., & Burrows E.H. (1989) The prognostic significance of the third ventricle and basal cisterns in severe closed head injury. *Clinical Radiology*, **40** (1), 13–16.

22 Teasdale, E., Cardoso, E., Galbraith, S., & Teasdale, G.M. (1984) CT scan in severe diffuse head injury: physiological and clinical correlations. *Journal of Neurology, Neurosurgery and Psychiatry*, **47** (6), 600–603.

23 (a) Perel, P., Arango, M., Clayton, T. *et al*. (2008) Predicting outcome after traumatic brain injury: practical prognostic models based on large cohort of international patients. *British Medical Journal*, **336** (7641), 425–429. (b) Dagi, T.F., Meyer, F.B., & Poletti, C.A. (1983) The incidence and prevention of meningitis after basilar skull fracture. *American Journal of Emergency Medicine*, **1**, 295–298.

24 Kakarieka, A. (1997) Review on traumatic subarachnoid hemorrhage. *Journal of Neurology Research*, **19** (3), 230–232.

25 Greene, K.A., Marciano, F.F., Johnson, B.A., Jacobowitz, R., Spetzler, R.F., & Harrington, T.R. (1995) Impact of traumatic subarachnoid hemorrhage on outcome in nonpenetrating head injury. Part I: a proposed computerized tomography grading scale. *Journal of Neurosurgery*, **83** (3), 445–452.

26 Vos, P.E., van Voskuilen, A.C., Beems, T., Krabbe, P.F., & Vogels, O.J. (2001) Evaluation of the traumatic coma data bank computed tomography classification for severe head injury. *Journal of Neurotrauma*, **18** (7), 649–655.

27 Ashikaga, R., Araki, Y., & Ishida, O. (1997) MRI of head injury using FLAIR. *Neuroradiology*, **39** (4), 239–242.

28 Lagares, A., Ramos, A., Perez-Nunez, A. *et al*. (2009) The role of MR imaging in assessing prognosis after severe and moderate head injury. *Acta Neurochirurgicaurgica (Wien)*, **151** (4), 341–356.

29 Marquez de la Plata, C.D., Ardelean, A., Koovakkattu, D. *et al*. (2007) Magnetic resonance imaging of diffuse axonal injury: quantitative assessment of white matter lesion volume. *Journal of Neurotrauma*, **24** (4), 591–598.

30 Scheid, R., Walther, K., Guthke, T., Preul, C., & von Cramon, D.Y. (2006) Cognitive sequelae of diffuse axonal injury. *Archive of Neurology*, **63** (3), 418–424.

31 Gentry, L.R., Godersky, J.C., Thompson, B., & Dunn, V.D. (1988) Prospective comparative study of intermediate-field MR and CT in the evaluation of closed head trauma. *AJR American Journal of Roentgenology*, **150** (3), 673–682.

32 Gentry, L.R., Godersky, J.C., & Thompson, B. (1988) MR imaging of head trauma: review of the distribution and radiopathologic features of traumatic lesions. *AJR American Journal of Roentgenology*, **150** (3), 663–672.

33 Doezema, D., King, J.N., Tandberg, D., Espinosa, M.C., & Orrison, W.W. (1991) Magnetic resonance imaging in minor head injury. *Annals of Emergency Medicine*, **20** (12), 1281–1285.

34 Provenzale, J.M. (2010) Imaging of traumatic brain injury: a review of the recent medical literature. *AJR American Journal of Roentgenology*, **194** (1), 16–19.

35 Firsching, R., Woischneck, D., Klein, S., Reissberg, S., Dohring, W., & Peters, B. (2001) Classification of severe head injury based on magnetic resonance imaging. *Acta Neurochirurgica*, **143** (3), 263–271.

36 Mannion, R.J., Cross, J., Bradley, P. *et al*. (2007) Mechanism-based MRI classification of traumatic brainstem injury and its relationship to outcome. *Journal of Neurotrauma*, **24** (1), 128–135.

37 Bigler, E.D. (2007) Anterior and middle cranial fossa in traumatic brain injury: relevant neuroanatomy and neuropathology in the study of neuropsychological outcome. *Neuropsychology*, **21** (5), 515–531.

38 Pierallini, A., Pantano, P., Fantozzi, L.M. *et al.* (2000) Correlation between MRI findings and long-term outcome in patients with severe brain trauma. *Neuroradiology*, **42** (12), 860–867.

39 Ding, K., Marquez de la, P.C., Wang, J.Y. *et al.* (2008) Cerebral atrophy after traumatic white matter injury: correlation with acute neuroimaging and outcome. *Journal of Neurotrauma*, **25** (12), 1433–1440.

40 Huisman, T.A., Sorensen, A.G., Hergan, K., Gonzalez, R.G., & Schaefer, P.W. (2003) Diffusion-weighted imaging for the evaluation of diffuse axonal injury in closed head injury. *Journal of Computed Assisted Tomography*, **27** (1), 5–11.

41 Kurca, E., Sivak, S., & Kucera, P. (2006) Impaired cognitive functions in mild traumatic brain injury patients with normal and pathologic magnetic resonance imaging. *Neuroradiology*, **48** (9), 661–669.

42 Hou, D.J., Tong, K.A., Ashwal, S., Oyoyo, U., Joo, E., Shutter, L., & Obenaus, A. (2007) Diffusion-weighted magnetic resonance imaging improves outcome prediction in adult traumatic brain injury. *Journal of Neurotrauma*, **24** (10), 1558–1569.

43 Goetz, P., Blamire, A., Rajagopalan, B., Cadoux-Hudson, T., Young, D., & Styles, P. (2004) Increase in apparent diffusion coefficient in normal appearing white matter following human traumatic brain injury correlates with injury severity. *Journal of Neurotrauma*, **21** (6), 645–654.

44 Liu, A.Y., Maldjian, J.A., Bagley, L.J., Sinson, G.P., & Grossman, R.I. (1999) Traumatic brain injury: diffusion-weighted MR imaging findings. *American Journal of Neuroradiology*, **20** (9), 1636–1641.

45 Schaefer, P.W., Huisman, T.A., Sorensen, A.G., Gonzalez, R.G., & Schwamm, L.H. (2004) Diffusion-weighted MR imaging in closed head injury: high correlation with initial glasgow coma scale score and score on modified Rankin scale at discharge. *Radiology*, **233** (1), 58–66.

46 Suskauer, S.J., & Huisman, T.A. (2009) Neuroimaging in pediatric traumatic brain injury: current and future predictors of functional outcome. *Developmental Disabilities Research Reviews*, **15** (2), 117–123.

47 Mittal, S., Wu, Z., Neelavalli, J., & Haacke, E.M. (2009) Susceptibility-weighted imaging: technical aspects and clinical applications, part 2. *American Journal of Neuroradiology*, **30** (2), 232–252.

48 Tong, K.A., Ashwal, S., Holshouser, B.A. *et al.* (2003) Hemorrhagic shearing lesions in children and adolescents with posttraumatic diffuse axonal injury: improved detection and initial results. *Radiology*, **227** (2), 332–339.

49 Tong, K.A., Ashwal, S., Holshouser, B.A., *et al.* (2004) Diffuse axonal injury in children: clinical correlation with hemorrhagic lesions. *Annals of Neurology*, **56** (1), 36–50.

50 Babikian, T., Freier, M.C., Tong, K.A. *et al.* (2005) Susceptibility weighted imaging: neuropsychologic outcome and pediatric head injury. *Pediatric Neurology*, **33** (3), 184–194.

51 Haacke, E.M., Xu, Y., Cheng, Y.C., & Reichenbach, J.R. (2004) Susceptibility weighted imaging (SWI). *Magnetic Resonance in Medicine*, **52** (3), 612–628.

52 Bazarian, J.J., Zhong, J., Blyth, B., Zhu, T., Kavcic, V., & Peterson, D. (2007) Diffusion tensor imaging detects clinically important axonal damage after mild traumatic brain injury: a pilot study. *Journal of Neurotrauma*, **24** (9), 1447–1459.

53 Benson, R.R., Meda, S.A., Vasudevan, S. *et al.* (2007) Global white matter analysis of diffusion tensor images is predictive of injury severity in traumatic brain injury. *Journal of Neurotrauma*, **24** (3), 446–459.

54 Lipton, M.L., Gellella, E., Lo, C. *et al.* (2008) Multifocal white matter ultrastructural abnormalities in mild traumatic brain injury with cognitive disability: a voxel-wise analysis of diffusion tensor imaging. *Journal of Neurotrauma*, **25** (11), 1335–1342.

55 Lipton, M.L., Kim, N., Park, Y.K. *et al.* (2012) Robust detection of traumatic axonal injury in individual mild traumatic brain injury patients: intersubject variation, change over time and bidirectional changes in anisotropy. *Brain Imaging and Behavior*, **6** (2), 329–342.

56 Xu, J., Rasmussen, I.A., Lagopoulos, J., & Haberg, A. (2007) Diffuse axonal injury in severe traumatic brain injury visualized using high-resolution diffusion tensor imaging. *Journal of Neurotrauma*, **24** (5), 753–765.

57 Paul, A.M., Hofman, S.Z., Stapert Marinus J.P.G. *et al.* (2001) MR imaging, single-photon emission CT, and neurocognitive performance after mild traumatic brain injury. *American Journal of Neuroradiology*, **22,** 441–449.

58 Bendlin, B.B., Ries, M.L., Lazar, M., et al. (2008) Longitudinal changes in patients with traumatic brain injury assessed with diffusion-tensor and volumetric imaging. *Neuroimage*, **42** (2), 503–514.

59 Nakayama, N., Okumura, A., Shinoda, J. *et al.* (2006). Evidence for white matter disruption in traumatic brain injury without macroscopic lesions. *Journal of Neurology, Neurosurgery, and Psychiatry*, **77**, 850–855.

60 Wilde, E.A., Chu, Z., Bigler, E.D. *et al.* (2006) Diffusion tensor imaging in the corpus callosum in children after moderate to severe traumatic brain injury. *Journal of Neurotrauma*, **23** (10), 1412–1426.

61 Wang, J.Y., Bakhadirov, K., Devous, M.D., Sr. *et al.* (2008) Diffusion tensor tractography of traumatic diffuse axonal injury. *Archives of Neurology*, **65** (5), 619–626.

62 Rutgers, D.R., Fillard, P., Paradot, G., Tadie, M., Lasjaunias, P., & Ducreux, D. (2008) Diffusion tensor imaging characteristics of the corpus callosum in mild, moderate, and severe traumatic brain injury. *American Journal of Neuroradiology*, **29**, 1730–1735.

63 Sidaros, A., Skimminge, A., Liptrot, M.G. *et al.* (2009) Long-term global and regional brain volume changes following severe traumatic brain injury: a longitudinal study with clinical correlates. *Neuroimage*, **44** (1), 1–8.

64 Gale, S.D., Baxter, L., Roundy, N., & Johnson, S.C. (2005) Traumatic brain injury and grey matter concentration: a preliminary voxel based morphometry study. *Journal of Neurology, Neurosurgery, and Psychiatry*, **76** (7), 984–948.

65 Warner, M.A., Youn, T.S., Davis, T. *et al.* (2010) *Regionally* selective atrophy after traumatic axonal injury. *Archives of Neurology*, **67** (11), 1336–1344.

66 Smith, S.M., Zhang, Y., Jenkinson, M. *et al.* (2002) Accurate, robust, and automated longitudinal and cross-sectional brain change analysis. *Neuroimage*, **17** (1), 479–489.

67 MacKenzie, J.D., Siddiqi, F., Babb, J.S. *et al.* (2002) Brain atrophy in mild or moderate traumatic brain injury: a longitudinal quantitative analysis. *American Journal of Neuroradiology*, **23** (9), 1509–1515.

68 Trivedi, M.A., Ward, M.A., Hess, T.M. *et al.* (2007) Longitudinal changes in global brain volume between 79 and 409 days after traumatic brain injury: relationship with duration of coma. *Journal of Neurotrauma*, **24** (5), 766–771.

69 Xu, Y., McArthur, D.L., Alger, J.R. *et al.* (2010) Early nonischemic oxidative metabolic dysfunction leads to chronic brain atrophy in traumatic brain injury. *Journal of Cerebral Blood Flow and Metabolism*, **30** (4), 883–894.

70 Xue, R., van Zijl, P.C., Crain, B.J., Solaiyappan, M., & Mori, S. (1999) In vivo three-dimensional reconstruction of rat brain axonal projections by diffusion tensor imaging. *Magnetic Resonance in Medicine*, **42** (6), 1123–1127.

71 Sluimer, J.D., van der Flier, W.M., Karas, G.B. *et al.* (2008) Whole-brain atrophy rate and cognitive decline: longitudinal MR study of memory clinic patients. *Radiology*, **248** (2), 590–598.

72 Fox, N.C., Freeborough, P.A., & Rossor, M.N. (1996) Visualisation and quantification of rates of atrophy in Alzheimer's disease. *Lancet*, **348** (9020), 94–97.

73 Bigler, E.D. (2001) Quantitative magnetic resonance imaging in traumatic brain injury. *The Journal of Head Trauma Rehabilitation*, **16** (2), 117–134.

74 Kim, J., Avants, B., Patel, S. *et al.* (2008) Structural consequences of diffuse traumatic brain injury: a large deformation tensor-based morphometry study. *Neuroimage*, **39** (3), 1014–1026.

75 Buckner, R.L., Sepulcre, J., Talukdar, T. *et al.* (2009) Cortical hubs revealed by intrinsic functional connectivity: mapping, assessment of stability, and relation to Alzheimer's disease. *Journal of Neuroscience*, **29** (6), 1860–1873.

76 Ross, D.E., Ochs, A.L., Seabaugh, J.M. *et al.* (2012) Progressive brain atrophy in patients with chronic neuropsychiatric symptoms after mild traumatic brain injury: a preliminary study. *Brain Injury*, **26** (12), 1500–1509.

77 Biswal, B., Yetkin, F. Z., Haughton, V.M., *et al.* (1995) Functional connectivity in the motor cortex of resting human brain using echo-planar MRI. *Magnetic Resonance in Medicine*, **34** (4), 537–5541.

78 Peltier, S.J., & Noll, D.C. (2002) T2* dependence of low frequency functional connectivity. *Neuroimage*, **16** (4), 985–992.

79 Quigley, M., Cordes, D., Turski, P. *et al.* (2003) Role of the corpus callosum in functional connectivity. *American Journal of Neuroradiology*, **24** (2), 208–212.

80 Johnston, J.M., Vaishnavi, S.N., Smyth, M.D. et al. (2008) Loss of resting interhemispheric functional connectivity after complete section of the corpus callosum. *Journal of Neuroscience*, **28**, 6453–6458.

81 Meythaler, J.M., Peduzzi, J.D., Eleftheriou, E., & Novack, T.A. (2001) Current concepts: diffuse axonal injury-associated traumatic brain injury. *Archives of Physical Medicine Rehabilitation*, **82** (10), 1461–1471.

82 Adams, J.H., Graham, D.I., Murray, L.S., & Scott, G. (1982) Diffuse axonal injury due to nonmissile head injury in humans: an analysis of 45 cases. *Annals of Neurology*, **12** (6), 557–563.

83 Ng, H.K., Mahaliyana, R.D., & Poon, W.S. (1994) The pathological spectrum of diffuse axonal injury in blunt head trauma: assessment with axon and myelin strains. *Clinical Neurology and Neurosurgery*, **96**, 24–31.

84 Amaral, D.G., Insausti, R., & Cowan, W.M. (1984) The commissural connections of the monkey hippocampal formation. *Journal of Comparative Neurology*, **224**, 307–335.

85 MacDonald, C.L., Schwarze, N., Vaishnavi, S.N. *et al.* (2008) Verbal memory deficit following traumatic brain injury: assessment using advanced MRI methods. *Neurology*, **71**, 1199–1201.

86 Buckner, R.L., Snyder, A.Z., Shannon, B.J. *et al.* (2005) Molecular, structural, and functional characterisation of Alzheimer's disease: evidence for a relationship between default activity, amyloid, and memory. *Journal of Neuroscience*, **25**, 7709–7717.

87 Firbank, M.J., Blamire, A.M., Krishnan, M.S. *et al.* (2007) Atrophy is associated with posterior cingulate white matter disruption in dementia with Lewy bodies and Alzheimer's disease. *NeuroImage*, **36**, 1–7.

88 Greicius, M.D., Srivastava, G., Reiss, A.L., & Menon, V. (2004) Default-mode network activity distinguishes Alzheimer's disease from healthy aging: evidence from functional MRI. *Proceedings of the National Academy of Science USA*, **101**, 4637–4642.

89 He, Y., Wang, L., Zang, Y. *et al.* (2007) Regional coherence changes in early Alzheimer's disease: a combined structural and resting-state functional MRI study. *NeuroImage*, **35**, 488–500.

90 Rombouts, S.A.R.B., Barkhof, F., Goekoop, R. *et al.* (2005) Altered resting state networks in mild cognitive impairment and mild Alzheimer's disease: an fMRI study. *Human Brain Mapping*, **26**, 231–239.

91 Sorg, C., Riedl, V., Mühlau, M. *et al.* (2007) Selective changes of resting-state networks in individuals with Alzheimer's disease. *Proceedings of the National Academy of Science USA*, **104**, 18760–18765.

92 Wang, L., Zang, Y., He, Y. *et al.* (2006) Changes in hippocampal connectivity in the early stages of Alzheimer's disease: evidence from resting state fMRI. *NeuroImage*, **31**, 469–504.

93 Greicius, M.D., Flores, B.H., Menon, V., & Glover, G.H. (2007) Resting-state functional connectivity in major depression: abnormally increased contributions from subgenual cingulate cortex and thalamus. *Biological Psychiatry*, **62**, 429–437.

94 Liang, M., Zhou, Y., Jiang, T. *et al.* (2006) Widespread functional disconnectivity in schizophrenia with resting-state functional magnetic resonance imaging. *NeuroReport*, **17**, 209–213.

95 Bluhm, R.L., Miller, J., Lanius, R.A. *et al.* (2007) Spontaneous low-frequency fluctuations in the BOLD signal in schizophrenic patients: anomalies in the default network. *Schizophrenia Bulletin*, **733**, 1004–1012.

96 Garrity, A.G., Pearlson, G.D., McKiernan, K.A. *et al.* (2007) Aberrant 'default mode' functional connectivity in schizophrenia. *The American Journal of Psychiatry*, **164**, 450–457.

97 Zhou, Y., Liang, M., Tian, L. *et al.* (2007) Functional disintegration in paranoid schizophrenia using resting-state fMRI. *Schizophrenia Research*, **97**, 194–205.

98 Pomarol-Clotet, E., Salvador, R. Sarró, S. *et al.* (2008) Failure to deactivate in the prefrontal cortex in schizophrenia: dysfunction of the default-mode network? *Psychology Medicine*, **38**, 1185–1193.

99 Marquez de la Plata, C.D., Garces, J., Shokri Kojori, E., *et al.* (2011) Deficits in functional connectivity of hippocampal and frontal lobe circuits after traumatic axonal injury. *Archives of Neurology*, **68** (1), 74–84.

100 Marquez de la Plata, C.D., Yang, F.G., Wang, J.Y. *et al.* (2011) Diffusion tensor imaging biomarkers for traumatic axonal injury: analysis of three analytic methods. *Journal of the International Neuropsychological Society*, **17** (1), 24–35.

101 Yuh, E.L., Mukherjee, P., Lingsma, H.F. *et al.* (2013) TRACK-TBI Investigators. Magnetic resonance imaging improves 3-month outcome prediction in mild traumatic brain injury. *Annals of Neurology*, **73** (2), 224–235.

102 Mayer, A.R., Mannell, M.V., Ling, J., Gasparovic, C., & Yeo, R.A. (2011) Functional connectivity in mild traumatic brain injury. *Human Brain Mapping*, **32** (11), 1825–1835.

103 Mori, S., Crain, B.J., Chacko, V.P., & van Zijl, P.C. (1999) Three-dimensional tracking of axonal projections in the brain by magnetic resonance imaging. *Annals of Neurology*, **45** (2), 265–269.

104 Wang, J.Y., Bakhadirov, K., Abdi, H. *et al.* (2011) Longitudinal changes of structural connectivity in traumatic axonal injury. *Neurology*, **77**, 818–826.

105 McAllister, T.W., Saykin, A.J., Flashman, L.A. *et al.* (1999). Brain activation during working memory 1 month after mild traumatic brain injury: a functional MRI study. *Neurology*, **53**, 1300–1308.

106 Stulemeijer, M., Vos, P.E., van der, W.S., Van, D.G., Rijpkema, M., & Fernandez, G. (2010) How mild traumatic brain injury may affect declarative memory performance in the post-acute stage. *Journal of Neurotrauma*, **27**, 1585–1595.

107 Mayer, A.R., Mannell, M.V., Ling, J. *et al.* (2009) Auditory orienting and inhibition of return in mild traumatic brain injury: a FMRI study. *Human Brain Mapping*, **30** (12), 4152–4166.

108 McAllister, T.W., Sparling, M.B., Flashman, L.A., Guerin, S.J., Mamourian, A.C., & Saykin, A.J. (2001) Differential working memory load effects after mild traumatic brain injury. *NeuroImage*, **14**, 1004–1012.

109 Kasahara, M., Menon, D.K., Salmond, C.H. *et al.* (2010) Altered functional connectivity in the motor network after traumatic brain injury. *Neurology*, **75** (2), 168–176.

110 McAllister, T.W., Flashman, L.A., McDonald, B.C., & Saykin, A.J. (2006) Mechanisms of working memory dysfunction after mild and moderate TBI: evidence from functional MRI and neurogenetics. *Journal of Neurotrauma*, **23**, 1450–1467.

111 Slobounov, S.M., Gay, M., Zhang, K. *et al.* (2011) Alteration of brain functional network at rest and in response to YMCA physical stress test in concussed athletes: rsFMRI study. *Neuroimage*, **55**, 1716–1727.

112 Shumskaya, E., Andriessen, T.M., Norris, D.G., & Vos, P.E. (2012) Abnormal whole-brain functional networks in homogeneous acute mild traumatic brain injury. *Neurology*, **79** (2), 175–182.

113 Stevens, M.C., Lovejoy, D., Kim, J., Oakes, H., Kureshi, I., & Witt, S.T. (2012) Multiple resting state network functional connectivity abnormalities in mild traumatic brain injury. *Brain Imaging Behaviour*, **6** (2), 293–318.

114 Biswal, B.B., Van Kylen, J., & Hyde, J.S. (1997) Simultaneous assessment of flow and BOLD signals in resting-state functional connectivity maps. *NMR in Biomedicine* **10** (4–5), 165–170.

115 Zuo, X.N., Di Martino, A., Kelly, C., *et al.* (2010) The oscillating brain: complex and reliable. *Neuroimage*, **49**, 1432–1445.

116 Jantzen, K.J., Anderson, B., Steinberg, F.L., & Kelso, J.A. (2004) A prospective functional MR imaging study of mild traumatic brain injury in college football players. *American Journal of Neuroradiology*, **25**, 738–745.

117 Damoiseaux, J.S., Rombouts, S.A., Barkhof, F. *et al.* (2006) Consistent resting-state networks across healthy subjects. *Proceedings of the National Academy of Science USA*, **103**, 13848–13853.

118 Greicius, M.D., Krasnow, B., Reiss, A.L., & Menon, V. (2003) Functional connectivity in the resting brain: a network analysis of the default mode hypothesis. *Proceedings of the National Academy of Science USA*, **100** (1), 253–258.

119 Andriessen, T.M., Jacobs, B., & Vos, P.E. (2010) Clinical characteristics and pathophysiological mechanisms of focal and diffuse traumatic brain injury. *Journal of Cellular and Molecular Medicine*, **14** (10), 2381–2392.

120 Raichle, M.E., & Mintun, M.A. (2006) Brain work and brain imaging. *Annual Review of Neuroscience*, **29**, 449–476.

121 Bigler, E.D. (2004) Neuropsychological results and neuropathological findings at autopsy in a case of mild traumatic brain injury. *Journal of the International Neuropsychological Society*, **10** (5), 794–806.

122 Vanhaudenhuyse, A., Noirhomme, Q., Tshibanda, L.J. *et al.* (2010) Default network connectivity reflects the level of consciousness in non-communicative brain-damaged patients. *Brain*, **133** (Pt1), 161–171.

PART II

Prehospital and ED care

CHAPTER 3

Out-of-hospital management in traumatic brain injury

Peter R.G. Brink

Trauma Center, Maastricht University Medical Center, Maastricht, the Netherlands

Introduction

In developed countries, the existence of organized trauma systems is the base for providing good care for trauma patients, from the scene of the accident through rehabilitation. Developing countries have adapted aspects of these systems, and further development of national or regional trauma management systems is likely to be a very cost-effective measure for reducing mortality and improving outcome for accident victims.

Trauma systems link organizations working in the field of acute care together, allowing uniformity of terminology and adapting the evidence-based guidelines. In most developed countries, well-trained paramedics are the backbone of the emergency medical system (EMS) and are responsible for the first part of the trauma chain, the prehospital phase. Under specific circumstances, paramedics are supported by physicians. In geographically dispersed regions, the use of helicopters helicopter emergency medical system (HEMS) as an adjunct for transportation is helpful.

The practice of medicine in the prehospital environment is quite different from what is encountered in the hospital. Potential risks from hazardous materials or environmental and climatic conditions must be considered, which could present risks for both patient and rescuer. In cases of entrapped patients, a multidisciplinary coordination between rescue and medical teams is mandatory. Paramedics or EMS personnel have a complex job, requiring intensive training in invasive procedures and decision making.

Focusing on the trauma patient with a traumatic brain injury (TBI), guidelines for the optimal protection of the damaged brain in the prehospital phase are evolving and are sometimes conflicting. In this chapter, generally accepted guidelines for the assessment and treatment of brain-injured patients as well as controversies will be discussed.

A high index of suspicion for the existence of a brain injury is required when paramedics start treating a trauma victim. In situations where paramedics encounter patients with a possible or obvious injury of the brain,

Traumatic Brain Injury, First Edition. Edited by Pieter E. Vos and Ramon Diaz-Arrastia.
© 2015 John Wiley & Sons, Ltd. Published 2015 by John Wiley & Sons, Ltd.

Box 3.1 Examples of mechanisms of injury suspecting high-energy impact.

Ejection from automobile
Death of victim in the same vehicle
Extrication time > 20 min
Fall > 20 ft (>5 m)
High-speed vehicle accident (40 mph/60 km/h) and deformity > 20 in (>50 cm)
Motorcycle accident (20 mph/30 km/h) or separation driver–motorcycle

guidelines are used to guide assessment of the patient on the spot. These guidelines are based on the probability of having a brain injury due to the mechanism of the injury. Penetrating injury of the skull and/or face is a simple clue indicating that injury of the brain is likely. High-energy impact, as is common in motor vehicle accidents, is an important factor for the existence of brain injury. In such cases (Box 3.1), brain injury should always be suspected, and measurements should be directed to create an optimal situation for the patient and the brain.

Other informations found during the initial physiological assessment of the patient gives further clues that the brain is injured in the accident. In all potentially traumatized patients, a simple algorithm is used assess the victim rapidly. The paramedic always starts his or her assessment by asking a simple question of the patient. If the answer is coherent and in a normal voice, it can be assumed that the airway is patent. If the patient does not answer, or his answer is inappropriate, further investigation into the level of consciousness is required. Increasing the intensity of the stimulus by talking louder and/or by administering a noxious stimulus is usually the next step in order to evaluate the level of consciousness.

The paramedic should categorize the patient as having a level of consciousness above or below a Glasgow Coma Scale (GCS) of 8. In patients with a GCS ≤ 8, the algorithm of the ABC starts with maintaining an open and secured airway according to the Manual of Prehospital Trauma Life Support [1]. This algorithm was developed during the early 1980s in the USA, was adopted by the American College of Surgeons in 1982, and has since become the international standard. The algorithm is revised every 4 years by an international group of experts, based on newly available evidence. In general, in patients with a GCS > 8, without other reasons for a compromised airway (facial or neck injury, inhalation injury), the focus on the airway is less prominent than in the group with a GCS ≤ 8.

The basic rules are always the same. The type and severity of the brain damage does not play a role in the initial assessment. The principle is "the best way to protect the injured brain is to optimize perfusion." Maintaining or restoring cardiopulmonary stability is the next critical step in order to improve perfusion and oxygenation of all organs, including the brain.

Box 3.2 Signs of physiological disorders, used for the assessment of trauma patients making this patient at risk. These signs are used for triage purposes in order to select the most appropriate hospital.

Respiratory rate <10 or >29 breaths/min
Systolic blood pressure < 90 mmHg
Signs of low dermal blood flow (pale, cold, wet)
GCS < 14

The ABCs are designed to assess and treat disorders in oxygen intake, ventilation (either hypo- or hypercapnia), and circulation. At the scene, only physiological parameters can be assessed (Box 3.2), whereas full evaluation of the level of consciousness takes time and pathoanatomic information is lacking until CT scanning is performed. This focused information allows the implementation of measures to optimize the condition of the patient and to prevent secondary brain damage, such as preventing hypoventilation and hypovolemia, which have clear detrimental effects on survival and quality of life [2–5].

Because in the ATLS doctrine the sequence of assessment is mandatory (first airway, followed by ventilation and then circulation), the focus on brain injury seems to be placed on the back row, usually for good reasons (Figure 3.1). In the primary survey, every significant disorder discovered needs direct action. That means when the airway is compromised, it needs corrective action before ventilation is assessed. The goal is to stabilize the patient by ensuring an open airway, sufficient ventilation, and adequate circulation within the shortest time possible. Part of this optimizing process is the delivery of high-flow oxygen ($100\% O_2$, 10 l/min flow rate) using a non-rebreathing mask, since all trauma patients experience a higher level of metabolism due to stress.

These steps to restore oxygen delivery to tissues support the brain. Only after the phase of resuscitation, when the airway is safe, oxygen is supplied (a systemic saturation between 95 and 100%), and the circulation is under control (bleeding is controlled and volume is prudently replaced), is it time to assess the damage to the brain. Roughly three levels of severity of brain damage are assessed, as they have consequences for transportation: mild, moderate, and severe. Each is discussed as follows.

Prehospital management of mild TBI (GCS 13–15)

Mild TBI characterizes approximately 80% of patients seen with a head injury [1]. Disorientation, amnesia, and/or temporary loss of consciousness are signals to the paramedics that the brain could be injured. Confounders like alcohol or drug intoxication could sometimes be a problem. Hypoxemia and/or hypovolemia may also mimic minor brain injury, but these should have been ruled out or

Box 3.3 Patient-related factors that play a role in estimating the relative risk for a patient after a trauma and the selection of the hospital level.

Age <5 or >55 years
Cardiac disease
Respiratory disease
Diabetes mellitus (insulin dependent)
Cirrhosis
Morbid obesity
Immunosuppression
Pregnancy
History of bleeding or the use of anticoagulants
Pacemaker
Medication like beta-blockers

treated within the first part of resuscitation. When signs of mild brain injury are present, unexpected deteriorations occur in about 3% of cases [1]. The mechanism of injury and patient-related factors plays a role. High-energy impact, direct blow on the head (fall or heavy object), or perforating injuries should be a clue demanding in-depth investigation by a specialist in a hospital. For the patient-related factors (Box 3.3), the use of anticoagulants is the most risky.

As a rule, patients with the suspicion of having a mild brain injury are transported to the emergency department (ED) of a nearby hospital. During transport, the patient is immobilized, is administered oxygen, and is observed for deterioration. Immobilization of the spine (with a stiff collar and headblocks for the cervical spine or a stiff long spine board for the thoracic and lumbar spine) is standard in prehospital management of all patients, as there is always a risk for potentially catastrophic spine injuries. There is controversy on this practice, as only a minority of patients with mild TBI have a spine injury, and not all spine injuries are unstable and at risk for secondary neurological deterioration, and undoubtedly, there is quite a lot overtreatment. Collars and long spine boards are unpleasant for patients, although soft-layered spine boards are on the market today. The general rule remains that every patient with an injury above the level of the clavicle is prone for a cervical spine injury. The ethical question of how many thousands of trauma patients should be unnecessarily immobilized to prevent one case of paraplegia cannot readily be answered. The slogan *do no further harm* in ATLS is the result of anecdotal disasters for individual patients.

Prehospital management of moderate TBI (GCS 9–12)

Ten percent of all head-injured patients have a moderate brain injury, with signs of confusion, restlessness, agitation, decreased consciousness, and/or focal neurological deficits. Of this group, 10–20% will deteriorate into the group of severe brain injuries (see later) [1]. The basic rules of the ABCs of resuscitation are the same and have priority over specific neurological investigations. Optimizing saturation and circulation can distinguish primary brain damage (as a result of the trauma of the head) from an altered level of consciousness due to hypoxemia or hypovolemia. If a moderate brain injury is suspected, *stay and play* at the scene of the accident is contraindicated, since information about the extent of brain damage through a CT scan is obligatory, and that is only available in the hospital. Because of the chance of deterioration, in particular in the presence of life-threatening intracranial hematomas, these patients are selected for transport to hospitals with available neurosurgical expertise. The rate of neurosurgical intervention is 10–15%, and appropriate expertise in intensive care management is mandatory. Upon stabilization of the ABCs on the scene of the accident, direct transport to an appropriate hospital with neurosurgical expertise is preferable to transient observation in a smaller hospital. Regional guidelines should specify which hospitals are equipped with appropriate expertise to facilitate making the correct decision as to where to transfer patients on the spot.

Prehospital management of severe TBI (GCS 3–8)

If the patient is unable to follow any commands after adequate cardiopulmonary resuscitation, the brain is probably severely damaged. The basic rules are the same as for the other two categories, but airway management takes on a more prominent role. As prescribed by the guidelines, all patients need an open and secured airway for oxygen delivery and prevention of hypercapnia. In case of insufficient spontaneous breathing, supported ventilation is mandatory in addition to supplying oxygen. Simple maneuvers start with the inspection of the mouth and the removal of obstructed material, followed by suction. In cases of fractures of the mandibula and/or midface, retraction of the depressed mandibula could restore an open airway temporarily. Chin lift and jaw trust are well-known techniques, used by paramedics, but all have only a temporary effect.

Although the need to perform an endotracheal intubation in all patients with a GCS ≤ 8 may appear obvious, there are conflicting studies on this issue [6–16]. The International Neurotrauma Research Organisation in Vienna, Austria, studied 396 patients with a GCS ≤ 8 and showed no effect of intubation for better survival [6]. Two other studies also did not show any difference between the intubated and nonintubated groups, in either adults or children [8, 9]. A large retrospective study in California in 13 625 patients even showed a decrease in the survival of intubated patients [7], even when the intubations were done by specially trained paramedics. These results were confirmed by other studies [10–15]. The only study where prehospital intubation improved survival was published in 1997 [16]. Despite this conflicting observational data, intubation in case of a compromised airway combined with a GCS ≤ 8 is still a standard protocol.

The intubation technique used in the prehospital setting differs from the intubation technique used in the operating room under optimal circumstances. As every patient with a TBI could have an injury of the cervical spine, hyperextension of the neck during the intubation procedure is not allowed. In-line stabilization, using two hands by a person standing besides the thorax of the patient, gives the optimal possibility for stabilization. A cervical collar should be removed temporarily in order to open the mouth adequately. After intubation and tube control, the cervical collar, combined with head blocks, is replaced to offer the best possible protection in case of an unstable cervical injury. Alternatives to endotracheal intubation include a laryngeal mask airway, which could be inserted blindly. This approach is useful but does not minimize the risk for aspiration. It can be used as a backup in case endotracheal intubation fails. Indications for a surgical airway are rare. This procedure is done in less than 1% of cases needing a free airway.

The use of a gastric tube in the prehospital phase is questionable. After endotracheal intubation, the risk of aspiration is very low. If a less occlusive method is used (such as mayotube, laryngeal mask airway), the introduction of a gastric tube could be a stimulus for vomiting and/or rise in the intracranial pressure. If the introduction of a gastric tube is mandatory, insertion should be through the mouth instead of the nose, avoiding the risk of intracranial malplacement of the tube in case of a fractured lamina cribrosa.

There is no debate about oxygen supply and ventilation control after creating an open and secured airway. The 10 l, 100% oxygen supply rule is one of the less controversial issues in prehospital care for trauma patients. Ambulatory pulse oximetry makes it possible to have information about ventilation/diffusion processes in the thorax. One should aim for a saturation rate of 95% or higher in head-injured patients. At least as important is the avoidance of both hypocapnia and hypercapnia. In a study (submitted for publication) in a cohort of 60 patients with severe TBI, pCO_2 was measured directly after admission on the ED. We found moderate hypercapnia (pCO_2 6.0 ± 2 kPa, 45 ± 15 mmHg) in all head-injured patients, but there was no significant difference between the intubated patients (5.6 ± 2.6 kPa, 42 ± 19 mmHg) and patients that were not intubated on arrival at the ED (5.8 ± 1.1 kPa). Patients in whom intubation was attempted but where the procedure failed in the prehospital setting were all hypercapnic (7.2 ± 1.3 kPa, $54 + 10$ mmHg) [17]. So there is a risk of hypoventilation in these patients. This may be in reaction to the former guidelines where hypocapnia was recommended in order to lower the intracranial pressure, but later shown to be detrimental by lowering cerebral perfusion due to vasoconstriction. Today normoventilation with an overdose of oxygen is the standard and should be practiced in every setting of primary trauma care.

Optimizing circulation in order to protect the damaged brain tissue seems logical and helps survival in severe traumatic brain-injured patients. Several studies confirm that patients with hypotension after severe TBI have a mortality rate twice that of normotensive patients [5, 18–20]. Several techniques are available, starting with the autotransfusion effect achieved by lifting the legs. A Trendelenburg position as the ultimate form of autotransfusion to the brain could have an opposite effect. The increased arterial blood flow combined with a decrease of the venous return can have a detrimental effect on brain perfusion. In the past, antishock garments (antishock trousers) were used in order to stop the bleeding in the abdomen, pelvis, and lower extremities. As this system works to elevate peripheral resistance, the effect is a rise of blood pressure in almost all cases. People with decreased consciousness due to brain hypoperfusion some-times became alert within 1 minute after inflating the garment. Today, the adverse effects on local tissue (such as compartment syndrome) and the risk of extra hemorrhage of thoracic origin resulting from the use of this garment have made it obsolete. But stopping the bleeding is still the main goal when dealing with a circulation problem. Even the use of tourniquets is recommended again to control massive blood loss. One should never overlook blood loss from a con-comitant scalp lesion, which, due to its anatomy, seldom stops hemorrhaging spontaneously and can result in substantial blood loss.

Almost all patients with severe head injuries require intravenous access. Large-bore needles (14 gauge) are inserted in order to deliver a bolus of fluid rap-idly. However, the routine practice of administering a 2l bolus should be ques-tioned. In case of normotension, acute overhydration of a head-injured patient could have a negative effect on the outcome. So titration of fluid, with blood pressure as a guide, is recommended. In case of the need of intravenous access for patients in deep shock, the use of bone needles could be very helpful. Paramedics should realize that getting access to the vein takes time and should be done dur-ing transportation. Sometimes, it is better to *scoop and run* when the hospital is nearby. It has been clearly demonstrated that critically injured patients have an improved outcome when the on-scene time of the paramedics is less than 20 minutes [21]. In a retrospective study of brain-injured patients with GCS ≤ 8, we found a tripling of the duration of on-scene time in the last 20 years (for intuba-tion, IV access, thorax drainage, etc.) without improvement in the survival rate [17]. There is an ongoing discussion about the fluids that should be administered to patients with severe head injuries. Probably a small bonus of hypertonic fluid (salt or starch) is better than isotonic saline, but until now, the evidence is weak. In case of acute care in the prehospital setting for trauma patients, one should rely on simple rules and a limited number of medication and fluids.

Especially in cases of severe head injury or suspected brain damage in poten-tially unstable patients, early choice for the proper hospital and early contact with the ED are mandatory. In order to give the receiving hospital time to arrange proper facilities optimizing the admission of the patient (informing the trauma team including the neurologist, neurosurgeon, radiologist), a direct contact bet-ween the personnel on the scene of the accident and the hospital is the essential. For professional assignment, a simple abbreviation (MIST) could be used (Box 3.4).

Box 3.4 MIST protocol for the assignment of trauma patients from the prehospital phase to the ED of the hospital.

M: Mechanism injury	Traffic accident, fall, perforating injury
I: Identified injuries	Obvious or highly suspected injuries
S: Signs	Symptoms according to the ABCD system
T: Therapy	What has been done already

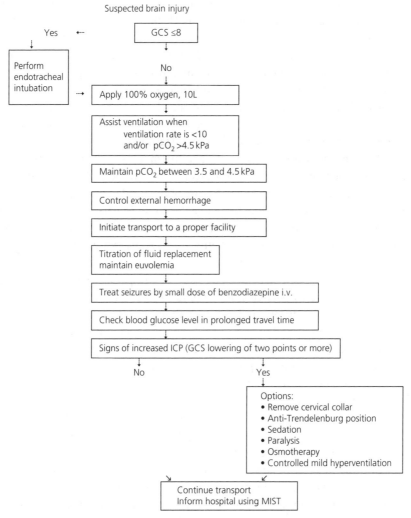

Figure 3.1 Algorithm for the prehospital management of traumatic brain injury (Source: Salomone and Frame [30]. Adapted with permission from McGraw-Hill).

Despite these ATLS management strategies, patients with severe TBI still have a high mortality rate, and many survivors suffer from persistent severe neurological disability [20, 22, 23, 24, 25]. It remains unproven whether these prehospital measures, all sound from a theoretical point of view, are actually beneficial to the patient. But they remain the best we have at present [20, 26, 27]. It may be that outcome from a severe TBI is determined by the injury itself and only modestly affected by optimal prehospital management, at least in hemodynamically stable patients.

The proposed ABC-based system of assessment and treatment is clear and understandable for those working in the prehospital environment and should be considered the standard until new studies present evidence that the protocol should be changed. The choice between basic life support (simple stabilization, *scoop and run*) and advanced life support (includes more invasive techniques and a prolonged stay at the scene of the accident *stay and play*) depends on several factors. In this respect, the physiological situation of the patient, the distance to a proper facility, and the skills of the paramedics/EMS personnel are important [20, 26–31]. The algorithm in Figure 3.1 can be used as a tool for decision making, but it is only a help for those who are working in the prehospital field, needing some guidelines.

References

1 National Association of Emergency Medical Technicians and American College of Surgeons Committee of Trauma. (2006) Manual of Prehospital Trauma Life Support, 7th edn. Mosby, St Louis.

2 Ghajar, J. (2000) Traumatic brain injury. *Lancet*, **356**, 923–929.

3 Bratton, S.L, Chestnut, R.M., Ghajar, J. *et al.* (2007) Guidelines for the management of severe traumatic brain injury. I. Blood pressure and oxygenation. *Journal of Neurotrauma*, **24** (Suppl), S7–S13.

4 Jones, P.A., Andrews, P.J., Midgley, S. *et al.* (1994) Measuring the burden of secondary insults in head injured patients during intensive care. *Journal of Neurosurgical Anesthesiology*, **6**, 4–14.

5 Marmarou, A., Anderson, R.L., Ward, J.D. *et al.* (1991) Impact of ICP instability and hypotension on outcome in patients with severe head trauma. *Journal of Neurosurgery*, **75**, S59–S66.

6 Lenartova, L., Janciak, I., Wilbacher, I. *et al.* (2007) Austrian Severe TBI Study Investigators Severe traumatic brain injury in Austria III: prehospital status and treatment. *Wiener Klinische Wochenschrift*, **119**, 35–45.

7 Davis, D.P., Peay, J., Sise, M.J. *et al.* (2005) The impact of prehospital endotracheal intubation on outcome in moderate to severe traumatic brain injury. *Journal of Trauma*, **58(5)**, 933–939.

8 Sloane, C., Vilke, G.M., Chan, T.C., Hayden, S.R., Hoyt, D.B., & Rosen, P. (2000) Rapid sequence intubation in the field versus hospital in trauma patients. *Journal of Emergency Medicine*, **19**, 259–264.

9 Gausche, M., Lewis, R.J., Stratton, S.J. *et al.* (2000) Effect of out-of-hospital pediatric endotracheal intubation on survival and neurological outcome: a controlled clinical trial. *JAMA: Journal of American Medical Association*, **283**, 783–790.

10 Murray, J.A., Demetriades, D., Berne, T.V. *et al.* (2000) Prehospital intubation in patients with severe head injury. *Journal of Trauma,* **49**, 1065–1070.

11 Eckstein, M., Chan, L., Schneir, A., & Palmer, R. (2000) Effect of prehospital advanced life support on outcomes of major trauma patients. *Journal of Trauma,* **48**, 643–648.

12 Floccare, D.J. (2003) Endotracheal intubation in the field does not improve outcome in trauma patients who present without an acutely lethal traumatic brain injury. Bochicchio GV, Ilahi O, Joshi M, Bochicchio K, Scalea TM. *Journal of Trauma,* **54**, 307–311.

13 Stockinger, Z.T. & McSwain, N.E. Jr. (2004) Prehospital endotracheal intubation for trauma does not improve survival over bag-valve-mask ventilation. *Journal of Trauma,* **56**, 531–536.

14 Wang, H.E., Peitzman, A.B., Cassidy, L.D., Adelson, P.D., & Yealy, D.M. (2004) Out-of-hospital endotracheal intubation with adverse outcome after traumatic brain injury. *Annals of Emergency Medicine,* **44**, 439–450.

15 Davis, D.P., Peay, J., Sise, M.J., et al. (2005) The impact of prehospital endotracheal intubation on outcome in moderate to severe traumatic brain injury. *Journal of Trauma,* **58 (5)**, 933–939.

16 Denninghoff, K.R., Griffin, M.J., Bartolucci, A.A., Lobello, S.G., & Fine, P.R. (2008) Emergent endotracheal intubation and mortality in traumatic brain injury. *The Western Journal of Emergency Medicine,* **9**, 184–189.

17 Winchell, R.J. & Hoyt, D.B. (1997) Endotracheal intubation in the field improves survival in patients with severe head injury: Trauma Research and Education Foundation of San Diego. *Archives of Surgery,* **132**, 592–597.

18 Aubuchon, M.M.F., Hemmes, B., Poeze, M., Jansen, J., & Brink, P.R.G. (2013) Prehospital care in patients with severe traumatic brain injury: does the level of prehospital care influence mortality? *European Journal of Trauma and Emergency Surgery,* **39**, 35–41.

19 Bullock, R.M., Chesnut, R.M., Clifton, G.L. *et al.* (2000) Management and prognosis of severe traumatic brain injury. *Journal of Neurotrauma,* **17**, 479–491.

20 Chesnut, R.M., Marshall, L.F., Klauber, M.R. *et al.* (1993) The role of secondary brain injury in determining outcome from severe head injury. *Journal of Trauma,* **34**, 216–222.

21 Salomone, J.P. & Frame, S.B. (2004) Prehospital care. In: E.E. Moore, D.V. Feliciano & K.L. Mattox (eds), *Trauma,* 5th edn. p. 118. McGraw-Hill Companies Inc, New York.

22 Demetriades, D., Chan, L., Cornwell, E.E. III. *et al.* (1996) Paramedic vs private transportation of trauma patients. *Archives of Surgery,* **131**, 133–138.

23 Fearnside, M.R., Cook, R.J., McDougall, P., & McNeil, R.J. (1993) The Westmead Head Injury Project outcome in severe head injury. A comparative analysis of pre-hospital, clinical and CT variables. *British Journal of Neurosurgery,* **7**, 267–279.

24 Khan, F., Bagualy, I.J., & Cameron, I.D. (2003) Rehabilitation after traumatic brain injury. *Medical Journal of Australia,* **17**, 290–295.

25 Hunt, J., Hill, D., Besser, M., West, R., & Roncal, S. (1995) Outcome of patients with neurotrauma: the effect of a regionalized trauma system. *Australian and New Zealand Journal of Surgery,* **65**, 83–86.

26 Cooper, D.J., Myles, P.S., McDermott, F.T. *et al.* (2004) Prehospital hypertonic saline resuscitation of patients with hypotension and severe traumatic brain injury: a randomized controlled trial. *JAMA: Journal of the American Medical Association,* **291**, 1350–1357.

27 Haas, B. & Nathens, A.B. (2008) Pro/con debate: is the scoop and run approach the best approach to trauma services organization? *Critical Care,* **12**, 224–234.

28 Liberman, M., Mulder, D., Lavoie, A., Denis, R., & Sampalis, J.S. (2003) Multicenter Canadian study of prehospital trauma care. *Annals of Surgery,* **237**, 153–160.

29 Smith, R.M. & Conn, A.K. (2009) Prehospital care—scoop and run or stay and play? *Injury,* **40**, S23–S26.

30 Chapleau, W. (2002) ALS vs BLS. *Emergency Medical Services,* **31**, 102–103.

31 van der Velden, M.W., Ringburg, A.N., Bergs, E.A., Steyerberg, E.W., Patka, P., Schipper, I.B. (2008) Prehospital interventions: time wasted or time saved? An observational cohort study of management in initial trauma care. *Journal of Emergency Medicine,* **25**, 444–449.

CHAPTER 4

Emergency department evaluation of mild traumatic brain injury

Noel S. Zuckerbraun[1], C. Christopher King[2], and Rachel P. Berger[3]

[1] *Division of Pediatric Emergency Medicine, Department of Pediatrics, Children's Hospital of Pittsburgh of UPMC, University of Pittsburgh School of Medicine, Pittsburgh, PA, USA*

[2] *Department of Emergency Medicine, Albany Medical Center, Albany, NY, USA*

[3] *Division of Child Advocacy, Department of Pediatrics, Children's Hospital of Pittsburgh of UPMC, University of Pittsburgh School of Medicine, Pittsburgh, PA, USA*

Millions of people sustain traumatic brain injuries each year and for those who seek care, the Emergency Department (ED) is the front line. There are over 1 million ED visits annually in the USA for traumatic brain injury (TBI), 70–90% are mild (mTBI). Almost all of these patients will be treated and released from an ED without an in-patient admission [1]. Although mTBI may be "mild" in comparison to more severe injuries, it can still result in cognitive, physical, psychological, and social dysfunction, which can interfere with school, work, family, and social relationships, and sport participation [2–4]. Early recognition of mTBI, appropriate ED evaluation and detailed follow-up plans may facilitate recovery and reduce the risk of long-term symptoms and complications [5].

Defining mTBI

The marked variability in the definitions of and terminology for mTBI has contributed to limitations in understanding and management [6]. It is important to understand the different definitions and terminology to formulate a diagnosis and treatment plan and to communicate these findings to other medical professionals and the patient.

Definition

While numerous definitions of mTBI exist in the literature, three of the most widely recognized and cited definitions are from the American Congress of Rehabilitation Medicine (ACRM), the Centers for Disease Control (CDC), and the World Health Organization (WHO) [6–8] (Table 4.1). The International Conference on Concussion in Sport proceedings offers a separate, but similar definition for sport-related concussion [9]. In all definitions, loss of consciousness (LOC) is not

Traumatic Brain Injury, First Edition. Edited by Pieter E. Vos and Ramon Diaz-Arrastia.

Table 4.1 Comparison of common mTBI definitions.

	LOC (<30 min)	Amnesia (<24 h)	Mental status changes	Other neurologic features	GCS
ACRM [8]	Yes	Yes	Any alteration in mental state	Focal neurologic deficits, transient or nontransient	GCS 13–15, >30 min postinjury
CDC [6]	Yes	Yes	Any transient confusion, disorientation, or impaired consciousness	Observed signs of neurological or neuropsychological dysfunction, such as seizures acutely following injury among very young children: irritability, lethargy, or vomiting following head injury and symptoms among older children and adults such as headache, dizziness, irritability, fatigue, or poor concentration, when identified soon after injury, can be used to support the diagnosis of mTBI	Not specified
WHO [7]*	Yes	Yes	Confusion or disorientation	Transient neurological abnormalities (focal signs, seizure, and intracranial lesion not requiring surgery)	GCS 13–15, >30 min postinjury

mTBI is defined by trauma to the head and one or more of the following features: (i) loss of consciousness (LOC), (ii) amnesia, (iii) mental status changes as specified in the following, and (iv) other neurologic features as specified in the following.

ACRM, American Congress on Rehabilitation Medicine; CDC, Centers for Disease Control; WHO, World Health Organization.

*WHO definition also states that manifestations of mTBI must not be due to drugs, alcohol, and medications; caused by other injuries or treatment for other injuries (e.g., systemic injuries, intubation); or caused by other problems (e.g., psychological trauma, language barrier).

necessary for a head injury to be diagnosed. Indeed, 80–90% of mTBI does not involve LOC [10] and a presence of LOC does not correlate with injury severity or outcome [11]. The primary difference in the ACRM, CDC, and WHO definitions relates to the subtleties of patient inclusion criteria on both ends of the mTBI spectrum. For the ED clinician, using a less restrictive definition makes sense. This is highlighted even more in children in whom returning to sports before a complete recovery may worsen symptoms and increase the risk of reinjury [12, 13].

Terminology

While the term *mTBI* is being used in the current chapter, various other terms are sometimes used, including a *concussion, ding* or *bell ringer, head injury, head trauma, closed head injury, closed head trauma, minor head injury,* and *minor head trauma* [14–16], leading to difficulty in comparing published studies. Furthermore, when speaking with patients and families, use of some of these terms may not clearly convey the brain injury. While the CDC supports the interchangeable use of the terms concussion and mTBI [17], a recent study found that when the term *concussion* was used, some families interpreted this to mean that there had been no brain injury [18]. Since premature return to sports is perhaps the highest risk for children with mTBI, this misunderstanding suggests that a minor terminology change may have significant clinical significance. If ED physicians use the term *concussion*, it is important to stress that there has been brain trauma.

Neuropathophysiology of mTBI

Unlike more severe TBI, which typically results in significant structural brain abnormalities, mTBI is assumed to primarily cause neurometabolic dysfunction. Studies suggest that mTBI is a complex cascade of neurometabolic changes which includes an abrupt, indiscriminate release of neurotransmitters, unchecked ionic shifts, impaired axonal function, and an alteration in glucose metabolism. This cascade can result in a metabolic "energy crisis" which can persist for weeks in rat models and is believed to result in many of the clinical symptoms of mTBI [19]. However, recent studies with advanced neuroimaging (usually with MRI) indicate that subtle structural abnormalities may result from mTBI in at least some cases, particularly in athletes who are exposed to multiple such injuries [20]. The significance of these findings remains to be established.

Epidemiology of mTBI

In adults less than 55 years of age, the primary causes of mTBI are motor vehicle collisions (MVC) [21]. In adults, 55 years of age and older, falls are the leading cause of mTBI. The incidence of mTBI in adults is greatest among males under 24 years of age and among men and women 65 years of age and older [22]. The leading mechanisms of mTBI in children less than 14 years of age are falls, MVC, and recreation/sports [21].

Sports-related mTBI occurs in 1.6–3.8 million adults and children annually in the USA [23]. Estimating the precise rate of sports-related mTBI is difficult due a variety of factors including underreporting by athletes and underrecognition by athletes, trainers, and clinicians [24]. Increasing access to recreational and organized sports coupled with better awareness and education in the medical, scholastic, and sport settings, will likely result in more injured athletes presenting for care in the ED [15].

Abusive head trauma (AHT)—sometimes referred to as shaken baby syndrome—accounts for over 1000 cases of TBI annually in the USA [25]. Although AHT is more frequently moderate or severe rather than mild, this is likely, in large part, due to poor recognition of AHT in its more mild forms [26]. Recognition of mild AHT in the ED can be difficult even for the experienced clinician. Misdiagnosis of AHT, even its mild forms, can have devastating consequences; it allows children to be returned to unsafe households where they can be reabused. Many of the children who ultimately die from AHT initially presented to an ED with mTBI [26].

ED diagnosis and management of mTBI

Not every patient seen in the ED with head injury will be diagnosed with TBI. Many patients present with a focal injury (e.g., scalp abrasion), but without neurologic impairment. All patients evaluated in the ED for a head injury or injury to the body with possible force transmitted to the head should be assessed for mTBI. Common conditions, which should be *trigger cues* to the physician to assess for mTBI, include high-speed activities (e.g., MVC or all-terrain vehicle crash), sports and recreation, falls from significant heights, assaults, and mechanisms with external face/head injuries [17].

In addition to the patient with a chief complaint of trauma, any patient presenting with typical mTBI symptoms (Box 4.1) should have an evaluation for the presence of recent trauma. Diagnosing delayed presentations of mTBI can be challenging, as symptoms are nonspecific (Box 4.1), and the onset may occur days or weeks after injury.

The initial approach to all patients with known or suspected head injury should be the same. In keeping with the American College of Surgeons Guidelines for Advanced Trauma Life Support (ATLS), the primary trauma survey should be performed with a focused assessment and stabilization of the ABCs, including cervical spine immobilization, as needed (see also Chapter 3) [27].

Use of the Glasgow Coma Scale score in mTBI

The Glasgow Coma Scale (GCS) is the most widely used scale to distinguish mild from moderate/severe TBI [28]. Use of the GCS in young children is challenging since the verbal score is difficult to assess. For this reason, there is a modified pediatric GCS for use in young children [29]. For the ED physician, the GCS score is most useful for the initial distinction of mTBI from moderate to severe

Box 4.1 Four categories of typical mTBI symptoms.

Physical

– Headache
– Nausea/vomiting
– Balance problems
– Dizziness
– Blurred vision
– Fatigue
– Sensitivity to light or noise
– Numbness/tingling
– Dazed or stunned

Cognitive

– Feeling mentally *foggy*
– Feeling slowed down
– Difficulty concentrating
– Difficulty remembering
– Forgetful of recent information or conversations
– Confused about recent events
– Answering questions slowly
– Repeating questions

Emotional/behavioral

– Irritability
– Sadness
– More emotional
– Nervousness

Sleep

– Drowsiness
– Sleeping more than usual
– Sleeping less than usual
– Trouble falling asleep

Source: Langlois [17].

TBI and for tracking neurologic status over time in the ED. Beyond this, its use in mTBI is limited [30].

Most ED patients with a head injury have a GCS score of 15. The role of the ED physician is to provide the necessary additional evaluation to determine which patients with head injury and a GCS score of 15 have mTBI. The algorithm in Figure 4.1 is designed to assist the ED physician in making this assessment. As discussed in the "Neuroimaging" section, not all patients who present to the ED with an mTBI will require a head CT, but those who do undergo CT can be classified as *complicated* or -*uncomplicated* based on the CT results [31].

Assessment of signs and symptoms

A thorough history includes a detailed account of mechanism of injury, time of injury, immediate injury characteristics (Box 4.2), and subsequent symptoms [17]. Immediate injury characteristics are seen immediately *or* early after the injury and may be transient. Thus, specific inquiry to the patient, witnesses, and emergency medical services personnel as to their presence prior to ED arrival is needed. Symptoms of mTBI can be separated into four categories (Box 4.1) [17]. Headache is the most common single symptom [31]. Symptom duration is highly variable, lasting from a few minutes to several months or longer.

It is also important to collect information about features of the patient's history or injury that could change the way in which the symptoms manifest, change the risk level for an intracranial injury (ICI), and/or predict the potential for a prolonged recovery. For example, a history that medication was administered after the injury that might affect the central nervous system

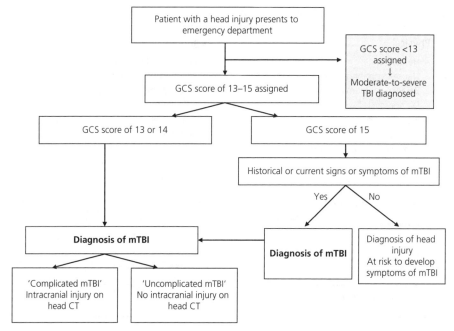

Figure 4.1 ED process for mTBI diagnosis: from initial GCS to diagnosis of mTBI.

Box 4.2 Immediate injury characteristics of mTBI.

LOC (and duration)

Amnesia
- Amnesia before (retrograde)

Are there any events just *before* the injury that the injured person has no memory of (even brief)?
- Amnesia after (anterograde)

Are there any events just *after* the injury that the injured person has no memory of (even brief)?

　　Other observed immediate or early mental status changes or neurologic features
- Altered mental state, confusion, or disorientation
  - Appears dazed or stunned
  - Answers questions slowly
  - Is confused about events
  - Repeats questions
  - Forgetful (recent information)
- Seizures

Source: Langlois [17].

(e.g., opioids) and/or a history of drug and alcohol use may lower the clinician's threshold for obtaining a CT scan. Risk factors for ICI including bleeding diathesis or known intracranial pathology should also be elicited. Finally, risk factors for prolonged recovery from mTBI should be assessed and include a history of concussion/mTBI, migraines, developmental disorders (e.g., attention deficit hyperactivity disorders) and/or psychiatric disorders [32–38].

Physical examination

The decision about whether to obtain a head CT in patients with mTBI is, in large part, reliant on a careful physical exam.

Particular attention should be directed at the head, eyes, ears, neurologic, and skin exams. Larger and nonfrontal scalp hematomas in young children are associated with skull fracture and ICI [39]. Scalp hematomas can be boggy and subtle, especially in children with thick or braided hair. Signs of a basilar skull fracture include retroauricular bruising, periorbital bruising, and CSF otorrhea or rhinorrhea. In infants, the anterior fontanel, if open, should be evaluated for bulging, a sign of increased intracranial pressure. A detailed neurologic examination should be performed to assess cranial nerve function, motor and sensory function, and deep tendon reflexes. All injuries should be documented, particularly in cases of suspected AHT since the ED physician may be the only person to visualize concerning bruises or abrasions which can quickly fade [40]. Any bruising in a premobile infant [41] or bruising of the trunk, ears, or neck in a young child [40] should prompt concern for AHT.

Neuroimaging

One of the most important clinical challenges for the ED physician is deciding whether neuroimaging is needed. A noncontrast CT is the most commonly performed neuroimaging test. Drawbacks of CT include the potential need for transporting patients outside the ED, cost, and exposure to ionizing radiation. Ionizing radiation is particularly concerning in pediatrics [42]. For the majority of patients with mTBI, neuroimaging will be normal and will contribute little to clinical management other than excluding ICI [17]. The goal is to perform the minimum number of head CTs while assuring that patients with potentially dangerous ICI are identified.

For adults, numerous studies have addressed clinical criteria that physicians can use to determine whether a patient with mTBI should undergo head CT. The two most commonly used clinical criteria are the New Orleans Criteria [43] and the Canadian CT Head Rule [44]. Follow-up studies have evaluated the effectiveness of these and other criteria in terms of sensitivity and specificity for identifying clinically significant ICI in adults [45, 46]. Based on the data available from these studies, the American College of Emergency Physicians (ACEP) and the CDC issued a clinical policy statement in 2008 regarding indications for obtaining head CT scans in adults with head trauma (Box 4.3) [47].

Box 4.3 Indications for head CT scan in adults (≥16 years of age) with head trauma from ACEP/CDC clinical policy statement.

Level A recommendation:*

Head CT is indicated for patients *with* LOC *or* posttraumatic amnesia only if one or more of the following are present:

1 Headache
2 Vomiting
3 Age > 60 years
4 Drug or alcohol intoxication
5 Deficits in short-term memory
6 Physical evidence of trauma above the clavicle
7 Posttraumatic seizure
8 GCS score < 15
9 Focal neurologic deficit
10 Coagulopathy

Level B recommendation:**

Head CT should be considered for patients without LOC or posttraumatic amnesia if one or more of the following are present:

1 Focal neurologic deficit
2 Vomiting
3 Severe headache
4 Age ≥ 65 years
5 Physical signs of a basilar skull fracture
6 GCS score < 15
7 Coagulopathy
8 Dangerous mechanism of injury (e.g., ejection from a motor vehicle, a pedestrian struck by a vehicle, or a fall from a height of more than 3 ft or 5 stairs)

Articles used in formulating the clinical policy statement were ranked in terms of quality from highest (Class I) to lowest (Class III).

---

*Level A recommendation defined as "generally accepted principles for patient management that reflect a high degree of clinical certainty"
**Level B recommendation defined as "recommendation for patient management that may identify a particular strategy or range of strategies that reflect moderate clinical certainty
Source: Langlois [17].

Less information is available to guide in the decision-making process for children. Up to 50% of pediatric patients in the USA evaluated in the ED for head trauma undergo head CT, the majority of whom have a GCS of 14–15, and less than 10% of which will have an abnormality on CT [48]. Neurosurgical intervention in pediatric patients with a GCS of 14–15 is extremely uncommon [48, 49].

Many pediatric studies have attempted to determine whether findings on history and physical examination can predict an ICI; none have been sensitive enough to diagnose all ICI, and all lack validation [50, 51]. However, a recent, large multicenter, prospective cohort study of 42 000 pediatric patients with mTBI

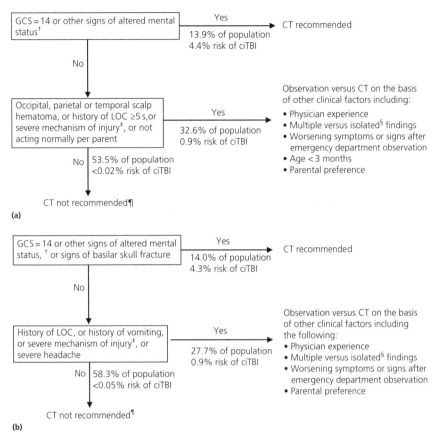

Figure 4.2 Suggested CT algorithm for children younger than 2 years (a) and for those aged 2 years and older. (b) with GCS scores of 14–15 after head trauma. †Other signs of altered mental status: agitation, somnolence, repetitive questioning, or slow response to verbal communication. ‡Severe mechanism of injury: motor vehicle crash with patient ejection, death of another passenger, or rollover; pedestrian or bicyclist without helmet struck by a motorized vehicle; falls of more than 0·9 m (3 ft) (or more than 1.5 m [5 ft] for panel b); or head struck by a high-impact object. §Patients with certain isolated findings (i.e., with no other findings suggestive of TBI, such as isolated LOC, isolated headache, isolated vomiting, and certain types of isolated scalp hematomas in infants >3 months, have a risk of ciTBI substantially lower than 1%. ¶Risk of ciTBI exceedingly low, generally lower than risk of CT-induced malignancies. Therefore, CT scans are not indicated for most patients in this group. GCS, Glasgow Coma Scale; ciTBI, clinically important TBI. LOC, loss of consciousness (*Source*: Kuppermann *et al.* [52]; reproduced with permission from Elsevier).

(GCS 14–15) derived and validated prediction rules to detect patients with a very low risk of a *clinically important* (ci) TBI. ciTBI was defined as an injury resulting in death, neurosurgical intervention, intubation more than 24 h, or hospital admission for more than 2 days [52]. Overall, the rate of ciTBI in the study was 0.9%. There were no deaths; 0.1% of patients required surgery. Figure 4.2 depicts the suggested CT algorithm suggested by the study authors. Despite some limitations, this algorithm is the best evidence-based approach to date. It is meant to inform, not replace, clinical decision making.

CT versus observation

Observation in the ED can be used as an alternative to CT in patients without altered mental status or signs of skull fracture (Figure 4.2) [52]. Additional factors that may play a role in the decision to observe include physician experience, the presence of risk factors, worsening symptoms, parental preference, and age less than 12 months, since infants are more difficult to examine, have an increased incidence of asymptomatic ICI, and are the group at highest risk of unsuspected child abuse [51]. The time period for this initial observation suggested by the American Academy of Pediatrics (AAP) is 4–6 h [53].

Hospitalization versus discharge

The decision about to discharge the patient with mTBI home from the ED or admit them to the hospital is based upon the same historical and examination findings that informed CT decision making, as well as the severity of symptoms, CT findings (if performed), and additional social issues. Delayed deterioration in patients with mTBI, a normal head CT, and a normal physical examination is extremely rare [52, 54]. Home observation is an option for those with a normal mental status, normal neurologic exam, and if CT performed, no ICI. If an ICI is identified, hospital admission for monitored observation is typically warranted. Pediatric patients or adult patients with mental limitations with mTBI should only be discharged from the ED with caretakers who have the ability to seek immediate medical attention if needed and understand instructions about what should prompt them to do so, such as seizures, extremity weakness/numbness, worsening headache, repeated vomiting, or behavior changes. Hospitalization may also be indicated for patients with persistent confusion, vomiting, or headache requiring pain management.

Establishing a system of care for the assessment of mTBI in the ED

Even patients with a normal GCS score, normal physical examination, and normal neuroimaging (if performed) can be at risk for prolonged mTBI recovery, especially if the mTBI is not diagnosed and managed properly from the onset. One of the most effective ways to ensure proper diagnosis and management is to incorporate a standardized mTBI assessment tool into the standard ED workflow and use for the evaluation of any patient with a head injury.

The acute concussion evaluation (ACE) is one of the few existing standardized assessment tools available to identify cognitive deficits in the acute medical care setting [17, 55]. This assessment tool is available free online as part of the CDC Heads Up Toolkit for Physicians [17]. The main ACE components prompt the clinician to:

1   Define the acute injury (Box 4.2).
2   Assess for the symptoms using a simplified version of the well-researched 22-item post-concussion scale [56].
3   Identify risk factors for prolonged recovery [32].
4   Make the diagnosis of mTBI and.
5   Provide a proper discharge plan including referral to primary care providers and specialists for ongoing evaluation [17].

Use of the ACE in the ED setting is currently being studied in the pediatric population (PI: G. Gioia, M. Collins; CDC 1U49CE001385). A recently published study found that the Graded Symptom Checklist reliably identified mTBI in children 6 years of age and older [30]. Using a standardized tool provides a consistent and individualized assessment to help the clinician determine whether to make a diagnosis of mTBI and serve as the basis for which the ED physician can speak with the family about the natural course of the injury, implications for recovery, and need for follow-up.

Providing patient education on mTBI: Understanding the natural history

In the hours to days that follow mTBI, many patients will have symptoms, and within weeks to months, most will make a complete recovery [31]. However, a significant fraction do not. In a recent study of children with mTBI, Yeates and colleagues demonstrated that 21% of patients had symptoms for greater than 3 months and patients with a higher number of acute clinical features were more likely to have persistent symptoms [57]. A large body of data from the sports literature describes the natural history of recovery in sports-related mTBI [15, 31]. Certain injury-related and noninjury-related risk factors are been associated with prolonged recovery including prior concussion, migraine, learning disorders and psychiatric disorders, younger age [58, 59], and genetic vulnerability (e.g., ApoE gene) [60].

After the ED visit: The importance of physical and cognitive rest

A discharge plan for patients with mTBI is the last critical piece of management for the ED physician. A useful resource for discharge instructions can be found in the CDC Heads Up Toolkit for Physicians [17]. These instructions provide clear indications for seeking immediate care, describe the natural course of the injury, discuss risk factors for prolonged recovery, and provide key strategies to potentially hasten recovery and prevent further injury [17]. This type of education has been shown to aid recovery [5, 61]. All patients should be instructed to obtain follow-up with a primary care provider, and in some cases, a concussion specialist [17]. Referral to a concussion specialist/neuropsychologist may be warranted for patients with symptoms lasting more than 7 days, with underlying learning/behavioral disorders, with a prior history of concussion, and/or returning to contact sports [9].

Many patients with mTBI report increased postconcussive symptoms with both physical and cognitive exertions [1]. These exertional effects are thought to be related to the inability of the brain to respond to the extra metabolic demands of physical or mental exertion during the period of metabolic crisis [19]. While physical rest has been the mainstay of concussion care for quite some time, cognitive rest is also crucial [12, 17]. In the pediatric population, cognitive rest may include temporary absence from school and/or shorted school days, limiting class workloads and/or allowing for more time to complete assignments and/or avoiding tests. Discharge instructions that include a *return to school* form can serve to communicate to school personnel regarding the injury's typical manifestations and the potential supports needed. For adults and older adolescents, considerations to driving restrictions should be made as well. Overall, emphasis should be on avoiding activities that produce symptoms.

Physical rest and return to sport

The concept of physical rest after mTBI is not new. It is well established in the sports-related mTBI literature that there is a period of increased vulnerability after a concussion; if returned to play during this period, athletes are four to six times more likely to have another concussion [62]. Consequences of repeat concussion may include increased symptoms and a more prolonged recovery (e.g., postconcussion syndrome [PCS]), second-impact syndrome (SIS), and potential chronic cognitive changes [36]. PCS is when patients have cognitive, physical, or emotional symptoms more than 1–2 weeks postinjury. SIS is very rare and is characterized by a sudden onset of brain edema at the time of a second, often minor, head injury. Although controversy remains as to causality, the existence of SIS highlights the importance of cautious management during recovery.

Children with mTBI should be removed from physical activity until they are fully asymptomatic at rest. With regard to return to play for athletes, the International Conference on Concussion in Sport (CIS) recommends against using the previously numerous graded classifications for sports-related concussions. Instead, they recommend using an individualized evaluation of the athlete's symptoms, neurocognitive functioning, and ability to balance [9]. Using this approach, the athlete is removed from play until asymptomatic at rest and with exertion, and neurocognitive function is normal. The athlete may then progress through levels of increasing physical and cognitive activity with 24 h between each step (steps: light aerobic activity, sport-specific activity, noncontact training, full contact practice, and, finally, game play). Patients should only return to activity and sport when cleared by a primary care provider or specialist.

For those in contact sports, recent CIS recommendations for return to play include both evaluation of symptoms and neurocognitive testing, if available. Several computerized neurocognitive tests are available commercially; all have demonstrated deficits in athletes with mTBI. The role in the ED in regard to neurocognitive testing remains referral of appropriate patients to a concussion specialist who can administer the tests.

Since the time needed for recovery from mTBI must be individualized and cannot be predicted at the time of the ED visit, the ED physician should refrain from making specific recommendations on time to return to play and instead emphasize the need for this decision to be made in follow-up. The focus at the time of the ED visit should be on the need for cognitive and physical rest and avoidance of activities that worsen symptoms or could lead to reinjury.

Summary

mTBI is a common injury encountered by the ED physician. All patients presenting with a history of a head injury as well as those with signs and symptoms suggestive of mTBI should be assessed for mTBI. The ED assessment should consist of an accurate and detailed history, which will guide decision making for neuroimaging. Making the diagnosis of mTBI in the ED is critical; early recognition of the injury, patient education, and active outpatient follow-up are keys to facilitating recovery and preventing reinjury. Ideally, the ED physician will incorporate a standardized mTBI assessment tool into the ED workflow to allow an individualized assessment of symptoms, timely diagnosis, and a patient-specific discussion on the natural course of mTBI and necessary outpatient management. Discharge instructions specific to mTBI are critically important and should include reasons to seek immediate care and instructions for both cognitive and physical rest, the mainstay of therapy. Emphasis on follow-up with a primary care provider or specialist should be made to ensure a safe return to school/work, activity, and sport.

References

1 Langlois, J.A., Rutland-Brown, W. & Thomas, K.E. (2004) *Traumatic Brain Injury in the United States: Emergency Department Visits, Hospitalizations, and Deaths.* Center for Disease Control and Prevention, National Center for Injury Prevention and Control (ed), Atlanta, GA.
2 Bazarian, J.J., Wong, T., Harris, M., Leahey, N., Mookerjee, S., & Dombovy, M. (1999) Epidemiology and predictors of post-concussive syndrome after minor head injury in an emergency population. *Brain Injury*, **13**, 173–189.
3 Thornhill, S., Teasdale, G.M., Murray, G.D., McEwen, J., Roy, C.W., & Penny, K.I. (2000) Disability in young people and adults one year after head injury: prospective cohort study. *British Medical Journal*, **320**, 1631–1635.
4 Yeates, K.O. & Taylor, H.G. (2005) Neurobehavioural outcomes of mild head injury in children and adolescents. *Pediatric Rehabilitation*, **8**, 5–16.

5 Ponsford, J., Willmott, C., Rothwell, A. *et al.* (2001) Impact of early intervention on outcome after mild traumatic brain injury in children. *Pediatrics*, **108**, 1297–1303.

6 Prevention, Centers for Disease Control and Prevention (ed). (2003) *Report to Congress on Mild Traumatic Brain Injury in the United States: Steps to Prevent a Serious Public Health Problem.* National Center for Injury Prevention and Control, Atlanta, GA.

7 Holm, L., Cassidy, J.D., Carroll, L.J. & Borg, J. (2005) Summary of the WHO Collaborating Centre for neurotrauma task force on mild traumatic brain injury. *Journal of Rehabilitation Medicine*, **37**, 137–141.

8 Kay, T., Harrington, D.E., Adams, R. *et al.* (1993) Definition of mild traumatic brain injury. *Journal of Head Trauma Rehabilitation*, **8**, 86–87.

9 McCrory, P., Meeuwisse, W., Johnston, K. *et al.* (2009) Consensus statement on concussion in sport—the Third International Conference on Concussion in Sport held in Zurich, November 2008. *Physician and Sportsmedicine*, **37**, 141–159.

10 Kelly, J.P. (2001) Loss of consciousness: pathophysiology and implications in grading and safe return to play. *Journal of Athletic Training*, **36**, 249–252.

11 Iverson, G.L., Lovell, M.R. & Smith, S.S. (2000) Does brief loss of consciousness affect cognitive functioning after mild head injury? *Archives of Clinical Neuropsychology*, **15**, 643–648.

12 Majerske, C.W., Mihalik, J.P., Ren, D. *et al.* (2008) Concussion in sports: postconcussive activity levels, symptoms, and neurocognitive performance. *Journal of Athletic Training*, **43**, 265–274.

13 Cantu, R.C. (1998) Second-impact syndrome. *Clinical Journal of Sports Medicine*, **17**, 37–44.

14 Lovell, M., Collins, M. & Bradley, J. (2004) Return to play following sports-related concussion, *Clinical Journal of Sports Medicine*, **23**, 421–441, ix.

15 Halstead, M.E. & Walter, K.D. (2010) American Academy of Pediatrics. Clinical report—sport-related concussion in children and adolescents. *Pediatrics*, **126**, 597–615.

16 Kirkwood, M.W., Yeates, K.O., Taylor, H.G., Randolph, C., McCrea, M. & Anderson, V.A. (2008) Management of pediatric mild traumatic brain injury: a neuropsychological review from injury through recovery. *Clinical Neuropsychology*, **22**, 769–800.

17 Langlois, J.A. *Heads Up: Facts for Physicians About Mild Traumatic Brain Injury.* Center for Disease Control and Prevention, National Center for Injury Prevention and Control (ed), Atlanta, GA.

18 Dematteo, C.A., Hanna, S.E., Mahoney, W.J. *et al.* (2010) My child doesn't have a brain injury, he only has a concussion. *Pediatrics*, **125**, 327–334.

19 Giza, C.C. & Hovda, D.A. (2001) The neurometabolic cascade of concussion. *Journal of Athletic Training*, **36**, 228–235.

20 Shenton, M.E., Hamoda, H.M., Schneiderman, J.S. *et al.* (2012) A review of magnetic resonance imaging and diffusion tensor imaging findings in mild traumatic brain injury. *Brain Imaging Behaviour*, **6**, 137–192.

21 Bazarian, J.J., McClung, J., Cheng, Y.T., Flesher, W. & Schneider, S.M. (2005) Emergency department management of mild traumatic brain injury in the USA. *Emergency Medicine Journal*, **22**, 473–477.

22 Holmes, J.F., Hendey, G.W., Oman, J.A. *et al* and for the NEXUS Group. (2006) Epidemiology of blunt head injury victims undergoing ED cranial computed tomographic scanning. *American Journal of Emergency Medicine*, **24**, 167–173.

23 Langlois, J.A., Rutland-Brown, W. & Wald, M.M. (2006) The epidemiology and impact of traumatic brain injury: a brief overview. *The Journal of Trauma Rehabilitation*, **21**, 375–378.

24 McCrea, M., Hammeke, T., Olsen, G., Leo, P. & Guskiewicz, K. (2004) Unreported concussion in high school football players: implications for prevention. *Clinical Journal of Sport Medicine*, **14**, 13–17.

25 Keenan, H.T., Runyan, D.K., Marshall, S.W., Nocera, M.A., Merten, D.F. & Sinal, S.H. (2003) A population-based study of inflicted traumatic brain injury in young children. *Journal of American Medical Association*, **290**, 621–626.

26 Jenny, C., Hymel, K.P., Ritzen, A., Reinert, S.E. & Hay, T.C. (1999) Analysis of missed cases of abusive head trauma. *Journal of American Medical Association*, **281**, 621–626.

27 Alexander, R.H. & Proctor, H.J. (eds) (1993) *Advanced Trauma Life Support Program for Physicians: ATLS.* American College of Surgeons, Chicago, IL.

28 Teasdale, G. & Jennett, B. (1974) Assessment of coma and impaired consciousness. A practical scale. *Lancet*, **2**, 81–84.

29 James, H.E. (1986) Neurologic evaluation and support in the child with an acute brain insult. *Pediatric Annals*, **15**, 16–22.

30 Grubenhoff, J.A., Kirkwood, M., Gao, D., Deakyne, S. & Wathen, J. (2010) Evaluation of the standardized assessment of concussion in a pediatric emergency department. *Pediatrics*, **126**, 688–695.

31 McCrea, M. (2008) *Mild Traumatic Brain Injury and Postconcussion Syndrome.* Oxford University Press, New York.

32 Ponsford, J., Willmott, C., Rothwell, A. *et al.* (1999) Cognitive and behavioral outcome following mild traumatic head injury in children. *The Journal of Head Trauma Rehabilitation*, **14**, 360–372.

33 Mooney, G., Speed, J., & Sheppard, S. (2005) Factors related to recovery after mild traumatic brain injury. *Brain Injury*, **19**, 975–987.

34 Mihalik, J.P., Stump, J.E., Collins, M.W., Lovell, M.R., Field, M. & Maroon, J.C. (2005) Posttraumatic migraine characteristics in athletes following sports-related concussion. *Journal of Neurosurgery*, **102**, 850–855.

35 Mather, F.J., Tate, R.L. & Hannan, T.J. (2003) Post-traumatic stress disorder in children following road traffic accidents: a comparison of those with and without mild traumatic brain injury. *Brain Injury*, **17**, 1077–1087.

36 Collins, M.W., Lovell, M.R., Iverson, G.L., Cantu, R.C., Maroon, J.C. & Field, M. (2002) Cumulative effects of concussion in high school athletes. *Neurosurgery*, **51**, 1175–1179; discussion 1180–1171.

37 Yeates, K.O., Luria, J., Bartkowski, H., Rusin, J., Martin, L. & Bigler, E.D. (1999) Postconcussive symptoms in children with mild closed head injuries. *The Journal of Trauma Rehabilitation*, **14**, 337–350.

38 Collins, M.W., Grindel, S.H., Lovell, M.R. *et al.* (1999) Relationship between concussion and neuropsychological performance in college football players. *Journal of American Medical Association*, **282**, 964–970.

39 Greenes, D.S. & Schutzman, S.A. (2001) Clinical significance of scalp abnormalities in asymptomatic head-injured infants. *Pediatric Emergency Care*, **17**, 88–92.

40 Pierce, M.C., Kaczor, K., Aldridge, S., O'Flynn, J. & Lorenz, D.J. (2010) Bruising characteristics discriminating physical child abuse from accidental trauma. *Pediatrics*, **125**, 67–74.

41 Sugar, N.F., Taylor, J.A. & Feldman, K.W. (1999) Bruises in infants and toddlers: those who don't cruise rarely bruise. Puget Sound Pediatric Research Network. *Archives of Pediatrics and Adolescent Medicine*, **153**, 399–403.

42 Brenner, D.J. (2002) Estimating cancer risks from pediatric CT: going from the qualitative to the quantitative. *Pediatric Radiology*, **32**, 228–223; discussion 242–224.

43 Haydel, M.J., Preston, C.A., Mills, T.J., Luber, S., Blaudeau, E. & DeBlieux, P.M. (2000) Indications for computed tomography in patients with minor head injury. *New England Journal of Medicine*, **343**, 100–105.

44 Stiell, I.G., Lesiuk, H., Wells, G.A. *et al.* (2001) Canadian CT head rule study for patients with minor head injury: methodology for phase II (validation and economic analysis). *Annals of Emergency Medicine*, **38**, 317–322.

45 Stiell, I.G., Clement, C.M., Rowe, B.H. *et al.* (2005) Comparison of the Canadian CT Head Rule and the New Orleans Criteria in patients with minor head injury. *Journal of American Medical Association*, **294**, 1511–1518.

46 Smits, M., Dippel, D.W.J., de Haan, G.G. *et al.* (2007) Minor head injury: guidelines for the use of CT—a multicenter validation study. *Radiology*, **245**, 831–838.

47 Jagoda, A.S., Bazarian, J.J., Bruns, J.J. Jr., *et al.*; Centers for Disease, C., and Prevention. (2008) Clinical policy: neuroimaging and decisionmaking in adult mild traumatic brain injury in the acute setting. *Annals of Emergency Medicine*, **52**, 714–748.

48 Palchak, M.J., Holmes, J.F., Vance, C.W., *et al.* (2003) A decision rule for identifying children at low risk for brain injuries after blunt head trauma. *Annals of Emergency Medicine*, **42**, 492–506.

49 Quayle, K.S., Jaffe, D.M., Kuppermann, N. *et al.* (1997) Diagnostic testing for acute head injury in children: when are head computed tomography and skull radiographs indicated? *Pediatrics*, **99**, E11.

50 Dunning, J., Daly, J.P., Lomas, J.P., Lecky, F., Batchelor, J. & Mackway-Jones, K. (2006) Derivation of the children's head injury algorithm for the prediction of important clinical events decision rule for head injury in children. *Archives of Disease in Child*, **91**, 885–891.

51 Greenes, D.S. & Schutzman, S.A. (1999) Clinical indicators of intracranial injury in head-injured infants. *Pediatrics*, **104**, 861–867.

52 Kuppermann, N., Holmes, J.F., Dayan, P.S. *et al.* (2009) Identification of children at very low risk of clinically-important brain injuries after head trauma: a prospective cohort study. *Lancet*, **374**, 1160–1170.

53 Committee on Quality Improvement, American Academy of Pediatrics Commission on Clinical Policies and Research, American Academy of Family Physicians. The management of minor closed head injury in children. *Pediatrics*, **104**, 1407–1415.

54 af Geijerstam, J.L. & Britton, M. (2005) Mild head injury: reliability of early computed tomographic findings in triage for admission. *Emergency Medicine Journal*, **22**, 103–107.

55 Gioia, G.A., Collins, M. & Isquith, P.K. (2008) Improving identification and diagnosis of mild traumatic brain injury with evidence: psychometric support for the acute concussion evaluation. *The Journal of Trauma Rehabilitation*, **23**, 230–242.

56 Lovell, M.R. & Collins, M.W. (1998) Neuropsychological assessment of the college football player. *The Journal of Trauma Rehabilitation*, **13**, 9–26.

57 Yeates, K.O., Taylor, H.G., Rusin, J. *et al.* (2009) Longitudinal trajectories of postconcussive symptoms in children with mild traumatic brain injuries and their relationship to acute clinical status. *Pediatrics*, **123**, 735–743.

58 Field, M., Collins, M.W., Lovell, M.R. & Maroon, J. (2003) Does age play a role in recovery from sports-related concussion? A comparison of high school and collegiate athletes. *Journal of Pediatrics*, **142**, 546–553.

59 Lovell, M.R. (2006) Is neuropsychological testing useful in the management of sport-related concussion? *Journal of Athletic Training*, **41**, 137–138; author reply 138–140.

60 Moran, L.M., Taylor, H.G., Ganesalingam, K. *et al.* (2009) Apolipoprotein E4 as a predictor of outcomes in pediatric mild traumatic brain injury. *Journal of Neurotrauma*, **26**, 1489–1495.

61 Wade, D.T., King, N.S., Wenden, F.J., Crawford, S. & Caldwell, F. E. (1998) Routine follow up after head injury: a second randomised controlled trial. *Journal of Neurology, Neurosurgery and Psychiatry*, **65**, 177–183.

62 Iverson, G.L., Gaetz, M., Lovell, M.R. & Collins, M.W. (2004) Cumulative effects of concussion in amateur athletes. *Brain Injury*, **18**, 433–443.

CHAPTER 5

In-hospital observation for mild traumatic brain injury

Pieter E. Vos[1] and Dafin F. Muresanu[2]

[1] *Department of Neurology, Slingeland Hospital, Doetinchem, the Netherlands*
[2] *Department of Neurology, University CFR Hospital, University of Medicine and Pharmacy "Iuliu Hatieganu," Cluj-Napoca, Romania*

Which patients should be admitted to the hospital?

Admission to hospital for MTBI depends on clinical and imaging findings. In general, patients with abnormal imaging results will be always admitted to the hospital. When imaging of the head is normal, it is usually safe to conclude that the risk of clinically important brain injury is very low (as long as coagulopathy is ruled out). The majority of all MTBI patients (>90%) show normal CT scan findings [1, 2]. In moderate TBI, lesions are more frequent (20%).

Patients with normal intracranial CT findings

Patients with a normal neurological examination and no risk factors (coagulopathy, drug or alcohol intoxication, other injuries, suspected nonaccidental injury, cerebrospinal fluid leak) and a normal CT can be safely discharged home from the ED. Well-done studies indicate that they are at very low risk of secondary deterioration due to delayed intracranial hematoma [3–5]. However, discharge instructions should provide counsel about the risk of persistent postconcussive syndrome, the need for physical and cognitive rest, graded resumption of activities and instructions for follow-up evaluation should postconcussive symptoms persist for longer than 1 week.

Even when imaging results are negative, other indications exist to observe patients including prolonged posttraumatic amnesia (PTA), drug or alcohol intoxication, cerebrospinal fluid (CSF) leakage, and systemic injuries (see Box 5.1).

Traumatic Brain Injury, First Edition. Edited by Pieter E. Vos and Ramon Diaz-Arrastia.
© 2015 John Wiley & Sons, Ltd. Published 2015 by John Wiley & Sons, Ltd.

Box 5.1 Criteria for hospital admission of MTBI patients.

> ### Clinically significant abnormal CT
>
> GCS < 15
> Focal neurological deficit
> Prolonged PTA/agitation
> Coagulation disorders
> Alcohol/drug intoxication
> Severe headache
> Persistent vomiting
> Skull (base) fracture—CSF leakage
> Multiple injuries (facial extremity fractures)
> Suspected nonaccidental injury
>
> ---
>
> Hospital admission criteria modified from NICE, ATLS, and Dutch guidelines [3, 6].

Patients with abnormal intracranial CT findings

Patients with abnormal CT results that do not require surgery or those with unresolved neurological signs usually require admission to the hospital for observation. Patients in coma (usually GCS ≤ 8) and those requiring immediate craniectomy for life-threatening hematoma will usually be admitted to the ICU of a neurosurgical center (see Chapter 6). Observation of mild and moderate TBI patients should occur until consciousness and anterograde memory are restored. In the UK, National Institute for Clinical Excellence (NICE) guidelines have extensively described standardized and protocolized procedures in observing patients with MTBI [3]. Implementation of these guidelines has resulted in improved patient care in the UK. Since the introduction of the guidelines, the number of CTs has increased but fewer patients require admission, because patients with normal imaging results, a normal consciousness, and no other signs and symptoms of concern to the clinician are discharged [4]. Adherence to these guidelines reserves in-hospital observation after TBI for patients with a more severe profile.

Role of specialized neurosurgical centers

Comparison of mortality following hospitalization for isolated head injury demonstrates significant differences among countries, depending on the level of organization of trauma services and whether patients are referred to a neurosurgical center. In the UK, a higher rate of mortality was found in severe TBI patients managed in nonneurosurgical centers compared to patients admitted to neurosurgical centers [5].

In a study of TBI admissions, 50–60 % were MTBI patients and risk-adjusted odds of mortality was higher in England/Wales than in Victoria, Australia [7]. A lower percentage of cases managed at neurosurgical centers in England and Wales has been suggested as an explanatory factor in this respect. These findings confirmed an earlier study that only 67% of British severe TBI patients were admitted to a neurosurgical center and only 53% of those initially arriving at a nonneurosurgical center were later transferred to a neurosurgical center [5]. Based on these findings, the NICE guidelines were changed and now recommend transfer of all severe TBI patients to hospitals with 24 h availability of neurosurgical services.

As the frequency of life-threatening hematoma in MTBI is low (<1%) and mortality is very low (<1%), transferral of patients from nonneurosurgical centers to neurosurgical centers is probably neither indicated nor feasible. The growing capacity in many hospitals to consult with neurosurgical experts by means of teleradiology further reduces the need for transfer. Because of concerns in the UK about the experience and skills of staff on general and orthopedic acute wards in TBI care, the Royal College of Surgeons of England in 1999 recommended that general and orthopedic surgeons should generally no longer be involved in the care of patients requiring a short period of observation for an isolated head injury (http://www.rcseng.ac.uk/publications/docs/report_head_injuries.html). In addition, the NICE guidelines (which first appeared in 2003 and were revised in 2007) cite evidence from a retrospective historical study involving medical and surgical (including head injury) patients that accident and emergency observation wards are more efficient and more cost-effective than general medical or surgical wards for managing short stay observation [3, 8] after trauma. Because patients' outcomes were not considered, in our opinion, no firm conclusion can be drawn regarding safety issues in relation to where to admit the patient. The indications for admitting patients who did not require initial neurosurgical intervention after mild-to-moderate TBI to a neurosurgical center have also been investigated in Italy. Observation in a neurosurgical unit was compared with observation in a peripheral hospital where a neurosurgeon could be consulted through teleradiology. In the peripheral hospital, 6% of 715 mild-to-moderate severe TBI patients required neurosurgical intervention during observation. Outcome was not different from 47/117 patients who were observed at a neurosurgical unit and subsequently required neurosurgical intervention. Hence, a model of care with observation in a peripheral hospital with neurosurgical consults by teleradiology, repeat CT scanning, and transfer times of 30–60 min to a neurosurgical center was not detrimental for subjects with initial nonneurosurgical lesions after mild-to-moderate head injury [9]. This study also indicates that direct assessment of the CT by a neurosurgeon via teleradiology reduces unnecessary transferrals [10, 11].

Observation of patients with mild and moderate TBI: Where to admit at which ward?

Irrespective of the type of hospital, alternatives exist for acute observation of mild and moderate TBI patients. These include accident and emergency ward, surgical ward, orthopedic ward, neurological ward, and neurosurgical ward. The choice of hospital service depends highly on country-specific resources, and the specific UK Royal College recommendations discussed here are probably difficult to generalize to other countries. Development of local protocols based on the organization of trauma systems and resources in each is essential (see also Chapter 3 on prehospital care). The NICE recommendation defines in general terms the criteria for observation *"in circumstances where a patient with a head injury requires hospital admission, the patient only be admitted under the care of a consultant who has been trained in the management of this condition during his/her higher specialist training. It is recommended that in-hospital observation of patients with a head injury, including all accident and emergency observation, should only be conducted by profes-sionals competent in the assessment of head injury"* [3]. Dutch guidelines, which were in part derived from NICE guidelines, advise to admit the patient at the ward where specialists are available with knowledge on the most vital threats to the patient. Interdisciplinary collaboration is of importance in this respect and sufficient education and skills for the minimal observations is required. In conclusion, it is not possible to generalize recommendations as to where to admit the MTBI patient. Rather, the use of local (defining also interdisciplinary collaboration within hospitals) and regional protocols for observation procedures of MTBI patients is necessary.

Observation in the hospital: Goals and procedures

The main purpose of observation is to detect secondary complications at an early stage. The probability of serious secondary complications, such as result from delayed hematoma, meningitis in patients with skull base fractures, and arterial dissection, is very low but finite. Given the large annual incidence of MTBI, secondary complications are regularly encountered.

General measures

During hospitalization, general measures can be undertaken to treat or prevent behavioral disturbances after TBI. Promoting the presence of family members, minimizing exposure to external stimuli (such as sounds and light) in the envi-ronment, clear communication, and a structured day program may all have a beneficial influence on the patient's behavior [12, 13]. Also pain and urinary retention can promote agitation after TBI, and adequate treatment of pain with analgesics is as effective as sedative treatment with hypnotics [14]. Specific medical and nursing expertise also has positive effects in the acute phase on the agitated/aggressive patient, reduces the incidence of delirium, and shortens the duration of hospitalization [15]. Based on a few studies of adequate methodolog-ical quality, Dutch guidelines recommend that haloperidol is probably effective

Table 5.1 In-hospital observation schedule and indications for repeat CT in mild and moderate TBI patients.

Modality	Frequency	Consider repeat CT
General	GCS = 15	1. Drop of one point in GCS level 2. Severe headache/vomiting 3. Agitation or abnormal behavior
Respiratory rate Heart rate/blood pressure Temperature Blood oxygen saturation	0–2 h: every 30 min* 2–6 h: every h >6 h: every 2 h	
Neurological GCS	GCS < 15 0–2 h: every 30 min*, hereafter every hour until GCS = 15	4. Any drop ≥ 2 points in GCS level
Pupil size, reactivity Limb movements Tendon reflexes Anterograde memory		5.Symptoms or signs pupil inequality or asymmetry of limb or facial movement 6. GCS = 15 not reached after 24 h

Modified from Refs. [3, 6].
*In general these observations will occur at the ED. Observations must be carried out by qualified personnel. NICE guidelines advice a second member of staff competent to perform observation to confirm deterioration before involving the supervising doctor. Every deterioration in neurological parameters should be discussed with the medical specialist and causes for deterioration explored.

in treating delirium caused by a general medical condition [15–18]. However, there are considerations based on animal studies that indicate that antipsychotics impair the recovery process and exacerbate TBI-induced behavioral deficits [19, 20]. When treatment is deemed necessary, see in the following for a treatment scheme that can be followed when a prompt result is required.

Observation

Specific observation measures consist of scheduled assessments of the patient aiming to detect complications at an earliest stage. See Table 5.1 for overview.

Complications

Anticoagulation

The use of anticoagulation in MTBI has been associated with increased mortality, in particular when the history of head injury is missed (see Figure 5.1). The international normalized ratio (INR) is positively correlated to mortality particularly in the setting of an intracranial hematoma [21]. Retrospective evidence in

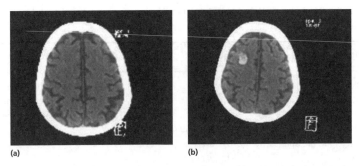

(a)   (b)

Figure 5.1 Delayed intracerebral hematoma in an 80-year-old MTBI patient on oral anticoagulation. CT on day 1 is normal (a); CT on day 2 shows intracerebral hematoma (b).

patients on anticoagulation with head trauma and a normal CT suggest that there is no increased risk for (delayed) intracranial hematoma [22]. A practical approach is then to question every patient with head injury about the use of anticoagulation therapy. All patients on anticoagulation therapy should have their INR checked and the indication for anticoagulation reviewed. These patients should be admitted for neurological observation. If CT demonstrates an intracranial hematoma, the INR should be corrected immediately [23]. Over-anticoagulation can be best corrected with fresh frozen plasma and vitamin K. If spontaneous coagulation disorders or additional injuries with bleeding exist, the decision to transfuse is complex, and consultation with a coagulation specialist should be considered. Transfusions are associated with well-recognized risks, and a recent retrospective study [24] indicates that in patients with moderate coagulopathy (INR 1.4–2.0) not resulting from anticoagulant therapy, transfusion with fresh frozen plasma was associated with worse neurologic outcome. In patients without any abnormalities on the CT and an INR in the therapeutic range, wait and see management under close clinical observation can be carried out. In case of a normal CT and an INR outside the therapeutic range, discontinuation of anticoagulants and vitamin K for several days until normalization of the INR seems rational [6]. The new oral anticoagulant medications including direct thrombin antagonists and factor Xa inhibitors work via different mechanisms and lack reliable laboratory tests to measure levels of anticoagulation. As long as no pharmacological antidote exists and there is no evidence how to best counteract intracranial hemorrhage, the care for patients taking these newer anticoagulants who experience intracranial hemorrhage remains difficult [25].

Behavioral complications in the acute phase

After TBI certain stages are recognized [26]. The first stage consists of loss of consciousness or coma, although this is not an obligatory phenomenon for MTBI. By definition, loss of consciousness, if present, lasts shorter than 30 min [27]. The second phase is characterized by a period of disorientation, memory disorders, and behavioral disturbances, also referred to as PTA. By (arbitrary) definition, PTA is under 24 h in MTBI, but can persist for days or weeks in moderate and severe TBI. The third phase is characterized by recovery of motor, cognitive, and behavioral disturbances. Particularly after moderate and severe TBI, where recovery can be incomplete, a fourth stage can be recognized that consists of acceptation of and compensation for the permanent sequelae.

Complaints like headache and dizziness are usually present in the second stage; in addition, other posttraumatic complaints like phono- and photophobia, poor concentration, sleep disturbances, irritability, and anxiety becoming more apparent during recovery or when resuming activities may last up to 3 months [28]. In moderate TBI, the acute phase is usually more protracted and encompasses the period of awakening from *stupor*, by definition the period with decreased consciousness (GCS 9–12), PTA, and related behavioral disturbances. In extreme cases, this period may last for weeks and require hospitalization.

Posttraumatic amnesia (PTA)

PTA is defined as the transient period of confusion, amnesia, and behavioral agitation after brain injury. PTA is an important factor in the day-to-day clinical management of all TBI patients, influencing decisions such as the moment of discharge and the start of rehabilitation. In severe TBI, duration of PTA is one of the best predictors of both short- and long-term functional, neurological, and cognitive outcomes [29]. After mild and moderate TBI, the presence of PTA is associated with an increased risk of intracranial hemorrhage and the need for neurosurgical intervention and is used to classify injury severity [22, 27, 30]. It is important to assess the PTA starting at the ED and continue evaluations at regular intervals during in-hospital observation.

Disorientation and anterograde amnesia are central elements of PTA. During PTA patients are unable to lay down new information, resulting in an inability to orient to unknown surroundings [31]. This bears an increased risk of falling and serious behavioral disturbances like agitation, and sometimes, frank aggression can be present. Several formal PTA scales exist that vary in the way PTA is tested [32–34]. Differences between scales can result in different conclusions about the duration of PTA. In the ED, testing for PTA includes assessment of orientation (time, place, person), attention, and a three-word recall test with immediate and delayed recall (as in the mini mental state examination). Such an assessment is simple and well accepted by physicians trained in multiple specialties. More detailed measures such as the Galveston Orientation and Amnesia Test (GOAT) are more appropriate for use in neurotrauma and rehabilitation units. At our department, we use a short examiner-independent, practical, and prospective PTA scale by selecting the most discriminative items from existing scales [35]. This scale was developed in a cohort of mild, moderate, and severe TBI patients and consists of seven items: age, name hospital, time, day, month, mode of transport, and three memory items (Box 5.2).

Box 5.2 The Nijmegen PTA scale.

1 What is your age?	[....]/1
2 Where are you now? (*name hospital*)	[....]/1
3 What time do you think it is? (margin of 30 min)	[....]/1
4 Which day of the week is it?	[....]/1
5 Which month of the year is it?	[....]/1
6 How did you get here? (*mode of transport*)	[....]/1

On day 1 end here and present three words as memory items (procedure see below); on day 2 and further continue:

7 Can you recall the three words you heard yesterday?
  If not: show the three words between six distracters (not used as target words before).
  Can you recognize which three of these words you heard yesterday? [....]/3
    – *If three words are recognized: give three new words not used as distracter before.*
    – *If less than 3 words are recognized: present the same three words that should have been remembered for this day as memory items.*
  While presenting the new words:
Can you repeat the words I am presenting you?
  Immediately after presenting the three words:
  Can you tell me the three words you just have heard?
  If not: present the words once more and let the patient repeat.
Score one point for every correct answer to the items 1–6 (maximum 6 points) and 1 point for every word correctly recalled or recognized.   [....]/9

Source: Jacobs *et al.* [35].

The advantage of the scale is that it is suitable both for testing PTA in mild TBI on the ED and follow-up and also for more severely injured TBI patients. Use of formal scales may improve the accuracy of the diagnosis and duration of PTA.

Although the exact neurobiologic substrate of PTA is not entirely known, anterograde memory impairment can occur from damage to the medial temporal lobe and diencephalic structures (mediodorsal thalamus and corpora mammillaria) or the connections between these structures (the mammillothalamic tract and the fornix) [36]. The temporal lobes are vulnerable to the effects of head injury due to its proximity to the sphenoid bone, and acute amnesia may be the result of structural medial temporal lobe damage. Alternatively, more diffuse injury to efferent and afferent connections between the prefrontal ventrolateral cortex and the mediotemporal lobe may result in amnesia, as has been demonstrated in recent studies using diffusion tensor imaging [37]. Interestingly, after mild-to-moderate TBI, single-photon emission CT within 72 h postinjury demonstrated an increased frequency of hypoperfusion in the temporal and frontal lobes with left temporal predominance in patients with PTA [38].

It is important to record details during the period of PTA, as other clinical relevant abnormalities are frequently present, such as attention deficits, agitation, or psychomotor alterations. Therefore, PTA might not be the best terminology to refer to this period, and some suggest that posttraumatic confusional state is more fitting [39]. Furthermore, this phase may also be considered a form of posttraumatic delirium or delirium when amnesia coincides with fluctuations in consciousness, attentional and cognitive disturbances, and sleep–wake cycle abnormalities [26, 40].

Agitation and aggression in the acute phase

The most frequently occurring complication in the third phase is delirium or prolonged PTA, as the patient may constitute a threat to himself or herself as a consequence of motor restlessness and behavioral disturbances that increase the risk of falling. Patients with MTBI have an increased risk for neuropsychiatric symptoms (Chapter 11). The most vulnerable period in this respect is that of confusion and disorientation during PTA. Sometimes, frank aggression may result in immediate danger to the patient, medical personnel, and family members. In the acute phase, altered psychomotor activity and agitation, especially in the presence of fluctuations in consciousness, are often present. Agitation has been defined by Sandel as a subtype of delirium unique to survivors of a TBI in which [2] the survivor is in the state of PTA and [3] there are excesses of behavior that include some combination of aggression, akathisia, disinhibition, and/or emotional lability [41]. General measures can be taken to prevent falls and agitation. When agitation and motor restlessness hamper vital diagnostic procedures or treatment despite general measures, it may become necessary to administer sedatives despite a possible negative influence on the brain. The necessity of urgent diagnostic procedures must be weighed against the possible side effects of sedative medication [42]. Every patient with a decreased consciousness, in particular when medication is given (anxiolytics, sedatives, analgesics, or a combination thereof), must be observed by specialized medical personnel [43]. When sedative medication is given, repeated monitoring of vital functions such as the GCS, pupil size and reactivity, limb movements, respiratory rate, heart rate, blood pressure, temperature, blood oxygen saturation is necessary.

Drug or alcohol intoxication may interfere with initial assessment since it can mimic signs and symptoms that are risk factors for intracranial complications (decreased consciousness, amnesia). However, alcohol intoxication is not an independent risk factor for intracranial injury, making a differential diagnosis difficult. In intoxicated patients, it may be necessary to first exclude life-threatening intracranial injury, before appointing alcohol or drugs as the cause of a decreased consciousness level or behavioral disturbances [44].

Although the term aggression is usually reserved for behavior in connection to personality changes in the chronic phase of TBI, aggression is occasionally observed during the acute phase. The frequency of aggression in MTBI is difficult to estimate because of varying definitions [45]. In particular, in the setting of delirium or PTA when cognitive functions are impaired and in patients with a history of mood disorder and alcohol or drug abuse, the likelihood of aggressive

Box 5.3 Treatment scheme for the acutely agitated patient.

> **1** Quetiapine (Seroquel®) 25–50 mg orally or via nasogastric/enteral tube. Can tritrate up
>   to a maximal dose of 200 mg every 12 h.
> *If insufficient effect:*
> **2** Add lorazepam 0.5–2 mg intramuscularly or intravenously,
> *or*
> **3** Midazolam 5 mg intramuscularly or intravenously.
> *If not sufficient: propofol (needs consulting an anesthesiologist or intensivist).*

behaviors [45] is increased, necessitating the use of sedative drugs, antipsychotic treatment, or even fixation (Box 5.3).

Akinetic mutism
Rarely, TBI patients do not produce speech or motor movement, though in principle they should be capable of doing so. This state of the so-called akinetic mutism can be misdiagnosed as decreased consciousness although the patient usually registers most of what is happening and forms memories. This condition, when present after trauma, is usually a temporary state associated with bilateral frontal lobe lesions with intact motor and sensory pathways. It can also be present in patients with MTBI (Table 5.2).

Delayed or expanding hematoma
In a retrospective study involving 110 patients with MTBI and a small intracranial hematoma less than 5 mm, none deteriorated during a 24 h observation period [46]. Hospital admission did not influence further management in these patients. Although no randomized controlled trials exist in how and where to observe patients with small intracerebral hematomas and no midline shift, guidelines in the Netherlands state that it is safe to admit such patients to local hospitals without consulting a neurosurgeon [24].

In case of epidural hematoma, evacuation of the hematoma is necessary in rapidly deteriorating patients because outcome is inversely related to the GCS motor score immediately before operation [47]. A small epidural hematoma that does not result in altered sensorium may resolve spontaneously and can be managed conservatively under certain conditions. In a study, 22 patients demonstrating a small asymptomatic epidural hematoma (defined as no clinical evidence of raised intracranial pressure and no evidence of focal neurological signs attributable to a space occupying lesion) were intensively observed and monitored for changes in neurological status and with repeat CT [48]. Only 32% of the patients, in particular those with skull fracture transversing a meningeal artery, vein, or major sinus or those diagnosed within 6 h, subsequently required evacuation of the epidural hematoma 1–10 days of the initial trauma. The conclusion from these studies is that patients with a small epidural or

Table 5.2 Overview of posttraumatic complications in mild and moderate TBI.

	Risk factor	Check
Delirium	Older age, infection, metabolic derangement, structural intracranial lesions	Laboratory results, urine analysis, retention
Early seizures	CACNA1A mutations Structural lesions, mass effect	Structural lesion
Electrolyte disturbances	Medication, alcohol, structural lesions	Medication, diencephalic lesions
Skull base fracture		Temperature
CSF leakage	Skull (base) fracture	β(2)-transferrin test
Meningitis	Skull base fracture	Temperature, neck stiffness, delirium
Carotid–cavernous fistula	Cervical spine trauma	Pulsating headache, exophthalmos, ophthalmoplegia
Arterial dissection	Cervical spine trauma	Horner's syndrome, miosis, and ptosis. Skull base fracture
Delayed hematoma	Coagulation disorders	Neurological examination
Anosmia	Frontal lobe injury, facial fracture	Anosmia tests

intracerebral hematoma may be managed conservatively because of a low risk of deterioration and only rarely require the explicit expertise and immediate presence of a neurosurgeon [49]. Referral to a neurosurgical center is only needed when neurosurgical treatment (intracranial operation or pressure monitoring) is necessary. For the frequency and type of observations see Table 5.1.

Meningitis

The diagnosis of skull base fracture is important as it bears an increased risk of CSF leakage and meningitis and, in case of simultaneous injury to the carotid artery, of developing carotid dissection or a carotid–cavernous fistula. Skull base fracture can affect the anterior fossa structures (frontal sinus, the cribriform plate, and ethmoid roof) or middle fossa structures (sphenoid sinus and the petrous bone). Skull base fracture is a clinical diagnosis. Rhinorrhea, bilateral periorbital ecchymosis, and anosmia are characteristic for anterior fossa fractures. Otorrhea, hematotympanum or blood in the external auditory canal, hearing loss, Battle sign (retroauricular hematoma), peripheral facial nerve palsy, and signs of vestibular dysfunction indicate middle fossa fractures. Current available evidence does not demonstrate a reduction in the frequency of meningitis with antibiotic prophylactic treatment after skull base fracture, although a Cochrane review concluded that the published studies in this respect are methodologically flawed [50]. The risk for meningitis is increased in the presence of cerebrospinal fluid leakage. Most (50–85%) traumatic CSF fistulae cease spontaneously within 48 h after injury (cf [51]). It seems therefore rational to observe patients at least for 48 h after skull base fractures and at discharge after this period to discuss the alarm signs and symptoms of meningitis and the fact that a small increased meningitis risk will last lifelong.

Traumatic cervical arterial dissection

Blunt cerebrovascular injury encompasses dissections, traumatic intracranial aneurysms, traumatic carotid–cavernous fistula, and venous sinus thrombosis. Dissection of cervical arteries (carotid and vertebral) is a rare and often underdiagnosed and potential serious complication after TBI, which carry a high risk of cerebral infarction. Delayed detection is in-built to late symptom manifestation and more likely in the presence of multiple injuries and failed suspicion after minor trauma to the head. Mortality associated with blunt carotid arterial injury is 15%, while morbidity in survivors is 16% [52]. Cervical artery dissection is associated with cervical spine injury and anterior or middle fossa skull base fractures. A study involving 2902 general trauma patients screening for cervical artery dissection yielded incidence of 0.86% [52]. Criteria that were used included an injury mechanism compatible with severe hyperextension or flexion and rotation of the neck; significant soft tissue injury of the anterior neck; cervical spine fracture; displaced midface fracture or mandibular fracture associated with a major injury mechanism; and basilar skull fracture involving the sphenoid, mastoid, petrous, or foramen lacerum. Patients asymptomatic at diagnosis had a better neurologic outcome than those who were symptomatic. The exact incidence of arterial dissection in MTBI is not known. Although risk factors for cervical artery dissection can be appointed, they are more or less nonspecific and cannot always be identified prior to onset of neurological symptoms [53]. Traumatic cerebral infarction can be the result of a dissection/intramural hematoma, intraluminal thrombus or raised intimal flap with luminal narrowing, a pseudoaneurysm, vessel occlusion, or vessel transection [54] (Figure 5.2).

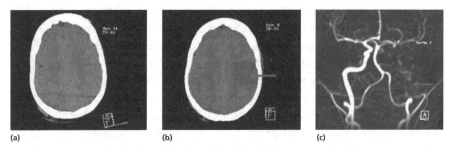

(a) (b) (c)

Figure 5.2 A 27-year-old patient with MTBI involved in a car accident. Initial CT was normal (a) after 10 h paralysis on the right side occurred and a CT showed middle cerebral artery infarction (b) caused by left-sided carotid artery dissection (c).

When to discharge from the hospital?

CT, which is sensitive in the detection of intracranial hematoma, is also a good technique to select patients for discharge home. In a review involving two prospective studies and 52 studies containing over 62, 000 patients investigating the safety of early CT in MTBI, only three cases were considered to have an early adverse outcome despite a normal initial CT, GCS = 15, and a normal neurological examination on presentation [55]. Only eight cases were identified in which the interpretation was unclear [55]. The conclusion was that the evidence available shows that a cranial CT, using modern CT scanners, is a safe way to triage patients for hospital admission.

One multicenter, pragmatic, noninferiority randomized trial involving 2602 patients aged ≥6 years with MTBI within the past 24 h, confirmed or suspected loss of consciousness or amnesia or both, normal results on neurological examination and a GCS of 15, and no associated injuries that required admission demonstrated that clinical outcomes are similar in those patients discharged home and those admitted for observation [56]. As no prospective studies exist evaluating the early discharge and home monitoring of patients with small intracranial hemorrhages, we advocate a restricted policy regarding early discharge. Only when patients are fully conscious—oriented in time, person, and space; free of severe headaches; and able to dress, feed, and walk independently—does it seem safe to discharge patients if they have a capable person for home observation. Although only very few MTBI patients will develop late complications, a system of high-quality discharge advice (oral and written with a scheduled follow-up outpatient clinic visit) and postdischarge observation by a caregiver is required to ensure that these patients receive appropriate care as soon as possible [3].

References

1 af Geijerstam, J.L. & Britton, M. (2003) Mild head injury—mortality and complication rate: meta-analysis of findings in a systematic literature review. *Acta Neurochirurgica*, **145**, 843–850.
2 Servadei, F., Teasdale, G. & Merry, G. (2001) Defining acute mild head injury in adults: a proposal based on prognostic factors, diagnosis, and management. *Journal of Neurotrauma*, **18**, 657–664.
3 National Institute for Clinical Excellence (2007) Head Injury: triage, assessment, investigation and early management of head injury in infants, children and adults. Nice Clinical Guideline No 56. www.nice.org.uk/CG056 [accessed on July 12, 2014].
4 Hassan, Z., Smith, M., Littlewood, S. *et al.* (2005) Head injuries: a study evaluating the impact of the NICE head injury guidelines. *Emergency Medicine Journal*, **22**, 845–849.
5 Patel, H.C., Bouamra, O., Woodford, M., King, A. T., Yates, D.W. & Lecky, F.E. (2005) Trends in head injury outcome from 1989 to 2003 and the effect of neurosurgical care: an observational study. *Lancet*, **366**, 1538–1544.

6 Vos, P.E., Alekseenko, Y., Battistin, L., et al. (2012) Mild traumatic brain injury. *European Journal of Neurology*, **19 (2)**, 191–198.

7 Gabbe, B.J., Lyons, R.A., Lecky, F.E. *et al.* (2011) Comparison of mortality following hospitalisation for isolated head injury in England and Wales, and Victoria, Australia. *PLoS One*, **6**, e20545.

8 Hadden, D.S., Dearden, C.H. & Rocke, L.G. (1996) Short stay observation patients: general wards are inappropriate. *Journal of Accident and Emergency Medicine*, **13**, 163–165.

9 Fabbri, A., Servadei, F., Marchesini, G., Stein, S.C. & Vandelli, A. (2008) Observational approach to subjects with mild-to-moderate head injury and initial non-neurosurgical lesions. *Journal of Neurology and Neurosurgery Psychiatry*, **79**, 1180–1185.

10 Ashkenazi, I., Haspel, J., Alfici, R., Kessel, B., Khashan, T. & Oren, M. (2007) Effect of tele-radiology upon pattern of transfer of head injured patients from a rural general hospital to a neurosurgical referral centre. *Emergency Medicine Journal*, **24**, 550–552.

11 Eljamel, M.S. & Nixon, T. (1992) The use of a computer-based image link system to assist inter-hospital referrals. *British Journal of Neurosurgery*, **6**, 559–562.

12 Fowler, S.B., Hertzog, J. & Wagner, B.K. (1995) Pharmacological interventions for agitation in head-injured patients in the acute care setting. *Journal of Neuroscience Nursing*, **27**, 119–123.

13 Plylar, P.A. (1989) Management of the agitated and aggressive head injury patient in an acute hospital setting. *Journal of Neuroscience Nursing*, **21**, 353–356.

14 Karabinis, A., Mandragos, K., Stergiopoulos, S. *et al.* (2004) Safety and efficacy of analgesia-based sedation with remifentanil versus standard hypnotic-based regimens in intensive care unit patients with brain injuries: a randomised, controlled trial [ISRCTN50308308]. *Critical Care*, **8**, R268–R280.

15 van der Mast, R.C., Huyse, F.J. & Rosier, P.F. (2005) Guideline 'Delirium'. *Nederlands Tijdschrift voor Geneeskunde*, **149**, 1027–1032.

16 Conn, D.K. & Lieff, S. (2001) Diagnosing and managing delirium in the elderly. *Canadian Family Physician*, **47**, 101–108.

17 Sharma, N.D., Rosman, H.S., Padhi, I.D. & Tisdale, J.E. (1998) Torsades de Pointes associated with intravenous haloperidol in critically ill patients. *American Journal of Cardiology*, **81**, 238–240.

18 American Psychiatric Association (1999) Practice guideline for the treatment of patients with delirium. *American Journal of Psychiatry*, **156**, 1–20.

19 Feeney, D.M., Gonzalez, A. & Law, W.A. (1982) Amphetamine, haloperidol, and experience interact to affect rate of recovery after motor cortex injury. *Science*, **217**, 855–857.

20 Bales, J.W., Wagner, A.K., Kline, A.E. & Dixon, C.E. (2009) Persistent cognitive dysfunction after traumatic brain injury: a dopamine hypothesis. *Neuroscience and Biobehavioral Reviews*, **33**, 981–1003.

21 Franko, J., Kish, K.J., O'Connell, B.G., Subramanian, S. & Yuschak, J.V. (2006) Advanced age and preinjury warfarin anticoagulation increase the risk of mortality after head trauma. *The Journal of Trauma*, **61**, 107–110.

22 Mina, A.A., Bair, H.A., Howells, G.A. & Bendick, P.J. (2003) Complications of preinjury warfarin use in the trauma patient. *The Journal of Trauma*, **54**, 842–847.

23 Vos, P.E., Battistin, L., Birbamer, G. *et al.* (2002) EFNS guideline on mild traumatic brain injury: report of an EFNS task force. *European Journal of Neurology*, **9**, 207–219.

24 Anglin, C.O., Spence, J.S., Warner, M.A., *et al.* (2013) Effects of platelet and plasma transfusion on outcome in traumatic brain injury patients with moderate bleeding diatheses. *Journal of Neurosurgery*, **118**, 676–686.

25 Awad, A.J., Walcott, B.P., Stapleton, C.J., Yanamadala, V., Nahed, B.V. & Coumans, J. (2013) Dabigatran, intracranial hemorrhage, and the neurosurgeon. *Neurosurgical Focus*, **34**(5), E7.

26 Rao, V. & Lyketsos, C. (2000) Neuropsychiatric sequelae of traumatic brain injury. *Psychosomatics*, **41**, 95–103.

27 Mild Traumatic Brain Injury Committee (1993) Definition of mild traumatic brain injury. *The Journal of Head Trauma Rehabilitation*, **8**, 86–87.

28 Kashluba, S., Paniak, C., Blake, T., Reynolds, S., Toller-Lobe, G. & Nagy, J. (2004) A longitudinal, controlled study of patient complaints following treated mild traumatic brain injury. *Archives of Clinical Neuropsychology*, **19**, 805–816.

29 Katz, D.I. & Alexander, M.P. (1994) Traumatic brain injury. Predicting course of recovery and outcome for patients admitted to rehabilitation. *Archives of Neurology*, **51**, 661–670.

30 Smits, M., Dippel, D.W., Steyerberg, E.W. *et al.* (2007) Predicting intracranial traumatic findings on computed tomography in patients with minor head injury: the CHIP prediction rule. *Annals of Internal Medicine*, **146**, 397–405.

31 Tate, R.L., Pfaff, A. & Jurjevic, L. (2000) Resolution of disorientation and amnesia during post-traumatic amnesia. *Journal of Neurology, Neurosurgery and Psychiatry*, **68**, 178–185.

32 Levin, H.S., O'Donnell, V.M. & Grossman, R.G. (1979) The Galveston Orientation and Amnesia Test. A practical scale to assess cognition after head injury. *The Journal of Nervous and Mental Disorder*, **167**, 675–684.

33 Fortuny, L.A., Briggs, M., Newcombe, F., Ratcliff, G. & Thomas, C. (1980) Measuring the duration of post traumatic amnesia. *Journal of Neurology, Neurosurgery and Psychiatry*, **43**, 377–379.

34 Shores, E.A., Marosszeky, J.E., Sandanam, J. & Batchelor, J. (1986) Preliminary validation of a clinical scale for measuring the duration of post-traumatic amnesia. *Medical Journal of Australia*, **144**, 569–572.

35 Jacobs, B., van Ekert, J., Vernooy, L.P., *et al.* (2012) Development and external validation of a new PTA assessment scale. *BMC Neurology*, **12**:69.

36 Gold, J.J. & Squire, L.R. (2006) The anatomy of amnesia: neurohistological analysis of three new cases. *Learning and Memory*, **13**, 699–710.

37 Wang, J.Y., Bakhadirov, K., Abdi, H. *et al.* (2011) Longitudinal changes of structural connectivity in traumatic axonal injury. *Neurology*, **77**, 818–826.

38 Gowda, N.K., Agrawal, D., Bal, C. *et al.* (2006) Technetium Tc-99m ethyl cysteinate dimer brain single-photon emission CT in mild traumatic brain injury: a prospective study. *AJNR American Journal of Neuroradiology*, **27**, 447–451.

39 Stuss, D.T., Binns, M.A., Carruth, F.G. *et al.* (1999) The acute period of recovery from traumatic brain injury: posttraumatic amnesia or posttraumatic confusional state? *Journal of Neurosurgery*, **90**, 635–643.

40 Nakase-Thompson, R., Sherer, M., Yablon, S.A., Nick, T.G. & Trzepacz, P.T. (2004) Acute confusion following traumatic brain injury. *Brain Injury*, **18**, 131–142.

41 Sandel, M.E. & Mysiw, W.J. (1996) The agitated brain injured patient. Part 1: definitions, differential diagnosis, and assessment. *Archives of Physical Medicine Rehabilitation*, **77**, 617–623.

42 Holger, J.S., Hale, D.B., Harris, C.R., Solberg, C. & Benfante, F. (1999) Sedation of intoxicated, agitated patients requiring CT to evaluate head injury. *American Journal of Emergency Medicine*, **17**, 321–323.

43 Knape, J.T. & van Everdingen, J.J. (1999) Guideline for administration of sedatives and analgesics by physicians who are not anesthesiologists. National Organization for Quality Assurance in Hospitals. *Nederlands tijdschrift voor geneeskunde*, **143 (21)**, 1098–1102. Dutch.

44 Stuke, L., Diaz-Arrastia, R., Gentilello, L.M., & Shafi, S. (2007) Effect of alcohol on Glasgow Coma Scale in head-injured patients. *Annals of Surgery*, **245 (4)**, 651–655.

45 Tateno, A., Jorge, R.E. & Robinson, R.G. (2003) Clinical correlates of aggressive behavior after traumatic brain injury. *The Journal of Neuropsychiatry and Clinical Neuroscience*, **15**, 155–160.

46 Schaller, B., Evangelopoulos, D.S., Muller, C. *et al.* (2010) Do we really need 24-h observation for patients with minimal brain injury and small intracranial bleeding? The Bernese Trauma Unit Protocol. *Emergency Medicine Journal*, **27**, 537–539.

47 Seelig, J.M., Marshall, L.F., Toutant, S.M. *et al.* (1984) Traumatic epidural hematoma: unrecognized high lethality in comatose patients. *Neurosurgery*, **15** (5), 617–620.

48 Knuckey, N.W., Gelbard, S. & Epstein, M.H. (1989) The management of "asymptomatic" epidural hematomas. A prospective study. *Journal of Neurosurgery*, **70**, 392–396.

49 Esposito, T.J., Reed, R.L., Gamelli, R.L. & Luchette, F.A. (2005) Neurosurgical coverage: essential, desired, or irrelevant for good patient care and trauma center status. *Annals of Surgery*, **242**, 364–370.

50 Ratilal, B.O., Costa, J., Sampaio, C. & Pappamikail, L. (2011) Antibiotic prophylaxis for preventing meningitis in patients with basilar skull fractures. *Cochrane Database of Systematic Review*, CD004884.

51 Rocchi, G., Caroli, E., Belli, E., Salvati, M., Cimatti, M. & Delfini, R. (2005) Severe craniofacial fractures with frontobasal involvement and cerebrospinal fluid fistula: indications for surgical repair. *Surgical Neurology*, **63**, 559–563.

52 Biffl, W.L., Moore, E.E., Ryu, R.K. *et al.* (1998) The unrecognized epidemic of blunt carotid arterial injuries: early diagnosis improves neurologic outcome. *Annals of Surgery*, **228**, 462–470.

53 Carrillo, E.H., Osborne, D.L., Spain, D.A., Miller, F.B., Senler, S.O. & Richardson, J.D. (1999) Blunt carotid artery injuries: difficulties with the diagnosis prior to neurologic event. *The Journal of Trauma*, **46** (6), 1120–1125.

54 Cothren, C.C., Biffl, W.L., Moore, E.E., Kashuk, J.L. & Johnson, J.L. (2009) Treatment for blunt cerebrovascular injuries: equivalence of anticoagulation and antiplatelet agents. *Archives of Surgery*, **144**, 685–690.

55 af Geijerstam, J.L. & Britton, M. (2005) Mild head injury: reliability of early computed tomographic findings in triage for admission. *Emergency Medicine Journal*, **22**, 103–107.

56 af Geijerstam, J.L., Oredsson, S. & Britton, M. (2006) Medical outcome after immediate computed tomography or admission for observation in patients with mild head injury: randomised controlled trial. *British Medical Journal*, **333**, 465.

PART III
In hospital

CHAPTER 6

ICU care: surgical and medical management—indications for immediate surgery

Peter S. Amenta and Jack Jallo

Department of Neurosurgery, Thomas Jefferson University Hospital, Philadelphia, PA, USA

Introduction

Within the industrialized world, traumatic brain injury (TBI) remains the most common cause of death in young adults, accounting for up to two-thirds of in-hospital deaths [1]. The overall mortality of trauma patients is three times higher in those afflicted with head injury in contrast to those without intracranial trauma. Death is attributed to the brain injury in 67.8% of cases [2]. Of those that survive, many suffer from poor quality of life and others fail to return to the same level of productivity as preinjury. Despite the magnitude of this devastating disease, treatment options remain limited.

The evolution in the understanding of the physiology and pathology of TBI has generated a shift in the manner in which this patient population is viewed and treated. Previous segregation of patients into operative and nonoperative categories has been replaced by a multidisciplinary approach in which medical and surgical interventions represent tools in a broader arsenal of general critical care. Although still a key component, neurosurgical intervention must be balanced with nonsurgical treatment alternatives. Medical therapy commonly comprises a major component of patient management. As a result, an understanding of surgical options is important not only to the neurosurgeon, but also to the neurologists and critical care specialists involved in the care of TBI patients.

This paradigm shift has led to increased reliance of medical decision making on evidence-based practices. The decision to operate, the indications for surgery, the approach used, the efficacy of alternative therapy, and the ultimate goal of surgery are all open to discussion. Within the current medical environment, each of these variables is examined to uncover the scientific data that support or contradict chosen interventions. Unfortunately, the nature of TBI does not lend itself easily to randomized prospective analysis and current approaches are largely based on decades of clinical experience. There are multiple clinical

Traumatic Brain Injury, First Edition. Edited by Pieter E. Vos and Ramon Diaz-Arrastia.
© 2015 John Wiley & Sons, Ltd. Published 2015 by John Wiley & Sons, Ltd.

scenarios in which intervention is obviously warranted, but little evidence-based data exist to define whether that intervention is medical or surgical. Neurosurgeons routinely employ operative intervention for clinical signs of herniation or impending devastating neurologic compromise, but no class I evidence exists to support these decisions. Further complicating the management of TBI are those patients with a normal and stable neurologic exam, but imaging that reveals what was traditionally viewed as a surgical lesion. As evidence-based practice continues to evolve, the literature must begin to answer these questions to optimize the management of this patient population.

The modern understanding of TBI and the role of surgical management begins with the publication of the findings of the International Coma Data Bank in 1975 [2]. This multicentered prospective analysis of 1000 comatose patients provided the data that made possible the Glasgow coma (GCS) and Glasgow outcome (GOS) scales. Building upon these data, the National Traumatic Coma Data Bank examined multiple clinical variables, including the quality of survival following severe head injury, the utility of measuring intracranial pressure (ICP), the impact of aggressive preadmission and emergency room care, and the identification of early predictors of clinical course and ultimate outcome [3].

The 1991 Traumatic Coma Data Bank represents one of the first attempts in the literature to define the role of surgical intervention in the management of TBI. The findings of this large multicenter data set highlighted the benefit of the evacuation of intracranial mass lesions, the importance of controlling ICP, and the deleterious effects of preadmission hypoxia and hypotension [4–6]. Based on these data, the Guidelines for the Management of Severe Traumatic Brain Injury was initially published in 1996, yet this comprehensive review of the literature provided no guidelines for surgical management [7]. It was not until 2006, with the release of the Guidelines for the Surgical Management of Traumatic Brain Injury that the role of surgery within the multidisciplinary approach to TBI was addressed [8]. This extensive review of the literature did not identify any data higher than class III evidence pertaining to the surgical management of five commonly encountered traumatic injuries: acute epidural hematomas, acute subdural hematomas, traumatic intraparenchymal lesions, posterior fossa mass lesions, and depressed skull fractures [8, 9]. The data do not represent well-proven standards of care, but instead are a collection of surgical options that provide a basis upon which to build clinical decision making. As a result, the importance of training, comfort level, and previous experiences and complications cannot be underestimated.

The following discussion is designed to feature the practice options detailed in the Guidelines for the Surgical Management of Traumatic Brain Injury, while also detailing important aspects of the pathophysiology of specific injuries. The information presented is intended to be of use to all practitioners involved in the care of the TBI patient. Additionally, neurosurgical intervention is highlighted within the broader context of a multidisciplinary approach to this patient population.

The pathophysiology of traumatic brain injury

TBI is best understood as a complex process that is composed of overlapping phases, including primary injury and its evolution, secondary injury, and recovery [10]. Primary injury represents a large category of insults that may be caused by multiple mechanisms, including, direct contact of the brain with the skull and shearing of the parenchyma as it stretches relative to the skull and dura [11]. This injury occurs at the time of insult and is directly proportional to the magnitude of the force applied to the brain. As a result, primary injury cannot be modified and is not amenable to treatment, but rather prevention. However, an accurate initial assessment of the primary injury is of the utmost importance as it assists in the determination of prognosis and overall outcome.

Secondary injury is defined as the constellation of cellular and biochemical processes that are set in motion by the primary injury and then evolve over the subsequent hours and days [12]. Many of these processes have been identified to include breakdown of the blood–brain barrier, release of excitatory amino acids, oxidative stress, and shifts in ion gradients [13, 14]. These changes manifest clinically as cerebral edema, increased ICP, and eventual cerebral infarction and neurologic deterioration. For these reasons, secondary injury is a significant contributor to posttraumatic neurological disability, and its prevention has become the focal point of the medical and surgical care of TBI patients [10] (Figure 6.1).

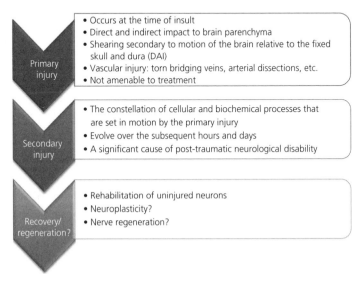

Figure 6.1 Phases of TBI (Data from Cernak [10], Lighthall and Anderson [11], McIntosh *et al.* [12], Lobato *et al.* [13], and Woie *et al.* [14]).

Preoperative evaluation and preparation

For those patients with an operative lesion at first presentation, rapid triage is coupled with emergent preoperative preparation. Labs are drawn and processed, including blood type and cross-matching, platelet count, and PTT/INR. The medication profile, with special attention to antiplatelet agents and anticoagulants, is reviewed and prompt reversal of these medications must be immediately initiated. The preoperative evaluation begins with an assessment of the standard ABCs of trauma care. If the GCS is 8 or less, the airway is secured via endotracheal intubation. If there is evidence of acutely increased ICP and incipient herniation, temporary moderate hyperventilation provides transient reduction until more definitive measures may be employed. However, prolonged hyperventilation may result in reduced cerebral blood flow and resulting ischemia. Medical intervention should be maximized in the moments before the definitive procedure in the operative theater. For patients without contraindications to being seated in the upright position, the head is positioned well above the heart with the neck in neutral position to maximize venous outflow from the head. In addition to temporary hyperventilation, a majority of tertiary care institutions routinely initiate hyperosmolar therapy with intravenous mannitol (0.25–1 g/kg), normal saline, and furosemide. The indications for placement of an ICP monitor have been detailed elsewhere and therefore will not garner further discussion. The authors routinely employ the use of ventriculostomy in situations where it may be placed accurately. In cases of medically refractory ICP, sedation, and paralysis, including the use of barbiturates may be used as a temporizing measure until surgical intervention.

It is important to include a determination of quality of life and salvageability in the preoperative evaluation of a patient with traumatic head injury. Family counseling and an informed discussion of prognosis are critical in this period, and factors such as advanced age, multiple medical comorbidities, and severity of intracranial and other traumatic injuries must be weighed when making the decision to proceed with surgical intervention (Box 6.1).

Extra-axial lesions

Extra-axial traumatic intracranial lesions, such as epidural and subdural hematomas, are among the most common pathologies seen in tertiary care centers. Management of these lesions is dependent upon multiple factors including some irreducible degree of clinical intuition. In patients with neurologic compromise and an intracranial mass lesion, the general assumption and accumulated clinical experience has been to surgically evacuate the lesion as quickly as possible. However, the guidelines are much less clear in neurologically intact patients or in those with only minimal neurologic findings [5].

Recent investigations into the management of extra-axial lesions have provided a set of guidelines for the nonoperative treatment of these hematomas.

Box 6.1 Computed tomographic appearance of common traumatic intracranial mass lesions.

Epidural hematomas

- Hyperdense
- Lenticular
- Respects suture lines
- Commonly temporoparietal
  - Up to 5–10% will lie both above and below the tentorium
- Commonly associated with overlying skull fracture

Acute subdural hematomas

- Hyperdense
  - Up to 10% appear isodense if identified within 72 h of the traumatic event
- Crescentic
- Does not respect suture lines
- Commonly associated with additional intracranial lesions

Contusions/intraparenchymal hematomas

- Hyperdense
- Commonly located in frontal and temporal lobes (contrecoup injuries)

Traumatic posterior fossa mass lesions

- Most commonly epidural hematomas
  - Subdural and intraparenchymal hematomas occur but far less frequently
- Important considerations
  - Brainstem compression
  - Fourth ventricular effacement or obstruction

Source: Adapted with permission from Chestnut [9]. © Thieme.

Fully conscious patients with extra-axial hematomas may be treated conservatively with close observation when imaging shows the hematoma to be less than 10 mm at its thickest point and to be the single dominant lesion. Imaging studies must also show no features of mass effect, such as midline shift greater than 3 mm or effacement of the basal cisterns (Box 6.2) [15, 16].

Epidural hematomas

Epidural hematomas are found in 6% of patients presenting with traumatic head injury and are often associated with an overlying skull fracture [17]. Regardless of the source of hemorrhage, epidural hematomas develop when blood accumulates between the periosteal layer of the dura matter and the inner table of the skull. The classic description is that of a skull fracture severing the anterior or posterior branch of the middle meningeal artery, resulting in a high-pressure arterial bleed in the temporoparietal region. Arterial sources of epidural bleeding are unlikely to tamponade and the natural history of these hematomas is to continuously expand. Epidural hematomas may also arise from a ruptured vein or venous sinus. Although venous bleeding is under relatively low pressure and

Box 6.2 Indications for immediate surgical evacuation: Epidural, subdural, intraparenchymal, and posterior fossa traumatic mass lesions.

Epidural hematomas

- Supratentorial EDH > 30 mL should be surgically evacuated regardless of the GCS
- Infratentorial EDH > 10 mL should be evacuated regardless of GCS
- Hematoma thickness > 15 mm and midline shift > 5 mm as measured on CT
- Data support rapid surgical evacuation in patients with a GCS < 9 and anisocoria

Acute subdural hematomas

- Acute SDH > 10 mm in thickness or midline shift > 5 mm regardless of GCS
- GCS < 9 and SDH < 10 mm in thickness and midline shift < 5 mm if:
  - GCS decreased by two or more points between time of injury and hospital admission
- Initial presentation with asymmetric or fixed/dilated pupils
- ICP > 20 mmHg

Intraparenchymal hematomas

- Parenchymal mass lesion
  - Signs of neurological deterioration referable to lesion or medically refractory ICP
- GCS 6–8 with frontal or temporal contusions > 20 mL
  - Midline shift ≥ 5 mm and/or cisternal compression
- Lesion volume > 50 mL

Posterior fossa traumatic mass lesions

- Neurological dysfunction or deterioration referable to the lesion
- The vast majority of hematomas associated with evidence of mass effect on CT require operative intervention [8, 9]
- Presence of obstructive hydrocephalus/effacement or obstruction of the fourth ventricle

Source: Adapted with permission from Chestnut [9]. © Thieme.

likely to tamponade without intervention, arterial and venous hemorrhage cannot be reliably differentiated by current imaging techniques. Thus, all epidural hematomas must be assumed arterial in nature and treated accordingly. The widespread availability and speed with which a CT scan can be obtained provides an efficient and reliable imaging modality by which to diagnose an epidural hematoma. These intracranial lesions will most commonly appear as biconvex hyperdense lesions bounded by the dural insertions into the cranial sutures. Up to 5–10% of these lesions can lie both above and below the tentorium.

Surgical decompression of an epidural hematoma has been found to be one of the most cost-effective of all procedures in terms of quality of life and years of productive life preserved [18]. This finding is due to the protection of the brain by the dura mater and the resultant relatively low incidence of underlying parenchymal injury. The prognosis associated with an epidural hematoma is largely dependent upon the neurological exam and level of consciousness at the time of surgery. Additional prognostic factors, such as age, time from injury to treatment, immediate coma versus lucid interval, presence of pupillary abnormalities, and postoperative ICP also influence neurologic recovery. A number of imaging characteristics found on CT at the time of presentation may also assist in determining prognosis and include hematoma volume, degree of midline shift, and the presence of an intradural lesion [19]. The resultant overall mortality rate for patients presenting with an epidural hematoma is 9% [17].

Craniotomy and evacuation of an epidural hematoma have long been the gold standard of treatment, yet the 2006 Guidelines for the Surgical Management of Traumatic Brain Injury were unable to identify any evidence greater than class III data to support surgical intervention. The study group was, however, able to provide a core set of treatment recommendations upon which to base current practices. The volume of the hematoma is one of the strongest indicators for surgical intervention and a supratentorial epidural hematoma greater than 30 mL should be surgically evacuated regardless of the GCS score. In the infratentorial compartment, any epidural hematoma with a volume greater than 10 mL should be evacuated. Hematoma thickness greater than 15 mm and midline shift greater than 5 mm as measured on CT were also found to be indications for surgical evacuation. Additionally, the study supported rapid surgical evacuation in patients with a GCS ≤ 9 and anisocoria. Multiple studies have also supported surgical evacuation of an epidural hematoma when found in the presence of additional intracranial lesions. Craniotomy continues to be the preferred method by which to achieve complete evacuation of an epidural hematoma, although no data were found to sufficiently support a particular surgical option [5, 8, 20, 21]. The guidelines for conservative nonoperative management of epidural hematomas are represented in the following table.

As with all disease processes, a consideration of the resources available to each individual practitioner must be factored into the decision for surgical intervention. While it is never desirable to perform unnecessary surgery, observation does risk neurologic deterioration beyond repair. When considering the relative speed and ease with which an epidural hematoma can be safely evacuated, many practitioners choose to err on the side of surgery to prevent such catastrophic events. In the instance where observation is chosen, the practitioner must be confident in the reliability in which serial neurologic exams and imaging studies can be performed within the institution [5, 18].

In most instances, the focal nature of epidural hematomas allows rapid evacuation via a limited incision and craniotomy. Craniotomy and clot evacuation are performed in the usual fashion with suction, irrigation, and resection of the hematoma. In cases of rapid deterioration, the first burr hole is placed over the thickest area of clot to promote immediate decompression. If there is suspicion for an associated subdural hematoma, the dura is opened and the subdural space is explored. In most instances, the bone plate may be replaced [5].

Acute subdural hematomas

Acute subdural hematomas represent the most common focal intracranial lesions in patients with severe closed head injury [4]. These lesions are also among the most deadly, with an average 50–60% mortality rate [17, 22, 23]. The underlying traumatic event is age dependent, with those aged 18–40 years most commonly being the victims of motor vehicle accidents, while those aged 65 years or older are most frequently the victim of falls [24]. Subdural hematomas develop when blood accumulates between the cortical surface of the brain and the dura mater. The bridging veins that traverse the subdural space en route to the dural venous sinuses represent the most common source of hemorrhage. The venous tear occurs when the mobile brain accelerates relative to the fixed dura and skull following the traumatic impact. Low-pressure venous bleeding will frequently tamponade without intervention. Subdural hematomas may also result from lacerated cortical blood vessels or eruption of a cortical contusion into the subdural space. Regardless of the source, acute subdural hematomas appear as hyperdense crescentic lesions that cross suture lines. Up to 10% of acute subdural hematomas appear isodense on CT if identified within 72 h of the traumatic event due to a low hemoglobin concentration [25]. Whether isolated or in conjunction with additional lesions, subdural hematomas lead to secondary injury by direct compression of adjacent structures, induction of edema formation, suppression of regional cerebral blood flow, and elevation of ICP. In turn, prolonged intracranial hypertension results in a reduction of cerebral blood flow and oxygenation [26].

A significant mechanical force is usually required to produce an acute subdural hematoma, resulting in up to 50% of patients presenting with an associated intraparenchymal lesion. As a result, the underlying parenchymal injury may prove to be the decisive factor in the determination of the ultimate outcome. Age is the most important variable in the determination of outcome, with higher mortality rates in patients aged greater than 65 years [24]. CT findings, particularly hematoma thickness and midline shift, are also reliable predictors of outcome in acute subdural hematomas. Acute subdural hematomas approaching 18 mm in thickness and causing 20 mm of midline shift are associated with a 50% survival rate. The survival rate progressively declines as shift exceeds hematoma thickness, dropping to 25% when shift exceeds hematoma thickness by 5 mm. The survival rate is 0% for hematomas resulting in over 25 mm of shift [27]. The presence of underlying edema, contusions, and effacement of the basal cisterns are additional variables associated with a poor prognosis [17, 28].

Multiple studies have proposed protocols for the nonoperative management of acute subdural hematomas [16, 29]. These studies are composed primarily of patients with high GCS scores, as those at the lower end of the spectrum are frequently taken to the operating room based on convention. Servadei *et al.* published favorable outcomes in two-thirds of comatose patients with subdural hematomas treated with nonoperative management [30]. All patients in this series had hematomas less than 10 mm in thickness and less than 5 mm of associated shift, experienced no neurologic deterioration, and were followed with an ICP monitor. Two of the fifteen patients eventually required craniotomy for intracranial hypertension and evolving intracerebral lesions.

When surgical evacuation of an acute subdural hematoma is necessary, the primary goal is the rapid evacuation of the life-threatening intracranial mass. With the realization that subdural hematomas frequently occur in combination with other systemic and intracranial lesions, large craniotomies often provide the best exposure for managing any pathology encountered. Adequate exposure should allow for rapid evacuation of the hematoma, grant access to most sources of bleeding, and, in the event of severe cerebral edema, provide room for the brain to swell. To assist in postoperative control of ICP, the bone flap is left out if the brain appears edematous (Figures 6.2 and 6.3).

Contusions and intraparenchymal hematomas

Most patients with severe head injury and 25% of those with moderate injury develop contusions or intracerebral hematomas. The majority of intraparenchymal hematomas are found in either the temporal or frontal lobes and are contrecoup injuries caused by the impact of the brain against the skull. Parietal and occipital hematomas are usually the result of a direct impact over the site of the lesion. In up to 50% of cases,{2269} serial imaging reveals enlargement of the lesion over the first few days due to increased swelling or continued bleeding. Most of the increase in contusion volume occurs in the first few hours. In the absence of surgical intervention, intraparenchymal hematomas resorb in 4–6 weeks by macrophage phagocytosis and gliosis.

The choice between evacuation and observation of intraparenchymal hematomas remains among the most difficult management decisions in the field of TBI. The Guidelines for the Surgical Management of Traumatic Brain Injury offers treatment recommendations regarding intervention [8]. Intraparenchymal

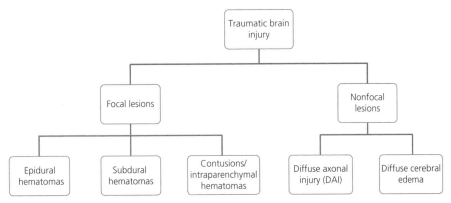

Figure 6.2 TBI: Focal and nonfocal pathology (Adapted with permission from Chestnut [9]. © Thieme).

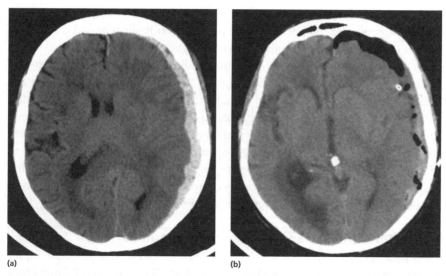

(a)   (b)

Figure 6.3 Acute subdural hematoma. A 76-year-old male status post fall from standing during a syncopal episode presents with progressive right upper and lower extremity weakness for 24 h. Admission head CT reveals an 11 mm left subdural hematoma with 6 mm of associated left-to-right midline shift (a). Patient was taken for left-sided craniotomy and clot evacuation (b). A subdural drain was placed at the time of surgery.

hematomas are particularly well suited for nonoperative management. The lack of a margin between salvageable brain and the hematoma and the inevitable need for dissection of uninjured brain to access the lesion represent significant risks of iatrogenic injury. As a result, decision making must be based on neurological exam, imaging, and clinical suspicion of future deterioration and development of intracranial hypertension. Serial CT is a valuable tool in monitoring intraparenchymal lesions and may aid in initial nonoperative management. CT scans revealing evidence of mass effect, including cisternal compression and midline shift, may be indicative of the need for surgical evacuation. Perhaps the most important guide in operative decision making is the attainment of an accurate admission GCS coupled with reliable serial evaluation and early recognition of clinical deterioration. ICP monitoring represents a useful tool in the management of this patient population, yet a significant number of patients will exhibit delayed neurologic deterioration without an associated increase in ICP [31]. When operative intervention is chosen, the goals of surgery are rapid evacuation of the mass lesion, acquisition of hemostasis, relief of mass effect, and reduction in ICP (Figures 6.4 and 6.5).

Posterior fossa mass lesions

Although relatively rare, accounting for only 3–5% of traumatic mass lesions, posterior fossa hematomas rank among the most lethal of injuries. Due to the dimensions of the posterior fossa and the close proximity of the brainstem,

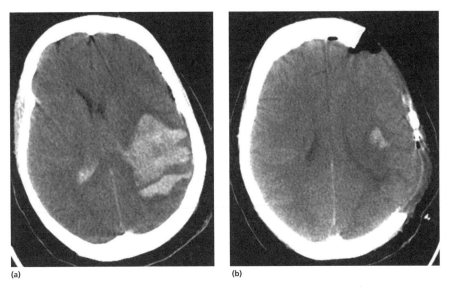

(a)   (b)

Figure 6.4 Traumatic intraparenchymal hematoma. A 55-year-old intoxicated female presents status post fall from standing with GCS 7. Admission INR 4.7 secondary to warfarin therapy for atrial fibrillation. Admission head CT reveals a $7 \times 4 \times 5$ cm intraparenchymal hematoma with intraventricular extension and 7 mm of left-to-right midline shift (a). The coagulopathy was reversed with factor IX and FFP. The patient was emergently taken for left-sided decompressive craniectomy and hematoma evacuation (b). A subgaleal drain was left at the time of the procedure.

neurologic compromise from an expanding posterior fossa lesion may be sudden, irreversible, and devastating. Epidural hematomas represent the most commonly encountered traumatic lesions of the posterior fossa and are frequently associated with overlying skull fractures. Signs of occipital trauma, such as scalp lacerations and open fractures, are present in over 80% of patients. Traumatic subdural and intraparenchymal hematomas, occurring with considerably lower frequency, pose identical risks of rapid and catastrophic neurologic deterioration. Standard ICP monitoring techniques are largely unreliable within the posterior fossa. As a result, imaging, particularly evidence of mass effect on CT, is the tool most heavily relied upon in deriving the recommendations for surgical management. As is the case with the surgical management of all traumatic lesions, no randomized prospective data currently exist to standardize medical and surgical intervention.

The current management of traumatic posterior fossa lesions is best understood if the various hematomas are viewed as a group unified by the unique anatomy of the posterior fossa. Patients presenting with traumatic posterior fossa lesions, but lacking signs of mass effect on CT and exhibiting no signs of neurologic dysfunction, may be managed with observation [8, 9]. These patients are monitored in the intensive care setting and it is critical that resources exist for reliable and consistent serial examination and imaging. High suspicion for

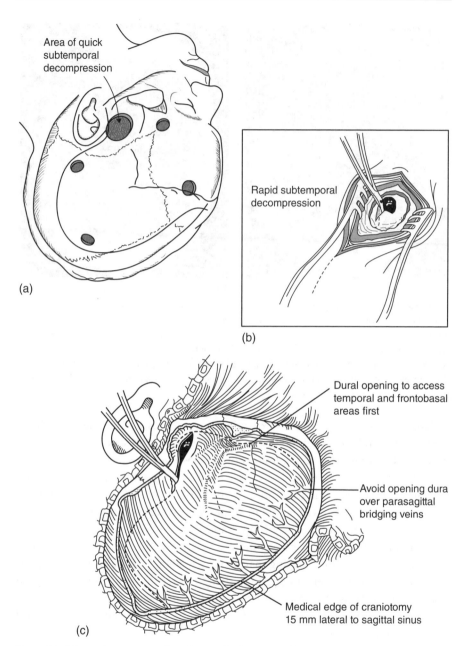

Area of quick
subtemporal
decompression

(a)

Rapid subtemporal
decompression

(b)

Dural opening to access
temporal and frontobasal
areas first

Avoid opening dura
over parasagittal
bridging veins

Medical edge of craniotomy
15 mm lateral to sagittal sinus

(c)

Figure 6.5 Schematic representation of a standard trauma craniotomy. Skin incision and suggested locations for burr hole placement (a). The inset shows rapid subtemporal decompression through a limited skin incision and evacuation of an intracranial hematoma (b). The dural incision is pictured (hash lines) along with underlying bridging veins that empty into the superior sagittal sinus (c). This standard craniotomy allows access to most subdural, epidural, and intraparenchymal hematomas (Reproduced with permission from Prabhu *et al.* [32]. © Elsevier).

deterioration must be maintained and changes in neurologic exam readily identified. In the event of neurological dysfunction or deterioration referable to the lesion, operative intervention is required immediately, as delay may result in disastrous consequences. The majority of hematomas associated with evidence of mass effect on CT require operative intervention [8, 9]. Mass effect in the posterior fossa manifests as midline shift, distortion or obliteration of the fourth ventricle, or compression or obliteration of the basal cisterns. These findings may present with, or subsequently lead to, the development of obstructive hydrocephalus via obstruction of cerebrospinal fluid (CSF) outflow through the fourth ventricle.

The majority of posterior fossa lesions are evacuated with a suboccipital craniectomy large enough to remove the hematoma and adequately decompress the fourth ventricle and brainstem. In almost all scenarios, the risk of acute obstructive hydrocephalus warrants readiness for the placement of a ventriculostomy. The ventriculostomy may be placed pre- or postoperatively via the frontal route or an occipital approach may be used intraoperatively with the patient in the prone position. Although the operative details of a suboccipital craniectomy are beyond the scope of this chapter, it is important to draw attention to a number of considerations unique to traumatic posterior fossa pathology. The presence of dural venous sinus injury must be considered for nearly all posterior fossa hematomas, as a torn sinus may bleed into the epidural, subdural, or intraparenchymal compartments. Preoperative planning includes the reversal of any coagulopathy, the preparation of packed red blood cells for potential transfusion, and the attainment of reliable large-bore intravenous access. Clinical stability permitting, preoperative vascular imaging via CT venogram or angiogram provides useful information regarding transverse sinus dominance and the presence of vascular injury. In planning the craniectomy, exposure must be wide enough to access and repair an injured sinus with the goal of maintaining sinus patency. The injured sinus may be sacrificed if irreparable, with special attention paid postoperatively to signs of venous outflow obstruction and intracranial hypertension (Box 6.3 and Figure 6.6).

Nonfocal intraparenchymal lesions

Management of nonfocal intraparenchymal lesions
Nonfocal intraparenchymal lesions, such as cerebral edema, disseminated swelling, and diffuse axonal injury (DAI), are relatively common and occur in isolation or in combination with focal lesions. DAI, the result of acceleration–deceleration and rotational forces applied to the mobile brain within the fixed skull and dura, is found in up to 90% of postmortem TBI specimens [33, 34]. Due to the lack of a well-delineated lesion amenable to resection, increased ICP secondary to nonfocal intraparenchymal injury is, at least initially, well suited for medical

Box 6.3 Considerations in the surgical management of traumatic posterior fossa pathology.

Obstructive hydrocephalus?

- Ventriculostomy placement
  - Pre- and postoperative placement via the frontal approach
  - Intraoperative placement via the occipital approach

Sinus injury?

- Preoperative vascular imaging
  - Computed tomographic venography
  - Angiogram
- Type and cross
  - Multiple units of blood readily available
  - Multiple large-bore IVs or central access for large-volume transfusion
- Repair of lacerated sinus
- Ligation of lacerated sinus
  - Postoperative signs and symptoms of venous outflow obstruction and intracranial hypertension?

Coagulopathy

- Reversal of coagulopathy
  - Antiplatelet agents: Platelet transfusion
  - Anticoagulation: Fresh frozen plasma, cryoprecipitate, factor IX

Suboccipital craniectomy

- Large exposure
- Removal of hematoma
- Resection of damaged cerebellum if excessively swollen/continued intracranial hypertension following clot resection
- Meticulous hemostasis
- Adequate dural closure
  - Prevention of CSF leak

Source: Adapted with permission from Chestnut [9]. © Thieme.

intervention. Critical care management of these patients begins with the goal of maintaining an ICP below 20–25 mmHg and a cerebral perfusion pressure (CPP) greater than 60 mmHg. Medical interventions for the control of ICP (see Chapter 6) consist of upright positioning and sedation to maximize cerebral venous outflow. Increasingly aggressive management includes the administration of hypertonic saline, mannitol, moderate hyperventilation, placement of an external ventricular drain, and high-dose pentobarbital. Although these maneuvers are frequently sufficient to maintain physiologic parameters, intracranial hypertension does not respond to maximal medical therapy in 10–15% of patients with severe head injury [6, 35, 36]. In these patients, multiple studies have repeatedly shown high morbidity and mortality rates. In 1982, Saul and

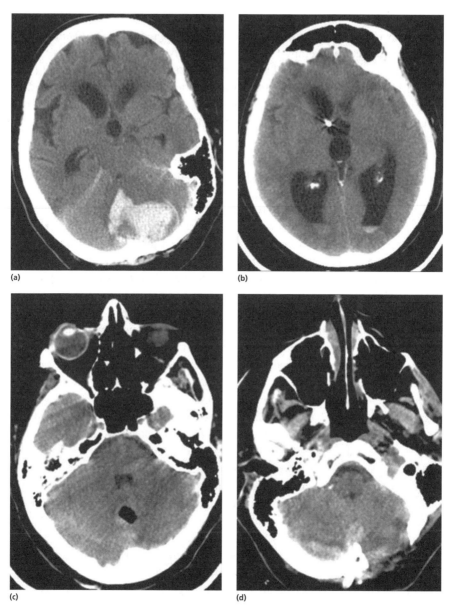

Figure 6.6 Traumatic posterior fossa intraparenchymal hematoma. A 65-year-old female on antiplatelet therapy for coronary artery stents presents status post striking occiput against steps. Patient found to be lethargic on arrival. Head CT showed $3 \times 3 \times 3$ cm cerebellar hematoma, effacement of the fourth ventricle, and acute obstructive hydrocephalus (a). After receiving platelets, a right frontal ventriculostomy was placed preoperatively at the bedside (b). The patient underwent emergent suboccipital craniectomy and hematoma evacuation. Postoperative CT demonstrating the re-expanded fourth ventricle (c) and the evacuation of the hematoma (d).

Ducker published an 84% mortality rate when ICP was ≥ 25 mmHg, and Miller *et al.* reported a 100% mortality rate when ICP greater than 20 mmHg was refractory to medical therapy [37, 38]. As recently as 2000, data analysis of the Selfotel trial revealed a mortality rate of 56.4% when an ICP ≥ 20 mmHg was detected before and during neurological deterioration [35]. Despite the clear enormity of the problem, treatment options for medically intractable intracranial hypertension remain limited. Research efforts have largely failed to uncover novel medications or additional interventions, thus leaving decompressive craniectomy as the remaining therapeutic option.

The supportive data related to decompressive craniectomy show that the incidence of major disability and persistent vegetative state has remained stable over the past four decades [39]. The literature reveals a gradual decrease in mortality rate, but this also reflects advances in imaging, prehospital care, and critical care management. There are sufficient data to show that decompressive craniectomy reduces ICP in TBI patients, yet there is a paucity of scientific evidence to support a significant improvement in outcome following the procedure [40–43]. Retrospective analyses, which compose the vast majority of the literature, have shown benefit from decompressive craniectomy. Aarabi *et al.* reported better-than-expected functional outcome following decompressive craniectomy in a retrospective analysis of 50 patients with malignant cerebral edema [39]. A study of 115 patients with severe closed head injury showed an 82.4% mortality rate in patients who failed medical therapy and pentobarbital coma, while the cohort undergoing subtemporal decompressive craniectomy exhibited a 40% mortality rate [44]. A meta-analysis of the literature from 1988 to 2006 collected data on 323 decompressive craniectomy patients and found a collective mortality rate of 22.3%, with 48.3% of patients achieving a good outcome [39, 42–50]. These results compare favorably when contrasted with the previously discussed data pertaining to prolonged medically refractory intracranial hypertension [35, 37–39].

The Early Decompressive Craniectomy in Patients With Severe Traumatic Brain Injury (DECRA) trial is a recently published randomized controlled trial of 155 adults with severe diffuse TBI and intracranial hypertension refractory to first-tier therapies [51]. Patients were randomized to undergo either bifrontotemporoparietal decompressive craniectomy or standard care (continued medical therapy). Unfavorable outcomes were defined as death, vegetative state, or severe disability as evaluated by the Extended Glasgow Outcome Scale (GOSE) at a point 6 months following the injury. Within the surgical group, patients experienced less time with an ICP above the treatment threshold, underwent fewer interventions for increased ICP, and spent fewer days in the intensive care unit. Unfortunately, patients randomized to surgery also exhibited poorer GOSE scores and displayed a greater risk of suffering an unfavorable outcome, thereby bringing into question the utility of decompressive craniectomy. The methodology, results, and conclusions of this study have been vigorously debated within the neurosurgical community, and the ultimate role for this therapy for refractory ICP remains to be established.

Future understanding of the role of decompressive craniectomy will be derived from multiple sources and must include prospective evaluation. The evolution of multimodality monitoring represents an attempt to define the significance of ICP monitoring in the context of additional variables. Of particular interest is the use of intracerebral oxygen partial pressure monitors, as the deleterious effects of prolonged hypoxia following TBI have been well documented [52–56]. Although requiring further study, the combined dual examination of both ICP and brain oxygen content may assist in the selection of those patients who will benefit from decompressive craniectomy (Table 6.1 and Figure 6.7) [52].

Depressed skull fractures

Skull fractures are commonly found in association with extra-axial and intraparenchymal injuries, and the presence of a fracture on physical exam is a strong predictor of an intracranial lesion [57–59]. Closed, nondisplaced skull fractures are often linear in nature, do not require surgery, and heal without any intervention. Depressed skull fractures, the majority of which are open, represent a class of injury associated with significant morbidity and a mortality rate as high as 19% [60–62]. Open fractures are defined by a breach in the galea aponeurotica in the region overlying the fracture. Common complications of open depressed skull fractures include an infection rate of 5–11% and the development of epilepsy in 15% of patients [60, 62–65]. In addition to the repair of cosmetic deformity, the goals of surgical management largely consist of limiting the incidence of these complications.

The widespread availability of CT has triggered an evolution in the surgical management of open depressed skull fractures. Prior to the advent of modern imaging techniques, almost all open skull fractures were treated surgically, as the existing data supported a strong link between these injuries and infection, epilepsy, and neurologic deficits [60, 63, 65]. These data, however, did not reflect the presence of underlying parenchymal lesions and their contribution to the development of a neurologic deficit remained unknown. The ability of CT to reliably rule out parenchymal injury has allowed for the nonoperative management of many open depressed skull fractures. Additionally, multiple studies have shown routine wound care and antibiotics to effectively prevent infection, while the data have failed to show a reduction in the incidence of epilepsy following elevation of depressed bone fragments [62, 66].

When operative intervention is required, the approach will vary significantly depending upon the location and associated intracranial injuries. However, there are specific considerations that should be applied to most situations. Whenever possible, the incision should incorporate scalp lacerations overlying the fracture so that devitalized scalp and contaminated tissues may be excised. Including these preexisting defects also assists in preserving the scalp blood supply by

Table 6.1 Decompressive craniectomy: Comparison of current prospective randomized studies.

	Randomised Evaluation of Surgery with Craniectomy for Uncontrollable Elevation of Intracranial Pressure (RESCUEicp)	Multi-centre Prospective Randomised Trial of Early Decompressive Craniectomy in Patients with Severe Traumatic Brain Injury (DECRA)
Age range	10–65 years old	15–60 years old
Inclusion criteria	Abnormal CT	Severe diffuse TBI defined as:
	Intracranial pressure (ICP) monitor placed with elevated ICP >25 mmHg for >1–12 h	GCS <9 and CT with any evidence of cerebral edema
	Refractory to initial medical therapy	
	Refractory to advanced medical therapy (does not include barbiturate coma)	GCS >8 before intubation and CT showing cisternal compression ± midline shift
	Patients may have an immediate operation to remove a mass lesion	ICP monitor *in situ*. EVD recommended
	Not an immediate decompressive craniectomy	*Refractory ICP* despite best conventional management
		Defined as spontaneous persistent increase in ICP despite optimal conventional ICU of >20 mmHg for more than 15 min (continuously or cumulative over 1 h)
Study groups	Continuation of optimal medical management with barbiturates versus surgical intervention	Early surgical intervention versus best current conventional management
Surgical intervention	Unilateral hemispheric swelling	Large bifrontotemporal decompressive craniectomy
	Unilateral frontotemporoparietal craniectomy	
	Bilateral diffuse hemispheric swelling	
	Bifrontotemporal decompressive craniectomy	
Timing of surgical intervention	Within 4–6 h of randomization	Within 6 h of presentation
Primary outcome measures	Outcome at discharge (Glasgow Outcome Score)	% favorable outcome (GOSE 5–8) 6 months postinjury
	Outcomes at six months (Extended Glasgow Outcome Score)	
Secondary outcome measures	Assessment of outcome using SF-3623 and SF-10 (for children)	Mean and maximum hourly ICP
	ICP control	Mean GOSE at 6 months and 12 months
	Length of ICU admission	Mortality at 6 and 12 months
	Health economic analysis	Length of ICU admission
	Outcome at 1 and 2 years	Brain metabolites measurements using microdialysis

Data from Whitfield et al. [50] and Cooper et al. [51].

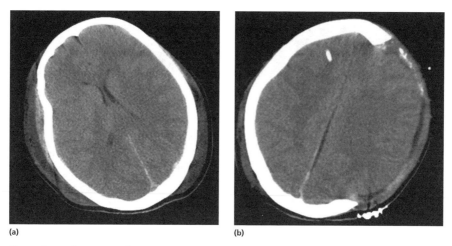

(a)   (b)

Figure 6.7 Malignant cerebral edema and medically refractory ICP. A 17-year-old female status post motor vehicle collision presents with GCS 6 and head CT revealing no focal lesion and the loss of the gray–white junction (a). Right frontal ventriculostomy placed on admission showed normal ICP. On hospital day 3, the patient developed intracranial hypertension refractory to maximal medical therapy and the patient was taken for an emergent left decompressive craniectomy (b).

avoiding intersecting lacerations. Additionally, the incision should be large enough to expose the entire fracture, so that fragments, foreign bodies, and macerated soft tissue can be effectively debrided. As with all surgery for TBI, meticulous hemostasis is required, with special attention paid to the control of bleeding from fractured bone edges.

Depressed skull fractures over venous sinuses represent a distinct class of fractures that present a number of unique management dilemmas. Closed depressed skull fractures overlying a venous sinus should not be elevated if there is no evidence of significant mass effect on the sinus. If the fractured bone fragment causes compression of the sinus, venous outflow obstruction may develop with subsequent increased ICP and neurologic deterioration [67]. In these cases, rapid elevation of the fracture and decompression of the sinus are necessary to restore venous outflow to the brain. When a fracture lacerates an adjacent sinus, profuse bleeding can result in the rapid formation of epidural, subdural, and intraparenchymal hematomas. Craniotomy and exploration of the sinus are necessary to evacuate the hematoma and to repair the injured sinus. In the event of an irreparable laceration, the injured sinus is ligated and the final outcome depends upon the dependence of the brain on the lost sinus. In a study of 78 Vietnam War casualties, Kapp showed ligation of the anterior 50% of the superior sagittal sinus to be generally tolerated, resulting in only one death [68]. Conversely, injury to the posterior 50% of the sagittal sinus was associated with a 24% mortality rate (Figure 6.8).

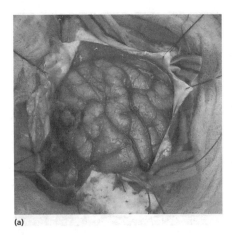
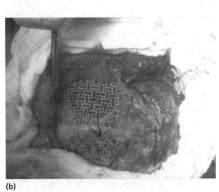

(a)   (b)

Figure 6.8 Repair of depressed skull fracture. A 21-year-old unrestrained male driver status post motor vehicle collision and ejection from the vehicle presents to the emergency room intubated with GCS 7 T. CT head and facial bones reveals right frontal intraparenchymal hematoma and associated open depressed skull fracture. Patient was taken for emergent evacuation of hematoma (a), cranialization of the frontal sinus, wound irrigation and debridement, and repair of the skull fracture with a plating system (b).

Penetrating brain injury

Penetrating brain injury is a broad category defined by various mechanisms of injury stemming from accidental, intentional, self-inflicted, and interpersonal traumas. Penetrating trauma also varies depending on the theater in which it occurs, with military and civilian injuries differing in projectile type and velocity. Regardless of the etiology, these injuries rank among the most devastating, with mortality rates estimated as high as 94% [69]. Stab and gunshot (GSW) wounds represent the most commonly encountered penetrating brain injuries, with a recent study of self-inflicted injuries showing 76.4% of GSW to involve the head [70]. Within this cohort, the mortality rate for a self-inflicted GSW to the head was 80%, a finding that is consistent with similar studies [71–73].

As with closed head injury, no prospective randomized data currently exist to guide the surgical management of penetrating brain injury. Management algorithms are based on the practice recommendations set forth in the Guidelines for the Management of Penetrating Brain Injury and individual clinical decision making [74]. There is extensive literature pertaining to the determination of prognosis, the majority of which is based on GSW to the head. Multiple prognostic indicators have been employed, including level of consciousness, the presence of motor release findings, pupillary abnormalities, and imaging characteristics [75–78]. The determination of outcome is complex, no one variable is definitive, and the reader is directed to the literature for a more extensive discussion of prognosis.

Standardized indications for surgical intervention in penetrating TBI do not exist and the techniques, timing of surgery, and ultimate goals are a topic of debate. Most neurosurgeons would agree that the acquisition of hemostasis, removal of significant intracranial hematomas, and revision of entrance and exit wounds to ensure scalp coverage are the primary goals of all interventions [77]. Additional goals include debridement of devitalized tissue, removal of foreign bodies, and dural repair [79]. Avoidance of infection is critical and all management algorithms should include broad-spectrum antibiotic therapy. The extent to which contaminated bone and metal fragments lodged in the parenchyma should be pursued is not clear. Previously, even when multiple explorations were required, the US military mandated removal of all intracranial bone and metal [80–83]. However, such aggressive debridement failed to result in improved morbidity and mortality when compared to less invasive approaches [32, 78, 84, 85]. Variations in current management protocols exist, but the majority of authors advocate thorough debridement of devitalized brain, removal of easily accessible bone and metal fragments, and evacuation of intracerebral hematomas. The data show a strong correlation between CSF leaks and infection, and it is imperative to achieve a watertight closure, often with the assistance of a dural graft [9, 74, 79]. Postinjury epilepsy is a common complication following penetrating brain injury, yet the effectiveness of aggressive debridement in the prevention of seizures is unclear (Box 6.4).

Box 6.4 Considerations in the surgical management of penetrating brain injury.

Prevention of infection

- Debridement of devitalized tissue
- Aggressive versus limited debridement
  - Extent of debridement remains controversial
- Broad-spectrum intravenous antibiotics

Scalp coverage

- Planning of incision to include preexisting lacerations
- Revision of missile entrance and exit wounds
- Undermining of scalp to facilitate closure

Dural closure

- Watertight closure
  - Prevention of CSF leak
  - Reduction in incidence of infection
- Close primarily or need for dural graft?

Associated hematomas

- Evacuation of readily accessible hematomas
  - Assists in control of ICP
- Acquire meticulous hemostasis

Data from Refs. [32, 8–85].

Conclusion

Within the modern multidisciplinary approach to TBI, neurosurgical intervention represents a treatment option within the broader context of comprehensive critical care. As a result, it is imperative that all members of the critical care team develop a working understanding of the role of surgery in the management of this patient population. Although immediate surgical evacuation of intracranial mass lesions is routinely employed in cases of active and anticipated neurologic decline, no class I evidence exists to support these maneuvers [1]. The Guidelines for the Surgical Management of Traumatic Brain Injury represents the most comprehensive review of the literature to date and offers detailed practice options that assist in clinical decision making. Future understanding of TBI pathophysiology and care must include prospective randomized studies to better define the utility, timing, and overall benefit of neurosurgical intervention.

References

1 Maas, A.I., Dearden, M., Teasdale, G.M. *et al.* (1997) EBIC-guidelines for management of severe head injury in adults. *Acta Neurochirurgica (Wien)*, **139**, 286–294.
2 Jennett, B. & Bond, M.R. (1975) Assessment of outcome after severe brain damage. *Lancet*, **1**, 480–484.
3 Marshall, L.F., Becker, D.P., Bowers, S.A. *et al.* (1983) The National Traumatic Coma Data Bank: part 1: design, purpose, goals, and results. *Journal of Neurosurgery*, **59**, 276–284.
4 Foulkes, M.A., Eisenberg, H.M., Jane, J.A. *et al.* (1991) The Traumatic Coma Data Bank: design, methods, and baseline characteristics. *Journal of Neurosurgery*, **75**, S8–S13.
5 Chesnut, R.M., Marshall, L.F., Klauber, M.R. *et al.* (1993) The role of secondary brain injury in determining outcome from severe head injury. *The Journal of Trauma*, **34**, 216–222.
6 Eisenberg, H.M., Frankowski, R.F., Contant, C.F. *et al.* (1988) High-dose barbiturate control of elevated intracranial pressure in patients with severe head injury. *Journal of Neurosurgery*, **69**, 15–23.
7 Bullock, R., Chestnut, R., & Clifton, G. (1996) Guidelines for the management of severe head injury. Brain Trauma Foundation, American Association of Neurological Surgeons, Joint Section on Neurotrauma and Critical Care. *Journal of Neurotrauma*, **13**, 639–734.
8 Bullock, M.R., Chesnut, R., & Ghajar, J. (2006) Guidelines for the surgical management of traumatic brain injury. *Neurosurgery*, **58**, S1–60.
9 Chestnut, R.M. (2009) Scientific surgical management. In: Jallo J & C.M. Loftus (eds), *Neurotrauma and Critical Care of the Brain*, pp. 255–274. Thieme, New York.
10 Cernak, I. (2005) Animal models of head trauma. *The Journal of the American Society for Experimental Neurotherapeutics*, **2**, 410–422.
11 Lighthall, J.W. & Anderson, T.E. (1994) In vivo models of experimental brain and spinal cord trauma. In: S.K. Salzman & A.I. Faden (eds), *The Neurobiology of Central Nervous System Trauma*, pp. 3–11. Oxford University Press, New York.
12 McIntosh, T.K., Smith, D.H., Meaney, D.F., Kotapka, M.J., Gennarelli, T.A., & Graham, D.I. (1996) Neuropathological sequelae of traumatic brain injury: relationship to neurochemical and biochemical mechanisms. *Laboratory Investigation*, **74**, 315–342.
13 Lobato, R.D., Sarabia, R., Cordobes, F. *et al.* (1988) Posttraumatic cerebral hemispheric swelling. Analysis of 55 cases studied with computerized tomography. *Journal of Neurosurgery*, **68**, 417–423.

14 Woie, K., Koller, M.E., Heyeraas, K.J., & Reed, R.K. (1993) Neurogenic inflammation in rat trachea is accompanied by increased negativity of interstitial fluid pressure. *Circulation Research*, **73**, 839–45.

15 Bullock, R. & Teasdale, G. (1991) Head injuries–surgical management of traumatic intracerebral hematomas. In: Vinken, P.J. Bruhn, G.W. Klawans, H.L. & Braakman R. (eds), *Handbook of Clinical Neurology, Vol 57: Head Injury*, pp. 249–298 Elsevier, London.

16 Mathew, P., Oluoch-Olunya, D.L., Condon, B.R., & Bullock, R. (1993) Acute subdural hematoma in the conscious patient: outcome with initial nonoperative management. *Acta Neurochirurgica (Wien)*, **121**, 100–108.

17 Marshall, L.F., Gautille, T., Klauber, M.R. *et al.* (1991) The outcome of severe closed head injury. *Journal of Neurosurgery*, **75**, S28–S36.

18 Pickard, J.D., Bailey, S., Sanderson, H., Rees, M., & Garfield, J.S. (1990) Steps towards cost-benefit analysis of regional neurosurgical care. *British Medical Journal*, **301**, 629–635

19 Servadei, F. (1997) Prognostic factors in severely head injured adult patients with epidural haematomas. *Acta Neurochirurgica (Wien)*, **139**, 273–278.

20 Chen, T.Y., Wong, C.W., Chang, C.N. *et al.* (1993) The expectant treatment of "asymptomatic" supratentorial epidural hematomas. *Neurosurgery*, **32**, 176–179.

21 Wong, C.W. (1994) The CT criteria for conservative treatment-but under close clinical observation-of posterior fossa epidural haematomas. *Acta Neurochirurgica (Wien)*, **126**, 124–127.

22 Wilberger, J.E., Harris, M., & Diamond, D.L. (1991) Acute subdural hematoma: mortality, morbidity and operative timing. *Journal of Neurosurgery*, **74**, 212–8.

23 Miller, J.D., Butterworth, J.F., Gudeman, S.K. *et al.* (1981) Further experience in the management of severe head injury. *Journal of Neurosurgery*, **54**, 289–299.

24 Howard, M.A., III, Gross, A.S., Dacey, R.G., Jr., & Winn, H.R. (1989) Acute subdural hematomas: an age-dependent clinical entity. *Journal of Neurosurgery*, **71**, 858–63.

25 Smith, W.P., Jr., Batnitzky, S., & Rengachary, S.S. (1981) Acute isodense subdural hematomas: a problem in anemic patients. *American Journal of Radiology*, **136**, 543–6.

26 Gopinath, S.P., Cormio, M., Ziegler, J., Raty, S., Valadka, A., & Robertson, C.S. (1996) Intraoperative jugular desaturation during surgery for traumatic intracranial hematomas. *Anesthesia and Analgesia*, **83**, 1014–1021.

27 Zumkeller, M., Behrmann, R., Heissler, H.E., & Dietz, H. (1996) Computed tomographic criteria and survival rate for patients with acute subdural hematoma. *Neurosurgery*, **39**, 708–712.

28 Massaro, F., Lanotte, M., Faccani, G., & Triolo, C. (1996) One hundred and twenty-seven cases of acute subdural haematoma operated on: correlation between CT scan findings and outcome. *Acta Neurochirurgica (Wien)*, **138**, 185–191.

29 Wong, C.W. (1995) Criteria for conservative treatment of supratentorial acute subdural hematomas. *Acta neurochirurgica*, **135(1–2)**, 38–43.

30 Servadei, F., Nasi, M.T., Cremonini, A.M., Giuliani, G., Cenni, P., & Nanni, A. (1998) Importance of a reliable admission Glasgow Coma Scale score for determining the need for evacuation of posttraumatic subdural hematomas: a prospective study of 65 patients. *The Journal of Trauma*, **44**, 868–873.

31 Bullock, R., Golek, J., & Blake, G. (1989) Traumatic intracerebral hematoma: which patients should undergo surgical evacuation? CT scan features and ICP monitoring as a basis for decision making. *Surgical Neurology*, **32**, 181–187.

32 Prabhu, S.S., Zauner, A., & Bullock, M.R. (2004) Surgical management of traumatic brain injury. In: R. Winn (ed). *Youmans Neurological Surgery*. pp. 5145–5180. Saunders, Philadelphia.

33 Adams, J.H., Graham, D.I., & Gennarelli, T.A. (1983) Head injury in man and experimental animals. Neuropathology. *Acta Neurochirurgica Supplement(Wien)*, **32**, S15–S30.

34 Gentleman, S.M., Roberts, G.W., Gennarelli, T.A. *et al.* (1995) Axonal injury: a universal consequence of fatal closed head injury. *Acta Neuropathology (Berlin)*, **89**, 537–543.

35 Juul, N., Morris, G.F., Marshall, S.B., & Marshall, L.F. (2000) Intracranial hypertension and cerebral perfusion pressure: influence on neurological deterioration and outcome in severe head injury. The Executive Committee of the International Selfotel Trial. *Journal of Neurosurgery*, **92**, 1–6.

36 Marmarou, A., Anderson, R.L., Ward, J.D., Choi, S.C., & Young, H.F. (1991) Impact of ICP instability and hypotension on outcome in patients with severe head trauma. *Journal of Neurosurgery (Supplement)*, **75**, S59–S66.

37 Saul, T.G. & Ducker, T.B. (1982) Effect of intracranial pressure monitoring and aggressive treatment on mortality in severe head injury. *Journal of Neurosurgery*, **56**, 498–503.

38 Miller, J.D., Becker, D.P., Ward, J.D., Sullivan, H.G., Adams, W.E., Rosner, M.J. (1977) Significance of intracranial hypertension in severe head injury. *Journal of Neurosurgery*, **47**, 503–516.

39 Aarabi, B., Hesdorffer, D.C., Ahn, E.S., Aresco, C., Scalea, T.M., & Eisenberg, H.M. (2006) Outcome following decompressive craniectomy for malignant swelling due to severe head injury. *Journal of Neurosurgery*, 2006; **104**, 469–479.

40 Coplin, W.M., Cullen, N.K., Policherla, P.N. *et al.* (2001) Safety and feasibility of craniectomy with duraplasty as the initial surgical intervention for severe traumatic brain injury. *The Journal of Trauma*, **50**, 1050–1059.

41 Dam Hieu, P., Sizun, J., Person, H., & Besson, G. (1996) The place of decompressive surgery in the treatment of uncontrollable post-traumatic intracranial hypertension in children. *Childs Nervous System*, **12**, 270–275.

42 De Luca, G.P., Volpin, L., Fornezza, U. *et al.* (2000) The role of decompressive craniectomy in the treatment of uncontrollable post-traumatic intracranial hypertension. *Acta Neurochirurgica (Supplement)*, **76**, 401–404.

43 Guerra, W.K., Gaab, M.R., Dietz, H., Mueller, M.J., Piek, J., & Fritsch, M.J. (1999) Surgical decompression for traumatic brain swelling: indications and results. *Journal of Neurosurgery*, **90**, 187–196.

44 Gower, D.J., Lee, K.S., & McWhorter, J.M. (1988) Role of subtemporal decompression in severe closed head injury. *Neurosurgery*, **23**, 417–422.

45 Albanese, J., Leone, M., Alliez, J.R. *et al.* (2003) Decompressive craniectomy for severe traumatic brain injury: evaluation of the effects at one year. *Critical Care Medicine*, **31**, 2535–2538.

46 Gaab, M.R., Rittierodt, M., Lorenz, M., & Heissler, H.E. (1990) Traumatic brain swelling and operative decompression: a prospective investigation. *Acta Neurochirurgica (Supplement)*, **51**, 326–328.

47 Polin, R.S., Shaffrey, M.E., Bogaev, C.A. *et al.* (1997) Decompressive bifrontal craniectomy in the treatment of severe refractory posttraumatic cerebral edema. *Neurosurgery*, **41**, 84–94.

48 Schneider, G.H., Bardt, T., Lanksch, W.R., & Unterberg, A. (2002) Decompressive craniectomy following traumatic brain injury: ICP, CPP, and neurological outcome *Acta Neurochirurgica (Supplement)*, **81**, 77–79.

49 Taylor, A., Butt, W., Rosenfeld, J. *et al.* (2001) A randomized trial of very early decompressive craniectomy in children with traumatic brain injury and sustained intracranial hypertension. *Childs Nervous System*, **17**, 154–162.

50 Whitfield, P.C., Patel, H., Hutchinson, P.J. *et al.* (2001) Bifrontal decompressive craniectomy in the management of posttraumatic intracranial hypertension. *British Journal of Neurosurgery*, **15**, 500–507.

51 Cooper, D.J., Rosenfeld, J.V., Murray, L. *et al.* (2011) Decompressive craniectomy in diffuse traumatic brain injury. *New England Journal Medicine*, **364**, 1493–1502.

52 Weiner, G.M., Lacey, M.R., Mackenzie, L. *et al.* (2010) Decompressive craniectomy for elevated intracranial pressure and its effect on the cumulative ischemic burden and therapeutic intensity levels after severe traumatic brain injury. *Neurosurgery*, **66**, 1–8.

53 Maloney-Wilensky, E., Gracias, V., Itkin, A. *et al.* (2009) Brain tissue oxygen and outcome after severe traumatic brain injury: a systematic review. *Critical Care Medicine*, **37**, 2057–2063.

54 Ho, C.L., Wang, C.M., Lee, K.K., & Ang, B.T. (2008) Cerebral oxygenation, vascular reactivity, and neurochemistry following decompressive craniectomy for severe traumatic brain injury. *Journal of Neurosurgery*, **108**, 943–949.

55 Jaeger, M., Soehle, M., & Meixensberger, J. (2005) Improvement of brain tissue oxygen and intracranial pressure during and after surgical decompression for diffuse brain edema and space occupying infarction. *Acta Neurochirurgica (Supplement)*, **95**, 117–118.

56 Reithmeier, T., Lohr, M., Pakos, P., Ketter, G., & Ernestus, R.I. (2005) Relevance of ICP and ptiO2 for indication and timing of decompressive craniectomy in patients with malignant brain edema. *Acta Neurochirurgica (Wien)*, **147**, 947–952.

57 Chan, K.H., Mann, K.S., Yue, C.P., Fan, Y.W., & Cheung, M. (1990) The significance of skull fracture in acute traumatic intracranial hematomas in adolescents: a prospective study. *Journal of Neurosurgery*, **72**, 189–194.

58 Hung, C.C., Chiu, W.T., Lee, L.S., Lin, L.S., & Shih, C.J. (1996) Risk factors predicting surgically significant intracranial hematomas in patients with head injuries. *Journal of the Formosan Medical Association*, **95**, 294–297.

59 Servadei, F., Ciucci, G., Pagano, F. *et al.* (1988) Skull fracture as a risk factor of intracranial complications in minor head injuries: a prospective CT study in a series of 98 adult patients. *Journal of Neurology, Neurosurgery and Psychiatry*, **51**, 526–528.

60 Braakman, R. (1972) Depressed skull fracture: data, treatment, and follow-up in 225 consecutive cases. *Journal of Neurology, Neurosurgery and Psychiatry*, **35**, 395–402.

61 Wylen, E.L., Willis, B.K., & Nanda, A. (1999) Infection rate with replacement of bone fragment in compound depressed skull fractures. *Surgical Neurology*, **51**, 452–457.

62 van den Heever, C.M., & van der Merwe, D.J. (1989) Management of depressed skull fractures: selective conservative management of nonmissile injuries. *Journal of Neurosurgery*, **71**, 186s–190s.

63 Jennett, B. & Miller, J.D. (1972) Infection after depressed fracture of skull. Implications for management of nonmissile injuries *Journal of Neurosurgery*, **36**, 333–339.

64 Mendelow, A.D., Campbell, D., Tsementzis, S.A. *et al.* (1983) Prophylactic antimicrobial management of compound depressed skull fracture. *Journal of the Royal College of Surgeons of Edinburgh*, **28**, 80–83.

65 Jennett, B., Miller, J.D., & Braakman, R. (1974) Epilepsy after nonmissile depressed skull fracture. *Journal of Neurosurgery*, **41**, 208–216.

66 Heary, R.F., Hunt, C.D., Krieger, A.J., Schulder, M., & Vaid, C. (1993) Nonsurgical treatment of compound depressed skull fractures. *The Journal of Trauma*, **35**, 441–447.

67 Taha, J.M., Crone, K.R., Berger, T.S., Becket, W.W., & Prenger, E.C. (1993) Sigmoid sinus thrombosis after ,closed head injury in children. *Neurosurgery*, **32**, 541–546.

68 Kapp, J.P. & Gielchinsky, I. (1972) Management of combat wounds of the dural venous sinuses. *Surgery*, **71**, 913–917.

69 C.D.C. (1997) Surveillance data on traumatic brain injury. *Morbidity and Mortality Weekly Report*, **46**, 8–11.

70 Bukur, M., Inaba, K., Barmparas, G. *et al.* (2010) Self-inflicted penetrating injuries at a Level I trauma center. *Injury*, **41**, 1013–1016.

71 Suddaby, L., Weir, B., & Forsyth, C. (1987) The management of 0.22 caliber gunshot wounds of the brain: a review of 49 cases. *Canadian Journal of Neurological Science*, **14**, 268–272.

72 Selden, B.S., Goodman, J.M., Cordell, W. *et al.* (1988) Outcome of self-inflicted gunshot wounds to the brain. *Annals of Emergency Medicine*, **17**, 247–253.

73 Pikus, H.J. & Ball, P.A. (1995) Characteristics of cerebral gunshot injuries in the rural setting. *Neurosurgery Clinics of North America*, **6 (4)**, 611–620.

74 Aarabi, B., Alden, T.D., & Chestnut, R.M. (2001) Guidelines for the Management of Penetrating Brain Injury. *The Journal of Trauma*, **51**, S1–S86.

75 Goodman, J.M. & Kalsbeck, J. (1965) Outcome of self-inflicted gunshot wounds of the head. *The Journal of Trauma*, **5**, 636–642.

76 Yashon, D., Jame, J.A., Martonffy, D., & White, R.J. (1972) Management of civilian craniocerebral bullet injuries. *Annals of Surgery* **38**, 346–351.

77 Byrnes, D.P., Crockard, H.A., Gordon, D.S., & Gleadhill, C.A. (1974) Penetrating craniocerebral missile injuries in the civil disturbances in Northern Ireland. *British Journal of Surgery*, **61**, 169–176.

78 Lillard, P.L. (1978) Five years experience with penetrating craniocerebral gunshot wounds. *Surgical Neurology*, **9**, 79–83.

79 Carey, M.E. (2004) Bullet wounds to the brain among civilians. In: H.R. Winn (ed). *Youmans Neurological Surgery*, 5th ed., pp. 5223–5242. Saunders, Philadelphia.

80 Martin, J. & Campbell, T.H. (1946) Early complications following penetrating wounds of the skull. *Journal of Neurosurgery*, **3**, 58–73.

81 Aarabi, B., Taghipour, M., Alibaii, E., & Kamgarpour, A. (1998) Central nervous system infections after military missile head wounds. *Neurosurgery*, **42**, 500–507.

82 Levi, L., Borovich, B., Guilburd, J.N. *et al.* (1990) Wartime neurosurgical experience in Lebanon, 1982–85, I: penetrating craniocerebral injuries. *Israel Journal of Medical Science*, **26**, 548–554.

83 Taha, J.M., Saba, M.I., & Brown, J.A. (1991) Missile injuries to the brain treated by simple wound closure: results of a protocol during the Lebanese Conflict. *Neurosurgery*, **29**, 380–383.

84 Grahm, T.W., Williams, F.C., Jr., Harrington, T., & Spetzler, R.F. (1990) Civilian gunshot wounds to the head: a prospective study. *Neurosurgery*, **27**, 696–700.

85 Raimondi, A.J. & Samuelson, G.H. (1970) Craniocerebral gunshot wounds in civilian practice. *Journal of Neurosurgery*, **32**, 647–653.

86 Benzel, E.C., Day, W.T., Kesterson, L. *et al.* (1991) Civilian craniocerebral gunshot wounds. *Neurosurgery*, **29**, 67–72.

CHAPTER 7

ICU care: surgical and medical management—neurological monitoring and treatment

Luzius A. Steiner

Department of Anesthesiology, University Hospital of Basel, Switzerland

Injury resulting from traumatic insults to the brain is typically divided into primary and secondary injury. Primary injury occurs at the moment of the trauma and currently cannot be influenced in the clinical setting. In contrast, secondary brain injury occurs at some time after the primary impact as a complication of primary injury and is potentially preventable and treatable. Secondary insults are classified as either intracranial or extracranial (Table 7.1) and have a major impact on outcome. The goal of neuromonitoring and neurological intensive care treatment in patients with traumatic brain injury (TBI) is to prevent, or if that is not possible, to rapidly recognize and treat secondary insults.

Neuromonitoring

Clinical neuromonitoring

Clinical deterioration is often the first sign of a secondary insult such as a rise in intracranial pressure (ICP) or developing intracerebral hematoma. This underlines the importance of repeated standardized neurological assessments to detect such a clinical deterioration as early as possible. Standardized scoring systems facilitate quantitative reporting of the neurological status and are indispensable if the neurological status needs to be compared to earlier assessments. The most widely used score is the Glasgow Coma Scale (GCS).Of the three components of the GCS, the motor score is considered to be the most important. Recently, a new coma scale has been introduced: the Full Outline of UnResponsiveness (FOUR score) [1]. It addresses some of the shortcomings of the GCS by including brainstem reflexes and respiration, allowing detection of subtle neurological changes and, thus, further classification of deeply comatose patients. A comparison between the GCS and the FOUR score is shown in Table 7.2. While such scores are

---

Traumatic Brain Injury, First Edition. Edited by Pieter E. Vos and Ramon Diaz-Arrastia.
© 2015 John Wiley & Sons, Ltd. Published 2015 by John Wiley & Sons, Ltd.

Table 7.1 Secondary brain insults following TBI.

Intracranial insults	Systemic insults
Intracranial hypertension	Hypoxia
Space-occupying lesion	Hypotension
Brain edema	Hypocapnia–hypercapnia
Seizures	Hypoglycemia–hyperglycemia
Vasospasm	Hyponatremia
Hydrocephalus	Hypo-osmolarity–hyperosmolarity
Cerebral infection	Hyperthermia
	Anemia
	Sepsis

rapidly administered and have a high interrater reliability, they cannot replace frequent in-depth neurological examinations.

Intracranial pressure and cerebral perfusion pressure monitoring

In contrast to most other organs the brain is protected by a stiff skull. A rise in ICP may therefore impede cerebral blood flow (CBF) and may cause ischemia. Elevated ICP is an important secondary insult and a predictor of poor outcome after TBI. Possible causes of raised ICP are intracranial mass lesions, disorders of cerebrospinal fluid (CSF) circulation, or brain edema. ICP is an important treatment endpoint and also used to calculate cerebral perfusion pressure (CPP), defined as the difference between mean arterial pressure (MAP) and ICP (CPP=MAP – ICP). CPP represents the pressure gradient across the cerebral vascular bed and is used as a therapeutic target for patients with TBI in most intensive care units (ICUs).

The gold standard for assessing ICP is an intraventricular drain inserted into one of the lateral ventricles and connected to an external pressure transducer [2]. The foramen of Monro or for clinical purposes the external auditory meatus is the reference point for zeroing the transducer. As patients are maintained in a 20–30° head-up position, the zero for arterial pressure should be set at the same height as for ICP to calculate CPP correctly. In addition to monitoring pressure, intraventricular catheters allow withdrawal of CSF to treat raised ICP. The main drawback of intraventricular catheters is the risk of infection that increases over time and may reach 20%. In many units CSF samples are analyzed on a daily basis to detect infection, although daily sampling itself may increase risk of infection. Moreover, the insertion of ventricular catheters may be difficult in patients with severe brain swelling. As an alternative, intraparenchymal probes are used. The infection rate of these probes is very low. An example of such a device is shown in Figure 7.1. The accuracy of subarachnoid, subdural, and epidural devices is lower than that of intraventricular or intraparenchymal sensors, and

Table 7.2 GCS and FOUR score [1]: A comparison.

FOUR score		GCS	
Eye response			
4	Eyelids open/opened, tracking, or blink to command	4	Spontaneous eye opening
3	Eyelids open but not tracking	—	—
2	Eyelids closed but open to loud voice	3	Eye opening to speech
1	Eyelids closed but open to pain	2	Eye opening to pain
0	Eyelids remain closed with pain	1	No reaction to pain
Motor response			
4	Thumbs-up, fist, or peace sign	6	Obeying commands
3	Localization to pain	5	Localization to pain
2	Flexion response to pain	4	Normal flexion to pain
—	—	3	Abnormal flexion to pain
1	Extension response to pain	2	Extension to pain
0	No response to pain or generalized myoclonus status	1	No response to pain
Verbal response			
Not assessed		5	Oriented
		4	Confused conversation
		3	Inappropriate words
		2	Incomprehensible sounds
		1	No response
Brainstem reflexes			
4	Pupil and corneal reflexes present		Not assessed
3	One pupil wide and fixed		
2	Pupil or corneal reflexes absent		
1	Pupil and corneal reflexes absent		
0	Absent pupil, corneal, and cough reflex		
Respiration			
4	Not intubated, regular breathing pattern		Not assessed
3	Not intubated, Cheyne–Stokes breathing pattern		
2	Not intubated, irregular breathing		

(Continued)

Table 7.2 (*Continued*)

FOUR score	GCS
1	Breathes above ventilator rate
0	Breathes at ventilator rate or apnea

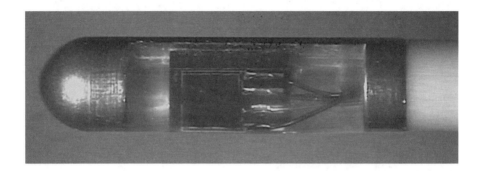

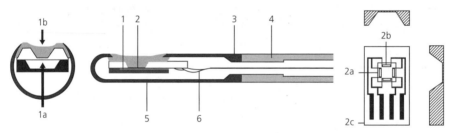

Figure 7.1 Intraparenchymal ICP monitoring device. 1a, Reference pressure, 1b, measured pressure; 1, reference pressure duct, chip with membrane; 3, catheter attachment; 4, polyurethane catheter; 5, titanium case; 6, connecting wires; 2a, pressure-sensitive resistor; 2b, membrane; 2c, pressure chip (Reproduced with permission from RAUMEDIC AG, Helmbrechts, Germany. ©RAUMEDIC AG).

they are rarely used in patients with TBI. Pressure measured in the lumbar CSF space is not a reliable estimator of ICP in brain-injured patients, and such measurements may be dangerous in patients with space-occupying lesions. ICP cannot be assumed to be evenly distributed in many pathological states and it is important to realize that with a ventricular catheter, uniformly distributed ICP will be observed only when CSF circulates freely between all its natural pools. Significant pressure gradients may exist in patients with intracranial hypertension, and an intraparenchymal probe measures only local pressure, which can be compartmentalized and is not necessarily identical with intraventricular pressure. Bilateral parenchymal ICP monitoring has demonstrated large ICP gradients between the two hemispheres.

Despite the broadly felt need of demonstrating the benefit of ICP monitoring, until recently, no randomized controlled trial was performed. In 2012, the BEST TRIP trial was published [3]. BEST TRIP is an acronym for Benchmark Evidence from South American Trials: Treatment of Intracranial Pressure. This study in Bolivian and Ecuadorian centers in collaboration with US neurosurgeons was designed to determine whether information derived from the monitoring of ICP in patients with severe TBI improves medical practice and patient outcomes. It was a multicenter, parallel-group trial randomizing patients with severe TBI for ICP monitoring or imaging and clinical examination. Randomization was stratified according to study site, injury severity, and age. The participating hospitals had ICUs that were staffed with intensivists, 24 h computed tomographic (CT) services, and neurosurgery coverage. The inclusion criteria were 13 years of age or older and GCS = 3–8 (with a score on the GCS motor component 1–5 if the patient was intubated) or a higher GCS score dropping to 3–8 within 48 h.

In the ICP monitoring group the treatment focused on keeping ICP below 20 mmHg.

A strength of this study was that outcome was determined at several time points and on various (as opposed to single) outcome domains. At the time of hospital discharge, measures of survival, duration, and level of impaired consciousness and orientation were obtained. At 3 months, functional status and orientation (GOS-E, the Disability Rating Scale, and GOAT) were measured. And at 6 months, a functional and neuropsychological battery of tests was administered including mental status, working memory, information-processing speed, episodic memory and learning, verbal fluency, executive function, and motor dexterity. A further asset of this study was that trained examiners unaware of the group assignments administered the tests at 3 and 6 months [3].

The results of the study demonstrated no significant differences in the 14-day mortality (30% in the imaging–clinical examination group vs. 21% in the pressure-monitoring group; hazard ratio, 1.36; 95% [CI], 0.87–2.11; $P=0.18$) or in the 6-month mortality (41% in the imaging–clinical examination group vs. 39% in the pressure-monitoring group, hazard ratio, 1.10; 95% CI, 0.77 to 1.57; $P=0.60$). Hence, the results of this long-awaited and important study do not support the superiority of management guided by ICP monitoring over management guided by neurologic examination and serial CT imaging in patients with severe TBI. Of interest further is that the length of stay in the ICU was similar in the two groups. Importantly, the same treatment options were available to both groups, but the imaging–clinical examination group compared to the pressure-monitoring group received hyperosmolar fluids and hyperventilation during more days (4.8 vs. 3.4, $P=0.002$). The distribution of serious adverse events was similar in the two groups [3].

However, this trial should not be used to justify abandoning ICP monitoring. The first author of this important paper points out: "The strongest clinical implication of the BEST TRIP trial is that we need to refine the role of ICP monitoring in sTBI management. Given its established ease and safety, we do not feel that diminished ICP monitoring should follow this report. Instead, clinical methods for interpreting ICP in the setting of individual patients must be developed [4]."

An observational study has even suggested that a CPP-/ICP-oriented therapy will increase treatment intensity and respirator days without an improvement in outcome [5]. Nevertheless, based on the available evidence the guidelines of the Brain Trauma Foundation conclude that ICP data are useful for guiding therapy [6]. These guidelines are accessible on the Internet (www.braintrauma.org). ICP monitoring is recommended in salvageable patients with a GCS of 3–8 and an abnormal CT defined as a scan showing hematomas, contusions, swelling, herniation, or compressed basal cisterns. ICP monitoring is also recommended in patients with a GCS of 3–8 and a normal CT scan provided at least two of the following criteria are fulfilled at admission: age greater than 40 years, unilateral or bilateral motor posturing or systolic blood pressure less than 90 mmHg [6]. Some clinicians will choose to adapt these recommendations and, for example, monitor patients with a GCS greater than 8 if they will undergo major noncranial surgery soon after admission.

CBF monitors

Rapid identification of episodes of low or high CBF would in principle allow timely intervention and possibly result in improved outcome. Methods for quantitative determination of CBF at the bedside based on measurements from the internal jugular vein have been developed but are rarely used [7, 8]. An intraparenchymal probe using thermal diffusion providing continuous quantitative real-time data that are in good agreement with values obtained by xenon CT for a volume of approximately $5\,cm^3$ around the tip of the probe has been used in brain-injured patients [9].

Transcranial Doppler is simple and noninvasive, and can be used repeatedly. Transcranial Doppler measures *blood flow velocity* in the basal cerebral arteries, not CBF, and the linear relationship between CBF and mean flow velocity is only present if neither the diameter of the insonated vessel nor the angle of insonation changes during the examination. This assumption is probably fulfilled for most situations where examinations of the basal cerebral arteries are performed. Transcranial Doppler is the simplest way to noninvasively obtain repeated real-time *estimates* of CBF. The clinical usefulness of transcranial Doppler lies mostly in its ability to quantify cerebrovascular pressure autoregulation and CO_2-reactivity, both of which have been linked to outcome.

The ability of all the aforementioned methods to detect episodes of critically low or excessive CBF is limited for technical reasons but also because the thresholds of ischemia and hyperemia are variable after head injury (Figure 7.2). Furthermore, manipulating CBF is difficult, and adjusting CPP or the arterial partial pressure of CO_2 ($PaCO_2$) does not necessarily have the desired effect. There is no convincing evidence that a strategy that attempts to manipulate CBF is superior to an approach using ICP or CPP to guide treatment. CBF monitoring is an option with unclear clinical benefit at the present time [10].

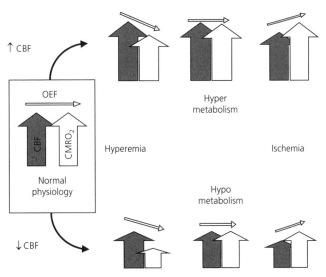

Figure 7.2 Diagram illustrating the relationship between cerebral blood flow (CBF), cerebral metabolic rate of oxygen (CMRO$_2$), and oxygen extraction fraction (OEF). Under physiological conditions, CBF and CMRO$_2$ are tightly coupled and OEF remains more or less stable. In TBI, an uncoupling of CBF and CMRO$_2$ may occur. With low CBF (lower half of diagram), CMRO$_2$ can remain coupled or decrease or increase. Accordingly, with low CBF, hyperemia, coupled with hypometabolism, or ischemia is possible. CBF values do not allow discriminating between these three states. However, OEF will rise or fall in response to the changing relationship between CBF and CMRO$_2$. With increased CBF, the same three scenarios are possible (Courtesy of Prof. D. Menon, Department of Anaesthesia, University of Cambridge, Cambridge, UK. Reproduced with permission).

Cerebral oxygenation monitoring

Due to the difficulties associated with CBF monitoring and treatment thresholds, the focus of interest has shifted to monitoring cerebral oxygenation. Ideally, changes in oxygen extraction fraction (OEF) should be monitored. Such a device is not readily available, but surrogate markers can be monitored.

Jugular bulb oxymetry

The placement of a catheter in the jugular bulb allows sampling of blood that almost exclusively drains from the intracranial circulation. Jugular bulb saturation (SJO$_2$) is measured either from blood that is sampled intermittently from such a catheter or continuously by a fiber-optic catheter. The arteriojugular oxygen content difference (AJDO$_2$) is calculated as the difference between the arterial and jugular oxygen content in paired blood samples. Normal values for SJO$_2$ range from 50% to 75%, and normal values for AJDO$_2$ from 4 mL·100 mL^{-1}to 9 mL·100 mL^{-1} [2]. Low CBF and ischemia raise oxygen extraction, decrease SJO$_2$, and increase AJDO$_2$. Hyperemia will lead to an increase in SJO$_2$ and a decrease in AJDO$_2$. Jugular oxymetry provides data on *global* cerebral oxygen extraction or the adequacy of *global* CBF in relation to metabolic demand. Despite the fact that blood is usually sampled from one jugular bulb only, it is assumed that the values relate to global CBF rather than hemispherical CBF. However, typically only two-thirds of the sampled blood is drained from the ipsilateral hemisphere, and there is a large interindividual variability of venous drainage of the brain. Therefore, methods relying on blood sampling from one of the jugular bulbs are prone to the influence of asymmetry of cerebral venous drainage. It is impossible to predict which side in a specific patient will give more important data, and there is no consensus on which side should be cannulated. Generally, the right internal jugular vein is preferred because it often is the dominant vessel. Alternatively, the side with the larger jugular foramen on the CT scan can be used or the side on which a compression of the jugular vein causes a greater increase in ICP. The catheter tip should lie at the level of the first or second cervical vertebral body, that is, above the point at which the jugular vein receives its first extracranial tributary, the facial vein. If samples are withdrawn too quickly ($>2\,mL \cdot min^{-1}$) falsely elevated values may be found because of retrograde aspiration of extracranial blood [2]. Too low or too high SJO_2 are associated with poor outcome. However, the question whether treatment directed at restoring normal SJO_2 improves outcome is unanswered [6]. This may also be due to the fact that sensitivity of SJO_2 to detect *regional* ischemia is low. A study in head-injured patients using positron emission tomography (PET) to quantify the ischemic brain volume found that on average 170 mL of brain tissue is ischemic at an SJO_2 of 50% [11].

Brain tissue oxygenation ($P_{bt}O_2$)

$P_{bt}O_2$ is the partial pressure of oxygen in the extracellular fluid of the brain and represents the balance between oxygen delivery and consumption [12]. Purpose-designed triple-lumen cranial access devices allow simultaneous monitoring of ICP, $P_{bt}O_2$, and microdialysis data (Figure 7.3). Recently, a single probe incorporating sensors for ICP, $P_{bt}O_2$, and temperature measurements has been developed [13]. Postinsertion CT confirmation of the probe position in the brain parenchyma is important for the interpretation of readings. Transiently increasing the FiO_2 and observing the corresponding $P_{bt}O_2$ increase are advised to exclude the presence of surrounding microhemorrhages or sensor damage at insertion. An equilibration time of up to a half hour is required before readings are stable. Most units use a threshold of 15–20 mmHg, below which therapy is initiated. $P_{bt}O_2$ sensors are extremely localized, with a sampling zone of only 15–22 mm². Accordingly, the position of the sensor is critical for the interpretation of the measurements. In *tissue at risk* regions near focal pathology, global assumptions cannot be made and the monitor is purely focal. When positioned in areas of seemingly normal tissue, or in areas of diffuse injury, the $P_{bt}O_2$ can be regarded as an indicator of global oxygenation [12]. $P_{bt}O_2$ measurements may contribute to the prevention of secondary injury after TBI and may allow adapting therapy to the specific needs of an individual patient by observing changes due to interventions such as CPP manipulation or hyperventilation [6].

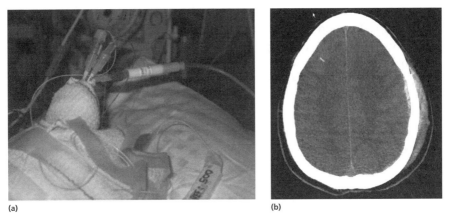

(a)   (b)

Figure 7.3 (a) Intracranial pressure (left), brain tissue oxygenation (right), and microdialysis catheter (center) inserted through a specifically designed triple-bolt access device. (b) Corresponding CT scan showing the tip of one of the three monitors in the right frontal lobe (Courtesy of Dr. M. Oddo, Adult Intensive Care Unit, University Hospital Center Lausanne, Switzerland. Reproduced with permission).

Near-infrared spectroscopy

This technique makes use of the fact that biological material, including the skull, is relatively transparent to light in the near-infrared range. The absorption and scatter of such light allows assessment of cerebral changes in oxyhemoglobin, deoxyhemoglobin, and cytochrome oxidase. Detection of transmitted light at two or more different distances from the light-emitting optodes, the so-called spatially resolved spectroscopy, allows monitoring of the ratio of absolute oxyhemoglobin concentration to total hemoglobin concentration, that is, the hemoglobin saturation, called *tissue oxygenation index* (TOI) or *regional oxygen saturation* (rSO$_2$) [14]. This value is a surrogate marker of cerebral venous saturation and hence oxygen extraction. Newer devices have been shown to have a good specificity and sensitivity for intracranial changes [15]. However, the precise location and size of the monitored brain volume remain unclear. Despite the advantage of being noninvasive and recent data suggesting that near-infrared spectroscopy (NIRS) may also allow noninvasive monitoring of cerebral blood volume and cerebrovascular autoregulation, this technology has yet to find its place in the management of TBI patients.

Cerebral biochemistry

Microdialysis allows detection of biochemical changes associated with hypoxia and/or ischemia. A dialysis catheter (Ø0.9 mm) is introduced into the brain parenchyma. A commercially available analyzer allows monitoring at the bedside with a short time delay between sampling and analysis. Cerebral extracellular levels of glucose, glutamate, lactate, pyruvate, and glycerol, the latter indicating loss of cellular structural integrity, are measured. The lactate–pyruvate ratio is calculated, yielding information on the brain's redox state, a marker of mitochondrial function. The lactate–pyruvate ratio is the most widely used microdialysis variable, and values greater than 20–25 are considered the critical threshold. There is some evidence that microdialysis has the potential to provide early warning of impending hypoxia or ischemia and neurological deterioration and high levels of this ratio have also been linked to chronic frontal atrophy after TBI. Therefore, microdialysis may allow timely implementation of neuroprotective strategies [16]. However, microdialysis reflects only local tissue biochemistry, and the accurate placement of the catheter is crucial. Interpretation of trend data is more important than individual values. Microdialysis has not yet been widely implemented into clinical practice and, at present, is considered primarily a research tool. However, because of its unique ability to contribute important information about the process of secondary brain injury, microdialysis has the potential to become a key component of multimodality monitoring in many forms of brain injury.

Electrical function monitoring: EEG and evoked potentials

The role of EEG monitoring in TBI is not clearly defined. While EEG monitoring is useful to detect nonconvulsive seizures or to titrate barbiturate therapy, interpretation depends on expert knowledge. Ideally, continuous monitoring should be used. This is technically feasible but interpretation and artifacts remain a major challenge [17]. Evoked potentials, particularly SSEPs, may be used for prognostication in patients with coma following TBI [18]. The role of EEG monitoring for the detection of posttraumatic seizures is discussed in more detail in this chapter.

Multimodality monitoring

The concept of multimodality monitoring assumes that combining several monitors for the detection of secondary brain insults will improve our chances of detecting relevant episodes of secondary injury. Despite the advantage of being able to integrate information from several monitors, results may be contradictory and a high degree of expertise is needed for interpretation (Figure 7.4). Multimodality monitoring requires specialized software allowing collecting and integrating data from the various monitors. Such software is commercially available [19] and indispensible when derived parameters such as pressure reactivity [20] or oxygen reactivity [21] are to be integrated into clinical algorithms. So far this concept has not been tested prospectively. Nevertheless, it provides a better understanding of pathophysiology after TBI and may be a key to optimizing therapeutic targets for individual patients.

Neuroimaging

Neuroimaging is an important component of neurocritical care in TBI. Noncontrast CT allows rapid assessment of the extent and type of brain pathology, which ensures that patients who require urgent surgical interventions receive

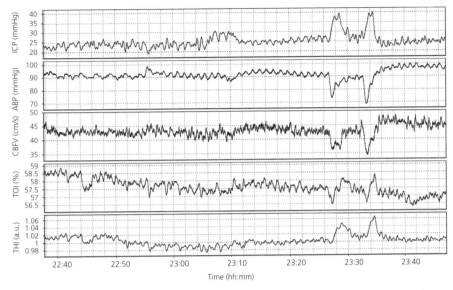

Figure 7.4 Example of multimodality monitoring data from a TBI patient. ICP, intracranial pressure; ABP, mean arterial pressure; CBFV, cerebral blood flow velocity measured by transcranial Doppler; TOI, tissue oxygenation index measured by NIRS; THI, tissue hemoglobin index, a marker of cerebral blood volume derived from NIRS data. Toward the end of the recording (23:27), two ICP waves can be seen triggered by a decrease in ABP and a consecutive increase in cerebral blood volume triggered by autoregulation and represented by an increase in THI. CBFV decreases due to the increase in ICP and TOI decreases as oxygen extraction increases (Reproduced with permission from Dr. M. Czosnyka and Dr C. Zweifel, Academic Neurosurgery, University of Cambridge, Cambridge, UK).

such care as early as possible. Despite the undisputable value of CT, intrahospital transport is required and is not without risk and complications [22]. Simple maneuvers such as lowering the head from a slight head-up position to 0° in the scanner may cause relevant increases in ICP, moving vasopressor pumps may cause subtle changes in infusion rates resulting in changes in CPP, and the unavoidable disconnections from the ventilator may change $PaCO_2$. CT imaging should therefore only be undertaken when it may be assumed that the result will influence clinical management.

Magnetic resonance imaging (MRI) and PET imaging have both been used in patients with acute TBI, albeit mainly for research purposes [23]. MRI requires specific MRI-safe ICP probes, respirators, and infusion pumps. It allows not only for the superior imaging of the posterior fossa and the brain stem, but methods such as diffusion tensor tractography also allow imaging of white matter and diffuse axonal damage, which may provide prognostic information. PET is the gold standard for the determination of CBF and cerebral metabolic data and has greatly improved our understanding of the pathophysiology of TBI. However, due to its complexity and cost its use is restricted to very few research centers.

Neurological treatment

Due to the many interactions of intracranial pathophysiology with extracranial variables, intensive care treatment of patients with TBI is complex. Guidelines that classify the current evidence and make recommendations for a systematic approach to these patients are available [6]. However, as there are only few evidence-based standards in the ICU treatment of TBI, there are many different opinions on how to approach these patients. What seems to be clear is that due to the complexity of the patients, irrespective of the interpretation of the available evidence, it is essential to implement structured protocols. Several studies document an improvement in outcome after the implementation of such a protocol despite remarkable differences in the used algorithms [24–27]. A generic example of such an algorithm is shown in Figure 7.5. Such algorithms usually intensify treatment in a stepwise fashion based on the results of neuromonitoring.

Level 1 interventions

On a first level of treatment intensity, physiological stability is achieved. At this treatment intensity, a $PaCO_2$ in the low normal range (4.5–5.0 kPa, 33–37 mm Hg) is targeted. Adequate oxygenation is essential. FiO_2 and perhaps PEEP are adjusted to achieve an arterial partial pressure of oxygen (PaO_2) in the high normal range, not only to compensate for a high oxygen extraction but also because a PaO_2 less than 8 kPa will lead to a vasodilatation and an increase in ICP. The use of PEEP to increase PaO_2 is much debated as the increase in intrathoracic pressure may impede venous drainage from the brain and increase ICP. However, in many TBI patients the gradient governing cerebral venous drainage is not the difference between arterial and central venous pressure but often between arterial pressure and ICP. Accordingly, ICP will often not rise if PEEP remains less than ICP. Nevertheless, this will have to be tested in an individual patient and a reduction of PEEP may be necessary.

Standard criteria for intubation and extubation are not always applicable in TBI patients. Typically, a GCS ≤ 8 is considered an indication for intubation. In patients with TBI, individual assessment is indispensible. Agitated patients may have to be intubated for imaging or ICP control irrespective of their GCS. The decision to extubate will depend not only on the standard criteria used for non-neurosurgical patients but also on whether the intracranial compliance will allow compensation for the rise in $PaCO_2$, which may occur during weaning and after extubation, and on cranial nerve dysfunction, which may interfere with airway protection.

Sedation is an important part of initial management in comatose patients. Sedation reduces cerebral metabolism and, provided coupling between cerebral metabolism and CBF is intact, leads to a reduction in CBF and hence cerebral blood volume. In the presence of a low intracranial compliance, this may reduce

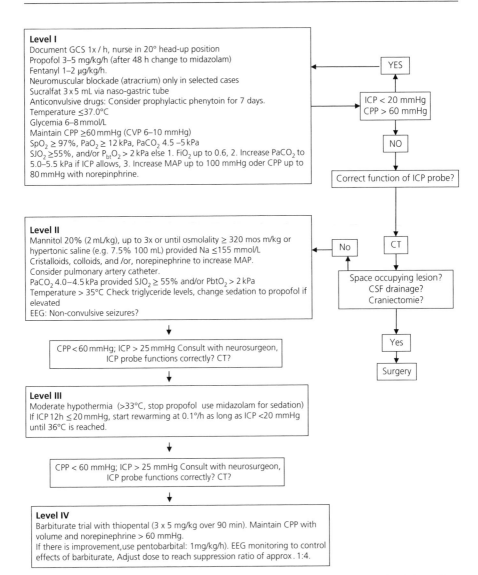

Level I
Document GCS 1x / h, nurse in 20° head-up position
Propofol 3–5 mg/kg/h (after 48 h change to midazolam)
Fentanyl 1–2 μg/kg/h.
Neuromuscular blockade (atracrium) only in selected cases
Sucralfat 3 x 5 mL via naso-gastric tube
Anticonvulsive drugs: Consider prophylactic phenytoin for 7 days.
Temperature ≤37.0°C
Glycemia 6–8 mmol/L
Maintain CPP ≥60 mmHg (CVP 6–10 mmHg)
SpO_2 ≥ 97%, PaO_2 ≥ 12 kPa, $PaCO_2$ 4.5 –5 kPa
SJO_2 ≥55%, and/or $P_{bt}O_2$ > 2 kPa else 1. FiO_2 up to 0.6, 2. Increase $PaCO_2$ to 5.0–5.5 kPa if ICP allows, 3. Increase MAP up to 100 mmHg oder CPP up to 80 mmHg with norepinphrine.

YES

ICP < 20 mmHg
CPP > 60 mmHg

NO

Correct function of ICP probe?

Level II
Mannitol 20% (2 mL/kg), up to 3x or until osmolality ≥ 320 mos m/kg or hypertonic saline (e.g. 7.5% 100 mL) provided Na ≤155 mmol/L
Cristalloids, colloids, and /or, norepinephrine to increase MAP.
Consider pulmonary artery catheter.
$PaCO_2$ 4.0–4.5 kPa provided SJO_2 ≥ 55% and/or $PbtO_2$ > 2 kPa
Temperature > 35°C Check triglyceride levels, change sedation to propofol if elevated
EEG: Non-convulsive seizures?

No

CT

Space occupying lesion?
CSF drainage?
Craniectomie?

CPP < 60 mmHg; ICP > 25 mmHg Consult with neurosurgeon, ICP probe functions correctly? CT?

Yes

Surgery

Level III
Moderate hypothermia (>33°C, stop propofol use midazolam for sedation)
If ICP 12h ≤ 20 mmHg, start rewarming at 0.1°/h as long as ICP <20 mmHg until 36°C is reached.

CPP < 60 mmHg; ICP > 25 mmHg Consult with neurosurgeon, ICP probe functions correctly? CT?

Level IV
Barbiturate trial with thiopental (3 x 5 mg/kg over 90 min). Maintain CPP with volume and norepinephrine > 60 mmHg.
If there is improvement,use pentobarbital: 1mg/kg/h). EEG monitoring to control effects of barbiturate, Adjust dose to reach suppression ratio of approx . 1:4.

Figure 7.5 Example of a generic protocol for the intensive care management of TBI. Intensity and the risk of complications of treatment increase with each level. Weighing of the available evidence and hence interventions in each level may differ from center to center, and adaptation to unit-specific standards is necessary (Adapted from Patel *et al.* [27], with permission from Springer-Verlag).

ICP considerably. Propofol and benzodiazepines are mostly used for this purpose. Accumulation of sedatives and the propofol infusion syndrome are concerns. The propofol infusion syndrome was initially observed in children but later also in adults. It is a rare but lethal syndrome associated with propofol infusions at doses greater than 4 mg/kg/h for more than 48 h [28]. The symptoms include severe metabolic acidosis, acute refractory bradycardia leading to asystole, and rhabdomyolysis. The cause of this syndrome has not been clearly identified but in vitro data suggest impaired mitochondrial function. Children must not be sedated with propofol on the ICU, and it has been suggested to limit the duration of propofol exposure in adults.

Seizures may lead to an increase in ICP and contribute to the ischemic burden. Seizures are frequent in TBI patients and categorized as *early* when they occur within the first 7 days after trauma. Up to 25% of patients have been shown to have early seizures after severe TBI [6], and it has been estimated that up to 20% of TBI patients have nonconvulsive seizures, which may be only detectable with continuous EEG monitoring [17]. Whenever ICP increases occur that do not have an apparent cause, seizures should be included in the differential diagnosis. Early seizures are a risk factor for late occurring seizures after TBI. However, early seizures are not associated with worse outcomes and side effects and benefits of a prophylaxis need to be considered. Nevertheless, early seizures should be treated and many experts recommend a prophylaxis [6]. Generally, phenytoin is used, although more recently levetiracetam has replaced it in many neurological ICUs. It is unknown whether levetiracetam or other modern anti-epileptic drugs offer clear benefits.

In addition to the general principles outlined earlier, CPP and ICP are the key components of treatment. Management of CPP and ICP are closely linked. Often, manipulation of one variable will influence the other. CPP is a frequently used target parameter in TBI. However, there is controversy as to which thresholds should be used. The current guidelines of the Brain Trauma Foundation suggest 50–70 mmHg in adults [6]. For pediatric TBI, specific guidelines with age-dependent thresholds are available [29]. Not only too low but also inappropriately high CPP is associated with poor outcome. The goal of any CPP augmentation is to improve CBF in brain regions where it is critically low. However, in general an increase in CPP will only lead to an increase in CBF when autoregulation has failed or CPP is below the lower limit or above the upper limit of autoregulation. In a normal brain, CBF is relatively constant in the CPP range of about 50–150 mmHg due to autoregulation. In the setting of TBI, autoregulation is frequently disturbed [30, 31], and there is a large interindividual variability of auto-regulatory failure. It may result in a shift of the autoregulatory plateau to the right or a shortening of the autoregulatory plateau. Some patients will completely lose autoregulation, that is, CBF will follow CPP passively [20]. Moreover, the degree of dysfunction will change with time. The effects of CPP augmentation on CBF and ischemic brain volume are therefore difficult to predict and may be small despite large increases in CPP [32, 33].There have been attempts to identify individual thresholds for CPP management. Microdialysis [34], brain tissue oxy-metry [35], and an index of pressure reactivity [20] and jugular bulb saturation may be used for this purpose. Optimization of intravascular fluid status is the critical first step in CPP management, after which norepinephrine is used by most clinicians. An altered blood–brain barrier may change the response of the cerebral vasculature to catecholamines, and differing effects on CBF of dopamine and norepinephrine at identical CPPs have been demonstrated [36]. The question whether and how excessively high CPP should be lowered has not been answered. Finally, it is important to keep in mind that CPP augmentation is not without risk. It has been suggested that the benefits of this strategy may be offset by adverse effects. Induced hypertension in head-injured patients has been associated with increased risk of adult respiratory distress syndrome (ARDS) [37].

In head-injured adults the ICP threshold above which outcome will be affected negatively lies between 20 and 25 mmHg [6]. Above this level, aggressive treatment is started in most units. There is controversy concerning critical thresholds for ICP in children [38]. Elevated ICP should be treated not only when it leads to an inadequately low CPP but also in the presence of an assumedly adequate CPP. If the patient's ICP remains less than 20 mmHg no further action is taken. If despite the measures described earlier the ICP exceeds 20 mmHg, the first step is to evaluate whether surgical treatment if necessary, in which case it is initiated as fast as possible. Therefore, unless there is reason to suspect incorrect function of the ICP probe, an emergent CT scan is usually the first step. If there are no surgical options, the patient moves to the next level of treatment intensity.

Level 2 interventions

Hyperosmolar therapy is often the first level 2 intervention (Figure 7.5). Mannitol and increasingly hypertonic saline are used for this purpose [39]. There is currently no consensus on the ideal concentration for hypertonic saline, and NaCl concentration in the level of 3–30% has been used as a crystalloid solution or as colloids with supplemental NaCl. A rebound phenomenon of ICP has been reported after administration of mannitol, but in human TBI, this has not been observed so far. Hypertonic saline may aggravate or induce pulmonary edema in patients with underlying pulmonary or cardiac disease [6]. In addition, moderate hyperventilation (target $PaCO_2$, 30–33 mm Hg) is often used on this level. There is controversy regarding target values for $PaCO_2$. Hyperventilation leads to a reduction in CBF that may be deleterious [40]. Monitoring of brain oxygenation is potentially useful to avoid hyperventilation-induced ischemia.

Level 3 and level 4 interventions

If second-level measures are inadequate to control ICP, more intensive therapy is required. Hypothermia to treat refractory intracranial hypertension is an emerging strategy. Prophylactic hypothermia is controversial and currently not recommended [6]. However, hypothermia exerts many beneficial effects on the injured brain [41] and is an efficient intervention to reduce ICP. In contrast to sedation that only reduces electrical activity, hypothermia also reduces the metabolic demand caused by the processes needed to uphold structural integrity. Whenever hypothermia is used, it is important to be aware of the many associated complications such as coagulopathy, electrolyte disorders, hypovolemia following hypothermia-induced diuresis, and changes in drug effects and metabolism [42]. Typically, temperatures of 33–34°C are regarded as adequate for the control of ICP. The question of how long hypothermia should be maintained has not been answered yet. One approach is to cool the patient until ICP is stable at less than 20 mmHg and then to increase temperature slightly and observe the ICP response. While induction of hypothermia with cold fluids and commercially available intravascular or surface cooling devices is convenient and straightforward, the rate of rewarming is critical. Too rapid rewarming may be detrimental to an injured brain, and very slow rates (0.1°C/h) have been recommended.

Irrespective of whether hypothermia is used, induction of a barbiturate coma is used as a last resort, although neurosurgical maneuvers such as decompressive craniectomy have recently been used (decompressive craniectomy is discussed further in Chapter 5).The goal of barbiturate coma is to achieve maximal metabolic suppression. If all electrical activity is abolished the metabolic demands of the brain are reduced by roughly 60% from the awake state. Unfortunately, this intervention is associated with many complications. Often, the hypotensive effect that is frequently observed after administration of barbiturates will offset the ICP-lowering effect on CPP, and a considerable increase in vasopressor doses may be needed to keep CPP stable. Moreover, barbiturates have a long half-life after tissue pools are saturated. Therefore, accumulation is inevitable and it is recommended to titrate the dose with EEG monitoring to a predefined suppression ratio. Nevertheless, extubation or diagnosis of brain death may be delayed. Barbiturates depress cardiac function and lower CPP. While barbiturates have been shown to control ICP even after all other medical and surgical treatments have failed, there is no evidence that this translates into improved outcome [6].

Lund concept

A somewhat different approach to TBI developed by investigators at the University of Lund in Sweden is referred to as the *Lund concept* [43]. It focuses on the physiological volume regulation of the intracranial compartments. The concept has two main goals: to reduce or prevent an increase in ICP and to improve perfusion and oxygenation around contusions. The Lund concept is based on the model that after TBI the blood–brain barrier will be partially disrupted. Transcapillary water exchange will then be determined by the differences in hydrostatic and colloid osmotic pressure between the intra- and extracapillary compartments. A high CPP accordingly increases intracapillary hydrostatic pressure and leads to increased intracerebral water content and an increase in ICP. A lasting reduction of ICP can be obtained by increased reabsorption of fluid over the capillary membrane. The therapeutic measures are manifold and include normalization of all essential hemodynamic parameters. In patients who are managed according to the Lund concept, normovolemia is mandatory and erythrocyte (target 125–140 g/L) and albumin infusions (target 35–42 g/L) are used. MAP is reduced using metoprolol or clonidine, typically to a CPP of 60–70 mmHg, but a CPP as low as 50 mmHg may be used in selected cases. A reduction of the intracranial blood volume is obtained by reducing cerebral energy metabolism through sedation; if necessary, as a last option before craniotomy is performed a further reduction of blood volume within the venous compartment may be obtained by dihydroergotamine. Normothermia and normocapnia are further goals. The intention of the treatment is to reach a slow and lasting reduction of ICP over hours to days. Clinical studies using the Lund concept have shown favorable results [25]. However, so far no prospective controlled randomized evaluation has been performed, and the Lund concept is not widely used outside of Sweden.

Further neuroprotective measures

Normobaric and hyperbaric hyperoxia to improve outcome after TBI have been investigated with conflicting results. Further studies are needed to confirm the usefulness of this simple intervention [44]. Steroids are not indicated in the acute care of TBI [6].

ICU discharge

The optimal time-point for ICU discharge will depend on the local structures. Typically, patients are discharged to a step-down unit once the intracranial situation is stable, that is, ICP is stably less than 20 mmHg, CPP is stable and adequate without vasopressor drugs, and intracranial monitors have been removed. However, many TBI patients suffer from a prolonged delirium, which may preclude transfer to an intermediate care unit. Many units have developed a follow-up clinic that reexamines all patients, for example, 6 months postinjury. This is an excellent way of collecting follow-up data that are essential for quality control and important as a feedback for the ICU staff who are typically confronted with these patients during a very unstable and difficult phase after TBI.

In summary, despite the absence of unequivocal evidence, the most important and widely used instrument is the ICP monitor. Brain oxygen and biochemical monitors are further options. However, their role is not yet clearly defined, and they are primarily used in the context of a multimodality monitoring strategy to individualize CPP and/or ICP treatment. Standard of care today is individualized treatment based on a unit-specific protocol that translates the available evidence into the everyday practice of a specific unit.

References

1 Wijdicks, E.F., Bamlet, W.R., Maramattom, B.V. *et al.* (2005) Validation of a new coma scale: the FOUR score. *Annals of Neurology*, **58**, 585–593.
2 Steiner, L.A. & Andrews, P.J. (2006) Monitoring the injured brain: ICP and CBF. *British Journal of Anaesthesia* **97**, 26–38.

3 Chesnut, R.M., Temkin, N., Carney, N. *et al.* (2012) A trial of intracranial-pressure monitoring in traumatic brain injury. *New England Journal of Medicine* **367 (26)**: 2471–2481.

4 Chestnut, R. (2013) Intracranial pressure monitoring: headstone or a new head start. The BEST TRIP trial in perspective. *Intensive Care Medicine* **39 (4)**: 771–774.

5 Cremer, O.L., van Dijk, G.W., van Wensen, E. *et al.* (2005) Effect of intracranial pressure monitoring and targeted intensive care on functional outcome after severe head injury. *Critical Care Medicine*, **33**, 2207–13.

6 Braintrauma Foundation. (2007) Guidelines for the management of severe traumatic brain injury. *Journal of Neurotrauma*, **24 (Suppl 1)**, S1–S106.

7 Melot, C., Berre, J., Moraine, J.J. *et al.* (1996) Estimation of cerebral blood flow at bedside by continuous jugular thermodilution. *Journal of Cerebral Blood Flow and Metabolism*, **16**, 1263–1270.

8 Wietasch, G.J., Mielck, F., Scholz, M. *et al.* (2000) Bedside assessment of cerebral blood flow by double-indicator dilution technique. *Anesthesiology*, **92**, 367–75.

9 Rosenthal, G., Sanchez-Mejia, R.O., Phan, N. *et al.* (2011) Incorporating a parenchymal thermal diffusion cerebral blood flow probe in bedside assessment of cerebral autoregulation and vasoreactivity in patients with severe traumatic brain injury. *Journal of Neurosurgery*, **114 (1)**, 62–70.

10 Steiner, L.A. & Czosnyka, M. (2002) Should we measure cerebral blood flow in head-injured patients? *British Journal of Neurosurgery*, **16**, 429–439.

11 Coles, J.P., Fryer, T.D., Smielewski, P. *et al.* (2004) Incidence and mechanisms of cerebral ischemia in early clinical head injury. *Journal of Cerebral Blood Flow and Metabolism*, **24**, 202–211.

12 Nortje, J. & Gupta, A.K. (2006) The role of tissue oxygen monitoring in patients with acute brain injury. *British Journal of Anaesthesia*, **97**, 95–106.

13 Purins, K., Enblad, P., Sandhagen, B. *et al.* (2010) Brain tissue oxygen monitoring: a study of in vitro accuracy and stability of Neurovent-PTO and Licox sensors. *Acta Neurochir (Wien)*, **152**, 681–688.

14 Greisen, G. (2006) Is near-infrared spectroscopy living up to its promises? *Seminars in Fetal and Neonatal Medicine*, **11**, 498–502.

15 Al-Rawi, P.G., Smielewski, P. & Kirkpatrick, P.J. (2001) Evaluation of a near-infrared spectrometer (NIRO 300) for the detection of intracranial oxygenation changes in the adult head. *Stroke*, **32**, 2492–2500.

16 Tisdall, M.M. & Smith, M. (2006) Cerebral microdialysis: research technique or clinical tool. *British Journal of Anaesthesia*, **97**, 18–25.

17 Moulton, R. (2005) Electrical function monitoring. In: P. L. Reilly & R. Bullock (eds), *Head Injury*, pp. 246–257. Hodder Education, London.

18 Houlden, D.A., Taylor, A.B., Feinstein, A. *et al.* Early somatosensory evoked potential grades in comatose traumatic brain injury patients predict cognitive and functional outcome. *Critical Care Medicine*, **38**, 167–174.

19 Smielewski, P., Czosnyka, M., Steiner, L. *et al.* (2005) ICM+: software for on-line analysis of bedside monitoring data after severe head trauma. *Acta Neurochirurgica Supplement* **95**, 43–49.

20 Steiner, L.A., Czosnyka, M., Piechnik, S.K. *et al.* (2002) Continuous monitoring of cerebrovascular pressure reactivity allows determination of optimal cerebral perfusion pressure in patients with traumatic brain injury. *Critical Care Medicine*, **30**, 733–738.

21 Jaeger, M., Dengl, M., Meixensberger, J., & Schuhmann, M.U. (2010) Effects of cerebrovascular pressure reactivity-guided optimization of cerebral perfusion pressure on brain tissue oxygenation after traumatic brain injury. *Critical Care Medicine*, **38**, 1343–1347.

22 Waydhas, C. (1999) Intrahospital transport of critically ill patients. *Critical Care*, **3**, R83–89.

23 Coles, J.P. (2007) Imaging after brain injury. *British Journal of Anaesthesia*, **99**, 49–60.

24 Clayton, T.J., Nelson, R.J. & Manara A.R. (2004) Reduction in mortality from severe head injury following introduction of a protocol for intensive care management. *British Journal of Anaesthesia*, **93**, 761–767.

25 Elf, K., Nilsson, P. & Enblad, P. (2002) Outcome after traumatic brain injury improved by an organized secondary insult program and standardized neurointensive care.*Critical Care Medicine*, **30**, 2129–2134.

26 Palmer, S., Bader, M.K., Qureshi, A. *et al.* (2001) The impact on outcomes in a community hospital setting of using the AANS traumatic brain injury guidelines. Americans Associations for Neurologic Surgeons. *The Journal of Trauma*, **50**, 657–664.

27 Patel, H.C., Menon, D.K., Tebbs, S. *et al.* (2002) Specialist neurocritical care and outcome from head injury. *Intensive Care Medicine*, **28**, 547–553.

28 Kam, P.C. & Cardone, D. (2007) Propofol infusion syndrome.*Anaesthesia*, **62**, 690–701.

29 Adelson, P.D., Bratton, S.L., Carney, N.A. *et al.* (2003) Guidelines for the acute medical management of severe traumatic brain injury in infants, children, and adolescents. Chapter 8. Cerebral perfusion pressure. *Pediatric Critical Care Medicine*, **4**, S31–S33.

30 Czosnyka, M., Smielewski, P., Piechnik, S. *et al.* (2001) Cerebral autoregulation following head injury. *Journal of Neurosurgery*, **95**, 756–763.

31 Hlatky, R., Furuya, Y., Valadka, A.B. *et al.* (2002) Dynamic autoregulatory response after severe head injury. *Journal of Neurosurgery*, **97**, 1054–1061.

32 Coles, J.P., Steiner, L.A., Johnston, A.J. *et al.* (2004) Does induced hypertension reduce cerebral ischaemia within the traumatized human brain? *Brain*, **127**, 2479–2490.

33 Steiner, L.A., Coles, J.P., Johnston, A.J. *et al.* (2003) Responses of posttraumatic pericontusional cerebral blood flow and blood volume to an increase in cerebral perfusion pressure. *Journal of Cerebral Blood Flow and Metabolism*, **23**, 1371–1377.

34 Nordstrom, C.H., Reinstrup, P., Xu, W. *et al.* (2003) Assessment of the lower limit for cerebral perfusion pressure in severe head injuries by bedside monitoring of regional energy metabolism. *Anesthesiology* **98**, 809–814.

35 Meixensberger, J., Jaeger, M., Vath, A. *et al.* (2003) Brain tissue oxygen guided treatment supplementing ICP/CPP therapy after traumatic brain injury. *Journal of Neurology, Neurosurgery, and Psychiatry*, **74**, 760–764.

36 Steiner, L.A., Johnston, A.J., Czosnyka, M. *et al.* (2004) Direct comparison of cerebrovascular effects of norepinephrine and dopamine in head-injured patients. *Critical Care Medicine*, **32**, 1049–1054.

37 Contant, C.F., Valadka, A.B., Gopinath, S.P. *et al.* (2001) Adult respiratory distress syndrome: a complication of induced hypertension after severe head injury. *Journal of Neurosurgery*, **95**, 560–568.

38 Adelson, P.D., Bratton, S.L., Carney, N.A. *et al.* (2003) Guidelines for the acute medical management of severe traumatic brain injury in infants, children, and adolescents. Chapter 6. Threshold for treatment of intracranial hypertension.*Pediatr Critical Care Medicine*, **4**, S25–S27.

39 Himmelseher, S. (2007) Hypertonic saline solutions for treatment of intracranial hypertension. *Current Opinion in Anaesthesiology*, **20**, 414–426.

40 Coles, J.P., Minhas, P.S., Fryer, T.D. *et al.* (2002) Effect of hyperventilation on cerebral blood flow in traumatic head injury: clinical relevance and monitoring correlates.*Critical Care Medicine*, **30**, 1950–1959.

41 Polderman, K.H. (2004) Application of therapeutic hypothermia in the ICU: opportunities and pitfalls of a promising treatment modality. Part 1: indications and evidence. *Intensive Care Medicine*, **30**, 556–575.

42 Polderman, K.H. (2004) Application of therapeutic hypothermia in the intensive care unit. Opportunities and pitfalls of a promising treatment modality—Part 2: practical aspects and side effects. *Intensive Care Medicine*, **30**, 757–769.

43 Grande, P.O. (2006) The "Lund Concept" for the treatment of severe head trauma—physiological principles and clinical application.*Intensive Care Medicine*, **32**, 1475–1484.

44 Kumaria, A. & Tolias, C.M. (2009) Normobaric hyperoxia therapy for traumatic brain injury and stroke: a review.*British Journal of Neurosurgery*, **23**, 576–584.

CHAPTER 8

ICU care: surgical and medical management—systemic treatment

Lori Shutter

Departments of Neurology and Neurosurgery, University of Pittsburgh Medical Center, Pittsburgh, PA, USA

Initial ICU evaluation of the traumatic brain injury patient

The initial evaluation of any patient with traumatic brain injury (TBI) upon arrival in the Intensive care unit (ICU) must include reassessment of the basic *airway, breathing, and circulation (ABCs)*. Intubated patients should have confirmation of endotracheal tube placement, oxygenation, and ventilation, while the ability to protect and maintain an adequate airway needs to be reassessed in nonintubated patients. Repeat vital signs should be performed promptly upon ICU arrival, with a focus on immediate management of hypoxia, hypotension, and adequate acute resuscitation with fluids and blood products. Isolated hypoxic or hypotensive events are frequently not well documented in the medical records; therefore, a thorough review of prehospital and emergency department records is crucial.

Hypoxia and hypotension

The adverse impact of hypoxia and hypotension on outcome after TBI has been well recognized, and multiple studies have shown that even a single episode of hypoxia or hypotension can have serious consequences and is to be avoided [1–4]. In 1978, Miller *et al.* reported on a prospective cohort of 100 consecutive patients with severe TBI. Hypotension, hypoxia, anemia, and hypercarbia were each found to be associated with increased morbidity and mortality. Hypotension in that study was defined as an isolated episode of systolic blood pressure (SBP) less than 95 mmHg [1]. Chesnut *et al.* evaluated the effect of hypotension in 717 consecutive TBI patients and found that it was an independent predictor of poor outcome. In addition, a single documented episode of hypotension was sufficient to double mortality and increase morbidity [2]. In a cohort study of 50 TBI patients transported by helicopter, hypoxia (defined as $SaO_2 < 90\%$) occurred in 55% of cases, while hypotension (defined as $SBP < 90\,mmHg$) occurred in 24% of cases. Both clinical factors exerted a negative impact on outcome [3]. Finally,

Traumatic Brain Injury, First Edition. Edited by Pieter E. Vos and Ramon Diaz-Arrastia.

in a study of 107 TBI patients, early episodes of hypotension but not hypoxia were found to predict mortality, with odds ratios increasing from 2.1 to 8.1 with repeat episodes of hypotension [4].

In summary, both hypotension and hypoxia adversely impact patient outcomes following TBI; therefore, prevention, rapid recognition, and correction of early episodes of hypoxia or hypotension be carried out while in the ICU in an effort to aggressively avoid any additional injury.

Basic ICU management

Severely ill TBI patients are often chemically sedated and bedbound during the course of their ICU stay and have nasal or oral feeding tubes, central venous catheters (CVC), bladder catheters, rectal pouches, and other invasive monitors to follow their hemodynamic and physiologic states. Management of these patients is complex and patients are particularly prone to developing any number of complications associated with ICU care. The next sections will discuss routine ICU care such as sedation and analgesia, ventilator management, temperature control, nutrition, prevention of infections, and other complications of care that could seriously complicate patient care and outcomes.

Sedation, analgesia, and neuromuscular blockade

Although these agents are commonly used in the patient with a TBI to assist in control of intracranial pressure (ICP), they actually have a much broader role in the ICU environment. Some of the additional indications include management of agitation, delirium, pain, seizures, withdrawal, and ventilator dyssynchrony. They may be used as individual bolus dosing or continuous infusions. Typical dosing regimens are shown in Table 8.1.

Sedation

Patients with a TBI may demonstrate agitation and physiological responses that may contribute to elevations in ICP. Sedation is frequently used to allow control of physiological parameters. The key is to find an appropriate balance that allows for adequate neurological examinations, but avoids excessive agitation. Short-acting sedatives, such as lorazepam, midazolam, or propofol, are frequently used to achieve this task. There are some concerns regarding the use of benzodiazepines due to their neurologic and respiratory depressant effects, prolongation of posttraumatic amnesia, and potential for accumulation of active metabolites. In addition, delayed elimination may occur in patients with renal failure, hepatic insufficiency, heart failure, and high body mass index and the elderly.

Propofol is widely used as a sedative in TBI patients due to the rapidity of onset, short duration of action, and potential neuroprotective effects by depressing cerebral metabolism and oxygen consumption. A study comparing

Table 8.1 Dosing of sedatives, analgesics, and neuromuscular blockade.

Sedatives	
Lorazepam	Bolus: 1–2 mg
	Infusion: 0.5–1 mg/h
Midazolam	Bolus: 1–2 mg
	Infusion: 0.01–0.1 mg/kg/h or 2–4 mg/h
Propofol	Bolus: 0.5–1.5 mg/kg
	Infusion: 10–100 µg/kg/min
	Notes: *not to exceed 5 mg/kg/h*
Dexmedetomidine	Bolus: 1 µg/kg
	Infusion: 0.2–0.7 µg/kg/h
	Notes: *monitor for bradycardia*
Analgesics	
Morphine Sulfate	Bolus: 2–5 mg
	Infusion: 0.5–4 mg/h
Fentanyl	Bolus: 25–100 mcg
	Infusion: 25–100 µg/h
Sufentanyl	Bolus: 10–30 mcg
	Infusion: 0.05—1 µg/kg/h
Remifentanil	Bolus: 1 µg/kg
	Infusion: 9–18 µg/kg/h
Neuromuscular blockade	
Vecuronium	Bolus: 0.1 mg/kg
	Infusion: 0.8–1.2 µg/kg/min
Cisatracurium	Bolus: 0.2 mg/kg
	Infusion: 0.5–5 µg/kg/min

propofol with midazolam found that both were equally effective for achieving the desired level of sedation, but the time needed to awakening was significantly shorter with propofol [5]. Enthusiasm for the use of propofol in this patient population must be tempered by the risk of propofol-related infusion syndrome (PRIS), which can occur with prolonged, high-dose infusions. Clinical features include hyperkalemia, hepatomegaly, lipemia, metabolic acidosis, myocardial failure, rhabdomyolysis, and renal failure resulting in death. The development of an unexplained lactic acidosis or hypertriglyceridemia may be early warning signs of PRIS [6]. In addition, ECG changes showing downsloping ST-segment elevation in precordial leads V1–V3 may indicate cardiac instability [7]. Propofol doses should be kept at less than 100 µg/kg/min, and extreme caution used with infusions beyond 48 h in critically ill adults [8].

The novel sedative–anesthetic dexmedetomidine may have a role in management of the patient with TBI, particularly when trying to concurrently manage agitation or withdrawal syndromes. Dexmedetomidine is an alpha2-agonist that is very short acting and provides sedation, anxiolysis, analgesia, and amnesia without suppressing respiratory function. Two recent randomized, controlled trials compared dexmedetomidine to benzodiazepines (lorazepam; midazolam) in mechanically ventilated ICU patients. Both found more days at goal sedation, fewer days of coma, and less delirium in the dexmedetomidine group [9, 10]. A single study using dexmedetomidine in neurosurgical patients has demonstrated safety and efficacy in this patient population [11]. While dexmedetomidine has characteristics that make it attractive for use in the TBI patient, there currently are only two case reports describing its use in this patient population [12, 13].

Analgesia

There are many possible indications for analgesia in a TBI patient in the ICU environment, including trauma-related pain, elevations in ICP, agitation, and dysautonomias. Although morphine sulfate is frequently used, there has been increasing use of synthetic narcotics such as remifentanil, fentanyl, and sufentanyl due to their shorter duration of action. There are limited studies comparing the efficacy of these agents in the TBI patient. Concerns have been raised about the use of synthetic narcotics as some studies have suggested that they may produce a slight elevation in ICP, particularly in patients with preserved autoregulation [14, 15]. ICP elevations can be minimized by slow titration of the agents [16]. A recent study comparing remifentanil, fentanyl, and morphine found that the synthetic agents allowed for faster and more predictable awakening for neurological assessments without any additional adverse effects [17].

There is increasing awareness that sedative and analgesic use in the ICU environment may contribute to delirium and mortality. Efforts to standardize protocols that allow individualized titration of sedation, analgesia, and delirium treatments have demonstrated reduced ventilator days, shorter ICU and hospital lengths of stay, and less dependency [18, 19]. Unfortunately, although one of these studies was specific to trauma patients, they excluded patients with a TBI. In contrast, there has been a recent report that the use of morphine sulfate early in the care of TBI patients may lower the risk of developing a posttraumatic stress disorder [20]. While the optimal agent for pain control in the TBI patient is not clear, it is apparent that pain control must be individualized based on the clinical needs of the patient.

Neuromuscular blockade

In general, the use of neuromuscular blockade agents has decreased in ICU settings as adequate sedation and analgesia should allow patients to tolerate mechanical ventilation. This is particularly relevant in patients after a TBI. Early prophylactic neuromuscular blockade in this patient population has been shown to be detrimental due to increases in the length of ICU stays, pneumonia, and sepsis [21]. Neuromuscular blockade may have a role when significant ventilator dyssynchrony affects systemic and cerebral oxygenation despite adequate sedation. If chemical paralysis is necessary, then short-acting agents such as vecuronium or cisatracurium are recommended. Patients should be monitored closely with *train of four* stimulation to assess the level of paralysis, with a therapeutic goal of maintaining the lowest dose that achieves ventilator synchrony.

Temperature management

Hypothermia has been studied as a possible neuroprotective agent for reducing secondary brain injury from various causes over the past 60 years. Its mechanism as a neuroprotectant remains a matter of debate. While hypothermia has been shown to be effective in reducing secondary injury following cardiac arrest [22, 23], no human studies have demonstrated an unequivocal benefit of hypothermia in TBI.

The National Acute Brain Injury Study: Hypothermia (NABIS:H) demonstrated no benefit from prophylactic hypothermia on patients with acute TBI [24]. Subsequently, the National Institutes of Neurological Disorders and Stroke (NINDS) funded NABIS:H II as a follow-up study that focused a specific subset of patients, but this study was terminated in June 2009 for futility [25]. There is evidence that therapeutic hypothermia may be beneficial for refractory ICP elevations [26–28].

Fever is common in TBI patients admitted to the ICU and is generally considered to be harmful to the injured brain [29]. General fever control practices in the ICU setting include identification and treatment of any infectious source and the use of antipyretics, fans, and ice packs. Neurogenic or central fevers may occur in TBI patients and have been attributed to injury or disruption of the hypothalamic thermoregulatory centers, with an incidence of 12%. Neurogenic fevers may produce very high temperatures that are often not responsive to conventional methods of fever management. Atypical medications that have been effective include bromocriptine, amantadine, dantrolene, and propranolol [30]. Another treatment option is the use of intravascular cooling methods, which have been shown to be more effective than conventional methods for fever control in the TBI patient [31–33]. In addition, induced normothermia has recently been shown to reduce fever burden and help maintain goal ICP parameters [33, 34]. While this information suggests that temperature control is warranted, currently there is no evidence that aggressive temperature control will improve clinical outcome. Further studies are indicated to determine what level of temperature management is beneficial in TBI patients.

Respiratory issues
Ventilator management

Respiratory failure is the most common nonneurologic organ dysfunction in patients with severe TBI and represents an ongoing challenge in their critical care management [35]. Despite this fact, relatively few studies have assessed ventilator management in TBI patients. The primary concern is the impact of ventilator mechanics on ICP and cerebral perfusion pressure (CPP). Positive end-expiratory pressure (PEEP) is a method that is frequently used in the ICU to improve oxygenation in patients with lung injury. The effect of PEEP on ICP is controversial, as studies have reported everything from ICP decreases to elevations in response to increases in PEEP [36–39]. The reason for these variations may relate to both cerebral and pulmonary compliance. Recent studies indicate that patients with either normal cerebral or pulmonary compliance can tolerate increases in PEEP without a detrimental effect on ICP or CPP, whereas those with poor brain and pulmonary compliance show adverse effects on ICP or CPP in response to increases in PEEP [37, 39]. A small prospective trial comparing zero positive end-expiratory pressure (ZEEP) versus $8\,cm\,H_2O$ PEEP in TBI patients showed abnormal respiratory mechanics consistent with low lung volume injury in the ZEEP group [40]. It should also be noted that something as simple as maintaining the head of the bed at 30–45° can decrease the impact of PEEP on ICP [41]. Based on this information, PEEP with appropriate neuro-monitoring and nursing care should be considered in TBI patients with lung injury.

There is very limited information providing guidance on other ventilator settings in patients with TBI. Pressure control inverse ratio ventilation has been reported to have minimal impact on ICP and CPP [42]. High-frequency jet ventilation (HFV) is used in settings of severe pulmonary compromise. There have been a few reports documenting a reduction in ICP after the start of HFV in TBI patients who were failing routine mechanical ventilation [43–45]. Inhaled nitric oxide has been used to improve oxygenation in patients with severe adult respiratory distress syndrome (ARDS) and has been used successfully in a very limited number of patients with TBI [46]. Finally, the transition from mechanical ventilation to starting spontaneous breathing trials must be undertaken with caution. A retrospective trial that monitored ICP and CPP while changing the mode of ventilation found that the majority of patients tolerated the transition. There was a smaller group who had higher baseline ICPs that showed significant ICP elevations from 25 to 33 mmHg. It is recommended that the initiation of spontaneous breathing trials should not be undertaken until ICP is normal [47]. Recent trials are beginning to focus on respiratory mechanics after TBI and the effect mechanical ventilation may have on outcome. In a prospective observational study of 137 isolated TBI patients ventilated for greater than 24 h, 31% of patients developed acute lung injury (ALI), which was independently predictive of mortality and poor neurologic outcomes [48]. At the present time, the best modes of ventilation to optimize respiratory mechanics and minimize risk of ALI in TBI are unknown and warrant clinical trials.

Ventilator-associated pneumonia

TBI is often associated with altered or loss of consciousness and recent alcohol use. These factors combine to increase the risk of aspiration and pneumonia in the mechanically ventilated patient with TBI. It is tempting to attribute this disease course as ventilator-associated pneumonia (VAP), but this may be misleading and incorrect. Commonly, patients with TBI suffer from early-onset pneumonia as a consequence of aspiration, and this pattern must be distinguished from hospital-acquired forms of VAP. The TBI patient continues to be at an ongoing risk in the ICU for the development of pneumonia due to multiple additional factors including coma, gastric ulcer prophylaxis, and use of nasogastric tubes. Bronchard *et al.* recently reviewed 109 patients with TBI over a 2-year period to evaluate risk factors for pneumonia. They found that nasal carriage of *Staphylococcus aureus* on admission, aspiration prior to intubation, and barbiturate use were independent risk factors for early-onset pneumonia in TBI. They also found important consequences of pneumonia in TBI patients. Patients with early-onset pneumonia had lower PaO_2/FiO_2, more febrile days, more frequent hypotension, and increased ICPs. These factors are known to adversely affect neurologic outcome [49].

VAP is common and contributes greatly to morbidity and mortality in critically ill patients [50]. Incidence rates of VAP have been estimated at 10–25% with mortality rates of 10–40%. In addition, hospital lengths of stays and cost are also increased in patients who develop VAP [50–53]. The challenge for the critical care team is to prevent pneumonia through elimination of risk factors, early diagnosis, and early, appropriate antibiotic treatment. The most important step in this process is to correctly identify those TBI patients who have pneumonia as their source of febrile illness versus any of the other causes for fevers in the ICU. Implementation of a VAP protocol that addresses a standard definition of the clinical criteria of pneumonia (fever, purulent sputum, CXR infiltrate, leukocytosis) combined with objective bacteriologic criteria and a standardized approach to antibiotic therapy is recommended. Fiber-optic bronchoscopy may be needed in this setting to acquire appropriate bronchial samples to guide therapy, but this procedure has been reported to produce ICP elevations that may not be blunted by optimal anesthetic methods [54]. Although the effect was temporary, caution should be used whenever fiber-optic bronchoscopy is performed in patients with ICP concerns.

VAP has been characterized as early (<4 days) or late (4 days or greater) based on the duration of mechanical ventilation. Early VAP should be treated with antibiotics that cover typical community organisms. Appropriate agents may include a macrolide (e.g., azithromycin) and third-generation cephalosporin (e.g., ceftriaxone). Late VAP, however, should be assumed to be caused by hospital-acquired organisms that carry a higher potential for resistance, as such much broader antibiotic coverage should be utilized. Empiric gram-positive coverage for methicillin-resistant *S. aureus* with vancomycin is appropriate; gram-negative coverage should cover for *Pseudomonas aeruginosa*, and some appropriate agents include cefepime, gentamicin, tobramycin, imipenem, and piperacillin/tazobactam. Some suggested antibiotic regimens for VAP are listed in Table 8.2, but the antibiotic selected should be determined based on the biogram

Table 8.2 Antibiotic recommendations for ventilator-associated pneumonia.

VAP < 4 days (presumed community acquired)	VAP ≥ 4 days (presumed hospital acquired)
Azithromycin plus third-generation cephalosporin (ceftriaxone/cefotaxime/ceftazidime)	Vancomycin or linezolid for methicillin-resistant *S. aureus* plus antipseudomonal agents listed in the following
Third-generation quinolones (levofloxacin, moxifloxacin)	Aminoglycosides (tobramycin, gentamicin)
Ampicillin/sulbactam	Fourth-generation cephalosporins (e.g., cefepime)
Ertapenem	Carbapenems (e.g., imipenem)
	Piperacillin/tazobactam

for an individual ICU. It has been shown that initial broad coverage that is then narrowed after the actual causative organism is identified as a safer and more effective way to treat VAP [55]. Few data are available regarding VAP in TBI patients in particular. In a prospective observational cohort study of 60 TBI patients with VAP, Zygun *et al.* reported a higher risk of VAP among patients with polytrauma compared to those with isolated TBI and a longer duration of mechanical ventilation, longer ICU and hospital length of stay, and more frequent tracheostomies in TBI patients who developed VAP compared with those who did not [56]. The next logical question is, "how do we prevent VAP"?

Preventive strategies for VAP have largely focused on minimizing oropharyngeal colonization and decreasing the risk of aspiration of oropharyngeal or gastric contents. Drakulovic *et al.* compared a semirecumbent or supine bed position and determined the incidence of VAP in a randomized clinical trial of 86 medical ICU patients [57]. Microbiologically confirmed pneumonia occurred in 5% of the semi-recumbent group compared with 23% of the supine group, although there was no difference in mortality. This low cost and relatively simple intervention may have a dramatic effect and should be practiced routinely. In addition to elevation of the head of the bed, sucralfate has been shown to decrease the risk of VAP compared with usual H2-blockers used for stress ulcer prophylaxis [58]. As such, sucralfate should be considered for stress ulcer prophylaxis in patients who are at low risk for gastrointestinal bleeding. Using the Center for Disease Control (CDC) Guidelines for Prevention of Nosocomial Pneumonia and aggressively auditing staff to ensure compliance, Cocanour *et al.* reported a decrease in VAP rates from 22.3–32.7 to 0 and 12.8 infections per 1000 ventilator days [59]. This demonstrates that prevention of VAP has to be an institutional commitment to achieve meaningful results. Simple things such as elevation of the head of the bed, washing/sanitizing of hands by healthcare providers, and appropriate antibiotic coverage once VAP is suspected may reduce patient morbidity, ICU cost, and length of stay. While no randomized trial has been performed, early tracheostomy is also gaining recent favor in TBI management.

Table 8.3 Patients to be considered for early (<7 days) tracheostomy [49, 50].

Glasgow Coma Score	≤8
Injury Severity Score	≥25
Anticipated length of mechanical ventilation	>7 days

Tracheostomy

Tracheostomy has long been used to facilitate secretion removal, airway management, and speed ventilator discontinuation in the TBI patient. Percutaneous tracheostomy at the bedside is emerging as an acceptable alternative to open tracheostomy in the operating room, but the appropriate timing of tracheostomy remains elusive. Seeking to develop criteria for TBI patients who would require tracheostomy, Gurkin *et al.* [60] performed a retrospective review of all TBI patients in their trauma registry over a 6-year period. Logistic regression analysis was used to identify GCS ≤ 8, injury severity score ≥ 25, and ventilator days greater than 7 as predictive of requiring tracheostomy. They suggested performing early tracheostomy to decrease morbidity and length of stay [60]. Another retrospective review of 55 patients found no difference in mortality, ventilator days, or VAP rates but found decrease ICU length of stay in early (<7 days) versus late (>7 days) tracheostomy patients [61]. A prospective randomized trial is warranted. Table 8.3 lists patient characteristics that may warrant early tracheostomy.

Catheter-related infections

CVCs are frequently used in the ICU to deliver fluids, nutrition, and drugs and to monitor hemodynamic status. Infection of these catheters results in increased morbidity, mortality, and duration of hospital stay. Catheter-related bloodstream infections (CBSIs) are associated with mortality rates of 10–20%, prolonged hospitalization, and medical costs of up to $10 000 per hospitalization [62, 63]. Unfortunately, patients in the ICU are generally ill enough that CVCs are needed as part of patient care; therefore, preventative measures must be part of routine critical care. As such, the emphasis of this discussion is to cover methods of preventing CBSIs in ICU patients.

CVC location has been associated with infectious and thrombotic complications. A randomized trial found that subclavian vein placement of a CVC was associated with lower rates of venous thrombosis and infection compared with femoral location [64]. Although jugular and subclavian locations have not been compared head-to-head in a trial, the available evidence suggests a lower thrombosis and infection rate in the subclavian location [65]. Antimicrobial-impregnated catheters have been studied for prevention of CBSIs. Chlorhexidine- and silver sulfadiazine-impregnated catheters were reported to lower the rate of CRIs from 7.6 per 1000 catheter days to 1.6 per 1000 catheter days [66]. Minocycline- and rifampin-coated catheters are likely even more effective than the chlorhexidine- and silver sulfadiazine-coated catheters in preventing CBSIs [67]. However, cost-effectiveness analyses indicate that anti-microbial-coated catheters should be reserved for instances where the infection rates are greater than 2% [68].

Catheters should be placed under maximal sterile barrier precautions, as this approach has been shown to reduce CBSIs and cost [69]. Chlorhexidine as the skin disinfectant prior to insertion has been shown to be superior to iodine or alcohol for preventing CBSIs [70]. Experienced care providers should either place or closely supervise placement of CVCs, since this can decrease risk of complications. Ultrasound guidance can be utilized when feasible but may not be particularly useful for placing a subclavian CVC. Catheters should be removed as soon as they are no longer required in the patient's care. There is no evidence favoring prophylactically changing a catheter after a prescribed period of time, although the risk of infection does increase after 3 days [62, 63]. A suspected CBSI should be investigated with blood cultures from the CVC and from a peripheral site. While positive cultures do not absolutely confirm a CBSI (since colonization of the catheter or contamination during blood draw may cause positive cultures), negative cultures have a 99% negative predictive value and almost certainly rule out the CVC as the source of infection [71]. Initial treatment of a suspected CVC infection should cover both gram-negative and gram-positive organisms. Treatment should then be narrowed or discontinued once an organism is identified or the cultures are negative, respectively.

Venous thromboembolism prophylaxis and treatment

Venous thrombosis occurs frequently in critically ill patients and may contribute to patient morbidity and poor outcomes by causing pulmonary embolism (PE). An incidence rate of 26–34% has been reported for development of deep venous thrombosis (DVT) in moderate-to-severe TBI patients [72]. However, distinctions are made about clinically relevant and irrelevant DVTs. It is generally thought that DVTs discovered in the calf veins as part of routine screening do not lead to clinically significant adverse events [73], while clots in more proximal veins are more likely to cause PE. Pulmonary emboli have been reported to occur in 1–2% of TBI patients during their hospital stay [74, 75]. However, the potential threat to life and inherent difficulties with anticoagulation in patients with intracranial injury make prevention of venous thromboembolism a priority in the ICU management of severe TBI.

Prevention of thromboembolism may be achieved using either mechanical compression or pharmacologically with heparinoid drugs. No randomized controlled trials have compared these two modalities for DVT prophylaxis in TBI or other cranial pathologies for that matter. A prospective observational study evaluated a pneumatic compression device for DVT prophylaxis in 523 neurosurgical patients, 89 of whom had TBI [76]. DVT rates were 0% in TBI and 3.8% in other patients in the study. Another prospective observational study evaluated enoxaparin use within 24 h of ED arrival in 150 TBI patients. While DVT rates were only 2%, the study protocol was changed to starting enoxaparin 48 h after ED arrival due to bleeding requiring craniotomy in 2 out of 24 patients [77]. In contrast, a retrospective analysis of 669 patients with traumatic intracranial hemorrhage who received enoxaparin for DVT prophylaxis early (<72 h; $n = 268$) versus late (>72 h; $n = 401$) found no difference in the rate of hemorrhagic progression after initiation of DVT prophylaxis [75]. While DVT prophylaxis remains a part of the ICU management of TBI, little evidence is available to guide clinicians. Pneumatic compression devices should be placed upon hospital admission, and then prophylactic heparinoids added as early as 24 h after admission once repeat head CTs have shown stabilization of intracranial hematomas. Current guidelines make grade III recommendations for using pneumatic compression devices and/or heparinoids for DVT prophylaxis but stated that there was insufficient literature evidence to make any recommendation regarding the appropriate timing of heparinoid initiation [78].

Transfusions in TBI

The concept that maintaining a hematocrit greater than 30% after TBI is needed to optimize cerebral oxygenation has little supportive evidence. In a subgroup analysis of 67 patients with moderate-to-severe TBI from the multicenter, randomized, controlled Transfusion Requirements in the Critical Care (TRICC) trial, no significant differences were found in 30-day mortality, ICU LOS, or hospital LOS between patients with targeted hemoglobin goals of 7–9 g/dL compared to those with goal hemoglobin of 10–12 g/dL [79]. In contrast, there is now evidence that transfusions can result in immunomodulation and ALI [80, 81] and are associated with poor long-term functional outcomes in patients with TBI [82]. This conflicting information may be related to patient-specific physiological parameters. Some recent studies have reported transfusion-related improvements in brain tissue oxygenation in anemic TBI patients, but there is no information regarding long-term outcomes [83–85]. Until further information is available, present management should limit transfusions unless there are clear signs of physiological compromise in volume status, hemodynamic state, EKG findings, cardiovascular disease, or brain tissue oxygen.

Fluids, nutrition, and glucose
Fluids

Intravenous fluids are used as part of the initial resuscitation after TBI, and then maintained as part of the supportive care in the ICU environment. This discussion will focus on the role of maintenance fluids. Volume abnormalities are common in TBI patients, with 59% of patients having an electrolyte abnormality at least once during the hospital stay [86]. Volume status has been shown to impact on clinical outcome. A subset analysis of 392 patients in a hypothermia study found

Table 8.4 Electrolyte components of common intravenous fluid.

IV Fluid	mOsm/L	Na⁺ (mEq/L)	Cl⁻ (mEq/L)	K⁺ (mEq/L)	Ca²⁺ (mEq/L)	Lactate (gm/L)	Mg²⁺ (mEq/L)	Acetate (mEq/L)	Gluconate (mEq/L)
Lactated ringers	275	130	109	4	3	28			
0.45% NaCl	154	77	77						
0.9% NaCl	308	154	154						
3.0% NaCl	1026	513	513						
Normosol	294	140	98	5			3	27	23

that the patients with a fluid balance of less than 594 mL at 96 h had worse outcomes independent of other physiological parameters [87]. Factors contributing to these abnormalities may include direct disruption of fluid balance systems in the brain, blood loss from other injuries, baseline medical condition of the patient, and iatrogenic causes related to the acute resuscitation. The optimal choice of maintenance fluids to use is not known, but it is generally felt that glucose-containing solutions should be avoided. The electrolyte makeup of different maintenance fluids must be considered (Table 8.4), and decisions should be based on the patient's individual needs. The infusion rate of maintenance fluids should strive to maintain normovolemia, and rates will need to be adjusted to account for additional insensible losses due to nasogastric or other drains, chest tubes, mechanical ventilation, or fevers.

Nutrition

Some recent studies are beginning to provide evidence-based guides for nutritional management of patients after a TBI. Hartl *et al.* reviewed nutritional data on 797 patients and found that early initiation of feeding (within 48 h) was associated with improved outcomes. In addition, the amount of caloric intake was important, as a significant increase in mortality was seen for every 10 kcal/kg decrease in caloric intake [88]. The method of feeding also impacts patient management. Transpyloric feeding has been shown to reduce the incidence of pneumonia and improve nutritional efficacy in severe TBI patients compared to gastric feeding [89]. To achieve full nutritional support with a trend toward better 6-month outcomes, the current guidelines recommend initiating nutrition within 72 h of injury [78]. The optimal formulation of nutritional supplementation remains uncertain.

No studies of various formulations of enteral or parenteral nutrition in isolated TBI patients have been published. To maintain adequate nitrogen balance, a greater than 15% protein content is recommended for most enteral formulations in trauma patients [78]. While branched-chain amino acids improve outcomes in septic patients and glutamine supplementation is believed to decrease infection rates [90], these findings have not been confirmed in TBI patients. Lastly, both hyperglycemia and hypoglycemia in the ICU environment have been associated with worse outcomes in TBI [91–94]. It remains debatable whether admission hyperglycemia is an inflammatory stress response and thus a marker of disease severity or an independent causative factor with regard to poor outcomes [95, 96].

Glucose

There have been a number of reports on the impact of glucose control in the ICU environment on patients with TBI. Recent studies have shown that tight glucose control may be beneficial in patients with TBI. Van den Berghe *et al.* reported on a subset of 63 patients with isolated TBI requiring 3 or more days of mechanical ventilation in the intensive insulin trial [97]. Patients in the intensive therapy arm had lower mean and maximum ICP compared with controls, achieved optimal CPP with lower vasopressor doses, and had fewer seizures. Yang *et al.* prospectively compared intensive versus conventional glucose control in 240 patients. The intensive therapy group had shorter ICU stays, decreased infection rates, and improved neurologic outcome at 6 months [98]. There was no difference in mortality between the treatment groups in either of these studies. Other groups have found minimal to no differences in outcome measurements when comparing intensive and conventional glucose control in TBI patients, but they have raised concerns regarding episodes of hypoglycemia in the intensive therapy group [99, 100].

Management decisions regarding glucose control may not be able to be easily categorized into one category or another, and the goal for glucose control may need to vary during the course of care in the ICU. Meier *et al.* compared TBI patients who had glucose maintained in a low glucose range (63–117 mg/dL) to a group that had a less restrictive range (90–144 mg/dL). During the first week after injury, ICPs were better in the group with higher glucose levels, but during the second week the group with lower glucose values had lower ICPs and fewer infectious systemic complications [101]. Interest in control of glucose has encouraged investigations on the physiological effects of systemic glucose levels on the brain using microdialysis technology. Two groups have independently shown that intensive glucose control results in lower brain glucose and increased markers of cellular distress (elevated lactate/pyruvate ratios and glutamate) [102, 103]. In addition, Oddo *et al.* found that lower brain glucose levels were associated with higher mortality [103]. It is apparent that more research is needed regarding the appropriate glucose range in patients with TBI, so at this time, it may be best to target an intermediate glucose range of 110–150 mg/dL.

In summary, general intensive care of TBI commonly involves a variety of factors that may seriously impact on patient outcomes. Special care must be taken to appropriately manage these issues and avoid complications that may compromise general ICU care. Protocols in the ICU provide a systematic approach that minimizes variability in the care provided to the severely ill TBI patient and improves patient outcomes and are recommended by current guidelines [78].

Neurologic syndromes in the ICU

A number of neurologic issues may develop in the severely ill TBI patient. Some of the more common ones will be discussed and management strategies presented.

Posttraumatic seizure prevention and detection
Seizure prevention

Seizures following TBI may occur at the time of injury (immediate), during the first week as a consequence of acute complications from the injury (early), or weeks to months after injury in the form of a posttraumatic seizure disorder (delayed). Among all patients with TBI, about 2% develop seizures (defined as any clinically evident seizure) but this number varies widely depending primarily on the severity of injury. In severe TBI patients, historical data suggest that about 12% develop early seizures [104, 105]. Antiepileptic drugs (AEDs) are routinely used prophylactically in severe TBI, as seizures may complicate ICU care, and prophylactic use of AEDs is effective in reducing clinically evident early seizures. However, prophylactic AED use does not prevent the occurrence of late posttraumatic seizures and does not improve clinical outcome. Thus, the question frequently arises as to whether or not to prophylactically treat TBI patients with AEDs in the acute period of injury and how long after injury the treatment will be continued. Practice patterns vary widely [106], but several well-done clinical trials and evidence-based guidelines provide a guide for clinicians.

In a randomized, double-blind, placebo controlled trial of 404 patients, severe TBI patients were treated for a year with placebo or phenytoin (PTN) beginning within 24 h of injury [107]. Serum PTN levels were maintained in the therapeutic range. Within 7 days of injury, 3.6% of the patients assigned to PTN had seizures, as compared with 14.2% of patients assigned to placebo (risk ratio 0.27, $p < 0.001$). Between day 8 and the end of the first year, 21.5% of the PTN group had seizures compared with 15.7% of the placebo group. By the end of year 2, 27.5% of the PTN group and 21.1% of the placebo group had seizures. The authors concluded that prophylactic PTN has a beneficial effect in reducing seizures only during the first week following severe TBI. Due to concerns about the sedating effects of PTN, other AEDs have been evaluated for seizure prophylaxis. A retrospective analysis of 32 patients treated with levetiracetam (LEV) for seizure prophylaxis reports equal efficacy for seizure prevention when compared to a historical cohort of 41 TBI patients treated with PTN [108]. A randomized, prospective study by Szaflarski *et al.* compared LEV to PTN for seizure prophylaxis, and performed continuous electroencephalography (cEEG) for 72 h to monitor for seizure activity. The LEV group had better long-term outcomes and fewer medication-related side effects. There was no difference in seizure frequency between the groups, but it was notable that all seizures identified were nonconvulsive [109].

Seizure detection

Questions have remained about the actual incidence and impact of seizures (clinical and subclinical) on morbidity and mortality following severe TBI. Two studies describe seizure incidence rates of 17 and 18% in TBI patients who had cEEG monitoring for 72 h or more. In both studies, all of the seizures were nonconvulsive and were diagnosed on the basis of cEEG alone [109, 110]. In a prospective observational study of 94 consecutive moderate-to-severe TBI patients monitored with cEEG for the first 14 days after injury, Vespa *et al.* report that convulsive and nonconvulsive seizures occurred in 22% of patients with status epilepticus occurring in six patients. More than half of the seizures were nonconvulsive. All six patients with status epilepticus died compared with a mortality rate of 24% in the nonseizure group [111]. Finally, early seizure activity in the first week after TBI has been associated with elevations in ICP and lactate/pyruvate ratios, as well as long-term hippocampal atrophy on follow-up MRI [112, 113]. Seizures occurred in all of these studies despite early use of prophylactic AEDs and maintenance of adequate drug levels.

Current recommendations for seizure prophylaxis following severe TBI are that AEDs should be started early after diagnosis of severe TBI and continued for 7 days, reflective of the aforementioned studies [78]. The use of newer AEDs for this purpose may be beneficial to minimize sedation and other medication side effects. Questions persist as to whether less severe cases of TBI would benefit from AED prophylaxis given the frequency of nonconvulsive seizures in the moderate-to-severe group mentioned earlier. Larger cEEG studies of TBI patients are warranted to better define patients who may benefit from seizure prophylaxis or who may warrant treatment beyond the currently recommended 7 days.

Pituitary dysfunction and electrolyte abnormalities

Sodium disturbance is common in the ICU, and normal sodium balance depends on many factors, including neuroendocrine functions, the renin–angiotensin system, osmoregulatory systems, and iatrogenic actions. TBI can alter the balance of these systems resulting in the direction of either hyponatremia or hypernatremia. Risk factors for neuroendocrine dysfunction after TBI include trauma affecting the frontal lobes, basilar skull fractures, and severe injury with greater than 24 h of posttraumatic amnesia. The posterior pituitary gland is involved with the regulation of fluid and sodium balance through release of antidiuretic hormone (ADH). Hyponatremia is the most common sodium abnormality after TBI, with a reported overall incidence of 9% [114]. It occurs in response to three different syndromes: the syndrome of inappropriate antidiuretic hormone (SIADH) secretion, cerebral salt wasting (CSW), or psychogenic polydipsia. Since fluid intake is generally monitored in the ICU setting, our discussions will focus on SIADH and CSW.

SIADH

SIADH is the most common cause of hyponatremia after TBI. The incidence ranges from 2 to 5%, with reports as high as 33% in severe TBI [115, 116]. Different mechanisms may prompt ADH release after TBI. These include increased ICP, hypercapnia, hypothalamic dysfunction, alterations in responsiveness of osmoreceptors, and medications. The clinical criteria for SIADH consist of hyponatremia with normovolemia, low serum osmolality, low urine output, high urine sodium, urine osmolality greater than serum osmolality, and high ADH levels. Treatment is primarily through fluid restriction and the avoidance of hypotonic IV fluids. In more severe or refractory cases, demeclocycline (300 mg every 6 h), fludrocortisone (0.1–0.2 mg/d), hypertonic saline (500 cm^3 over several hours), or salt by mouth or gastric tube may be necessary.

Cerebral salt wasting

Hyponatremia after TBI may also be due to CSW [115]. The mechanism is probably related to an increased release of atrial natriuretic factor and renal sodium loss. The clinical picture consists of hyponatremia with hypovolemia, high urine output and normal to increased serum osmolality. A comparison of the clinical findings in SIADH and CSW is reviewed in Table 8.5. Daily body weights can help in assessing the patient's volume status. At this time, treatment should focus on hydration and salt supplementation. Conivaptan is an arginine vasopressin antagonist that is being studied in a medical patient population for treatment of hyponatremia in euvolemic and hypervolemic patients [117]. This agent may play a future role in the management of hyponatremia in TBI, as there has been one case report describing the use of convaptin to successfully treat hyponatremia in a TBI patient [118].

Diabetes insipidus

Diabetes insipidus (DI) is relatively uncommon after TBI, but can be seen in patients with severe injuries or damage along the hypothalamic–pituitary axis resulting in the inadequate secretion of ADH. The patient will demonstrate hypernatremia with polyuria, polydipsia, hypovolemia, increased serum

Table 8.5 Comparison of clinical findings in SIADH and CSW.

Parameter	SIADH	CSW
Serum sodium	Decreased	Decreased
Serum osmolality	Decreased	Normal–increased
Urine sodium	Increased	Increased
Urine output	Decreased	Increased
Volume status	Normovolemia	Hypovolemia
Body weight	Increased	Decreased

osmolality, and low urine osmolality. Diagnosis can be made with careful fluid deprivation followed by vasopressin. DI will respond to treatment with pitressin, vasopressin, and fluid supplementation.

Iatrogenic hypernatremia

The use of hypertonic saline or mannitol with or without furosemide for ICP management can result in elevations of serum sodium. Insensible fluid loss through an endotracheal tube or tracheostomy, fever, or sweating can increase sodium. Phenytoin, captopril, Narcan, and ethanol can inhibit ADH secretion. Enteral tube feedings can have high levels of sodium. Any of these factors can result in iatrogenic hypernatremia. Correction can be accomplished by adjusting fluid and electrolyte intake.

Other electrolyte abnormalities

Potassium regulation can be affected after brain injury. Many mechanisms can produce hypokalemia. Aldosterone secretion in response to physical stress leads to an increase in potassium excretion. Hyperventilation produces respiratory alkalosis, which drives potassium intracellular and lowers serum levels. Diet, nausea, vomiting, and medications such as diuretics, mannitol, antibiotics, or corticosteroids may result in hypokalemia. Clinical symptoms of hypokalemia include cardiac conduction abnormalities, weakness, and hyporeflexia. Treatment should focus on resolution of the underlying cause and potassium supplementation. Hyperkalemia usually results from metabolic acidosis, renal failure, or hypoadrenalism. Glucose or insulin administration will increase cellular absorption of potassium.

Hypomagnesemia can result from excessive urinary excretion, alkalosis, sepsis, diuretics, and aminoglycosides. The relationship between magnesium and calcium suggests that hypomagnesemia increases the risk of secondary injury by worsening calcium-related excitotoxicity. The clinical findings include weakness, tetany, hyperreflexia, and cognitive changes. Either enteral or intravenous supplementation can be used for treatment.

Agitation in the ICU

Patients with TBI often develop a variety of neurobehavioral changes in the early stages after injury, which is frequently disruptive to patient care, distressing to family members, and potentially harmful to the patient. It has been suggested that posttraumatic agitation is a unique subtype of delirium that occurs during the period of amnesia after TBI and is characterized by excessive behaviors [119]. Others feel that these behaviors may be due to an increased sympathetic drive, resulting in the classic *fight or flight* response. Different descriptive terms have been used to define posttraumatic agitation, resulting in variable incidence rates ranging from 11 to over 50% [120–123]. The majority of posttraumatic agitation is reactive and in response to pain, overstimulation, and frustration with the demands of the environment. Other behaviors may be nonreactive agitation that occurs without obvious provocation. Both types of behaviors can be further characterized as *directed* toward a specific external stimulus or *nondirected* generalized responses. Patients will have a diminished ability to process new information or environmental stimuli during this period; thus, the surroundings can actually contribute to their confusion, aggression, motor restlessness, disinhibition, or emotional lability. Awareness of these differences can be useful in guiding the management of agitated behaviors.

The behavioral changes pose some of the greatest challenges in the medical care of brain-injured patients. Posttraumatic agitation may have a negative impact on patient care and is often managed by the initiation of psychopharmacologic interventions, which can influence the initiation of rehabilitation services and affect the speed of recovery. Many commonly used medications to manage agitation have potentially harmful effects on recovery after brain injury (Box 8.1) [124]. A retrospective study found that 72% of patients with TBI received one or more of these agents during their acute hospitalization [125]. The use of any pharmacologic agent in the patient with TBI must be considered carefully with increased awareness of the risk/benefit ratio. Tools have been validated for use in the ICU to objectively assess for both agitation (Richmond

Box 8.1 Medications reported to have adverse effects on recovery after TBI.

Anticholinergics
  Scopolamine
Anticonvulsants
  Phenytoin
  Phenobarbital
Antihypertensives
  Clonidine
  Prazosin
Benzodiazepines
  Diazepam
  Lorazepam
  Muscimol
Dopamine antagonists
  Antipsychotics
    Chlorpromazine
    Haloperidol
    Thioridazine
  Antiemetics
    Droperidol
    Metoclopramide
H2 receptor antagonists
  Cimetidine
  Ranitidine
Neuromuscular blockade

Agitation–Sedation Score (RASS)) and delirium (Cognitive Assessment Method in the ICU (CAM-ICU)) [126–129].

Delirium

There has been an increased awareness regarding the prevalence and impact of delirium in the ICU environment. In this setting, delirium presents with fluctuating changes in consciousness and cognition that can develop over a very short time as a result of the illness prompting ICU care, or as a complication of medical care. Two forms have been described: hyperactive with agitation and hypoactive with blunting of responsiveness. Hypoactive delirium has a reported prevalence of 60% in trauma patients in the ICU [130]. Currently, there is no information regarding the incidence of ICU delirium specific to patients with TBI, but delirium has a very high incidence in TBI patients admitted to a rehabilitation setting [131]. Exposure to midazolam while in the ICU has been reported to be an independent risk factor for the development of delirium in a trauma ICU [132].

Management of agitation and delirium in the ICU should focus on environmental factors in addition to pharmacological interventions. Recently, it has been proposed that a group of evidence-based practices should be used in an effort to minimize or prevent the development of ICU delirium. These include *a*wakening and *b*reathing *c*oordination, *d*elirium monitoring, and *e*xercise/*e*arly mobility (ABCDE) [133]. Efforts should also be made to provide structured environments and reassurance in order to minimize uncertainty and fear. Consistent staffing, frequent reorientation, and daily schedules should be maintained as much as possible. Environmental cues should be provided to assist with orientation. Attention should be paid to the lighting and noise levels to reflect a diurnal pattern and help restore normal sleep–wake cycles. When a patient is medically stable, *sleep holidays* can be initiated. A normal sleep cycle is typically 60–120 min, so changing neurological assessments overnight from every hour to every 2–4 h may allow a more normal sleep pattern. Pharmacological interventions should be used primarily to address patient and staff safety issues, and dosing should be minimized. Haloperidol can be used at 0.5–2.0 mg every hour if needed. Low doses of antipsychotics preferentially block presynaptic dopamine autoreceptors, which potentially results in a beneficial dopaminergic effect on the motor system, whereas higher doses can accumulate, prolong the anti-dopaminergic effects, and worsen a hypoactive state. Another option for acute control of agitation in patients with TBI may be loxapine, which is a tricyclic antipsychotic drug with sedating properties that is available in an intravenous form. Lescot *et al.* report that in two patients, clozapine was effective for control of agitation, lowered ICP, and did not affect MAP or cerebral blood flow [134]. Longer-acting anxiolytic and antipsychotic medications such as trazodone and quetiapine may help with behavioral issues and restoration of normal sleep–wake cycles.

Dysautonomias/paroxysmal sympathetic hyperactivity

Autonomic nervous system activation is a normal response after traumatic injuries. The resultant tachypnea, tachycardia, increased blood pressure, and increased blood flow to muscle, organs, and brain strive to maintain oxygen perfusion to support vital functions. The increased activation will continue as the body experiences secondary challenges such as pain and inflammation. Unfortunately, if the pathways controlling this process have been injured, the response can become excessive and contribute to additional morbidity. The underlying pathophysiology may be due to damage of inhibitory brainstem/ diencephalic centers, thus releasing excitatory spinal cord processes, which has been called the excitatory–inhibitory ratio (EIR) model [135]. Clinical presentation may fall along a continuum, with 24–33% of TBI patients displaying transient, self-limiting symptoms and 8–11.3% developing prolonged and severe symptoms [136]. Symptoms may be characterized as relatively pure sympathetic overactivity or they may present with mixed parasympathetic/ sympathetic features. Many terms have been applied to this process including dysautonomias, surging and sympathetic storms, and diencephalic seizures, which has led to confusion regarding the syndrome. Currently, the term paroxysmal sympathetic hyperactivity (PSH) has been recommended as a more clinical relevant and appropriate term [137].

Although hyperthermia frequently accompanies PSH, it should still prompt a complete workup to assess for an infectious source, presence of a DVT, or a drug fever. PSH-related hyperthermia can present as mild-to-moderate fever or severe and labile temperature fluctuations. Treatment primarily involves antipyretics and cooling blankets. Propranolol and bromocriptine have reported benefit in the treatment of persistent central fever [138, 139]. A recent case series of six patients suggested potential benefit with gabapentin [140]. Management of other PSH symptoms is largely based on anecdotal reports, case studies, or small case series, and is largely aimed at symptom control. Current evidence would suggest gabapentin, opioids, benzodiazepines, β-blockers, and centrally acting α-agonists as first-line therapy, with bromocriptine as a second-line treatment. Intrathecal baclofen may be useful in cases that are more severe, prolonged, or resistant to oral medication [136, 137].

Critical illness polyneuropathy/myopathy

Critical illness neuropathy/myopathy (CIPNM) is a continuum of a syndrome that in the past decade has been increasingly recognized as a serious consequence of prolonged ICU care. Neuromuscular weakness during ICU stay has traditionally been thought to be due to muscle atrophy or fatigue, but electrophysiologic and muscle biopsy studies suggest a distinct pathophysiology that is generally underrecognized in the ICU setting.

CIPNM is estimated to occur in 25–42% of patients who have been mechanically ventilated for 1 week [141, 142]. Other risk factors include sepsis and multiorgan system failure. Clinical features of CIPNM consist predominantly of distal muscle weakness and wasting, worse in the lower extremities. Facial weakness is rarely present. Thus, the development of distal weakness or a decrease in motor responsiveness with obvious facial grimace and decreased deep tendon reflexes should raise suspicion of CIPNM. Laboratory tests are not diagnostic although creatine kinase levels may be mildly elevated. Nerve conduction and electromyography studies show both motor and sensory axonal dysfunction in the upper and lower extremities, although sensory nerve potentials may be normal [143, 144]. No uniform diagnostic criteria exist for CIPNM, but its potential impact on patient outcomes warrants consideration of the diagnosis in the appropriate patient. Limited data are available to assess methods of adequately preventing or treating CIPNM. Good glucose control may be beneficial, as the rate of CIPNM fell from 52 to 29% in the Van den Berghe study of intensive insulin therapy [97]. The prognosis of CIPNM is poorly understood and methods adequately treating the ailment once identified are also lacking at this time. However, in the ICU environment where difficulties may arise with liberation from the ventilator and patient disposition is dependent upon this, recognizing CIPNM may have direct implications for patient care and utilization of resources.

In summary, neurologic syndromes in the severely ill TBI patient may lead to prolonged ventilatory dependence, increased length of hospital stay, and worse outcomes. Care must be taken to identify and treat these syndromes in order to optimize the potential for good patient outcomes.

Conclusion

Severely ill TBI patients are a special population requiring particular expertise to appropriately manage. The goal of the neurointensivist in the care of these patients is to prevent secondary brain injury while addressing common issues that afflict critically ill patients. The initial assessment focuses on evaluation of the ABCs and avoidance of hypotension and hypoxia. Subsequently, basic ICU care must be optimized; infections prevented or quickly recognized and treated; thromboembolism prevented or recognized and treated; and other complications of ICU care routinely screened for, identified, and treated. The care of these patients is complicated and institutions should develop protocols to standardize care in order to avoid lapses in assessment and treatment.

References

1 Miller, J.D., Sweet, R.C., Narayan, R., & Becker, D.P. (1978) Early insults to the injured brain. *Journal of American Medical Association*, **240**, 439–442.

2 Chesnut, R.M., Marshall, L.F., Klauber, M.R. *et al.* (1993) The role of secondary brain injury in determining outcome from severe head injury. *The Journal of Trauma*, **34**, 216–222.

3 Stochetti, N., Furlan, A. & Volta, F. (1996) Hypoxemia and arterial hypotension at the accident scene in head injury. *The Journal of Trauma*, **40**, 764–767.

4 Manley, G., Knudson, M., Morabito, D., Damron, S., Erickson, V. & Pitts, L. (2001) Hypotension, hypoxia, and head injury: Frequency, duration, and consequences. *Archives of Surgery*, **136**:1118–1123.

5 Sanchez-Izquierdo-Riera, J.A., Caballero-Cubedo, R.E., Perez-Vela, J.L., Ambros-Checa, A., Cantalapiedra-Santiago, J.A. & Alted-Lopez, E. (1998) Propofol versus midazolam: safety and efficacy for sedating the severe trauma patient. *Anesthesia and Analgesia*, **86**, 1219–1212.

6 Otterspoor, L.C., Kalkman, C.J., Cremer, O.L. (2008) Update on the propofol infusion syndrome in ICU management of patients with head injury. *Current Opinion in Anaesthesiology*, **21 (5)**, 544–551.

7 Vernooy, K., Delhaas, T., Cremer, O.L. *et al.* (2006) Electrocardiographic changes predicting sudden death in propofol-related infusion syndrome. *Heart Rhythm*, **3 (2)**, 131–137.

8 Kang, T.F. (2002) Propofol infusion syndrome in critically ill patients. *Annals Pharmacotherapy*, **36**, 1453–1456.

9 Pandharipande, P.P., Pun, B.T., Herr, D.L. *et al.* (2007) Effect of sedation with dexmedetomidine vs lorazepam on acute brain dysfunction in mechanically ventilated patients: the MENDS randomized controlled trial. *Journal of American Medical Association*, **298 (22)**, 2644–2653.

10 Riker, R.R., Shehabi, Y., Bokesch, P.M. *et al.* (2009) Dexmedetomidine vs midazolam for sedation of critically ill patients: a randomized trial. *Journal of American Medical Association*, **301 (5)**, 489–499.

11 Aryan, H.E., Box, K.W., Ibrahim, D., Desiraju, U. & Ames, C.P. (2006) Safety and efficacy of dexmedetomidine in neurosurgical patients. *Brain Injury*, **20 (8)**, 791–798.

12 Goddeau, R.P. Jr., Silverman, S.B. & Sims, J.R. (2007) Dexmedetomidine for the treatment of paroxysmal autonomic instability with dystonia. *Neurocritical Care*, **7 (3)**, 217–220.

13 Tang, J.F., Chen, P.L., Tang, E.J., May, T.A. & Stiver, S.I. (2010) Dexmedetomidine controls agitation and facilitates reliable, serial neurological examinations in a non-intubated patient with traumatic brain injury. *Neurocritical Care*. **15 (1)**, 175–181.

14 Albanese, J., Durbec, G., Viviand, X., Potie, F., Alliez, B., & Martin, C. (1993) Sufentanyl increases intracranial pressure in patients with head trauma. *Anesthesiology*, **74**, 493–497.

15 deNadal, M., Ausina, A. & Sahuquillo, J. (1998) Effects on intracranial pressure of fentanyl in severe head injury patients. *Acta Neurochirurgica*, **71**, 10–12.

16 Lauer, K.K., Connolly, L.A. & Schmeling, W.T. (1997) Opioid sedation does not alter intracranial pressure in head injured patients. *Canadian Journal of Anaesthesiology*, **44**, 929–933.

17 Karabinis, A., Mandragos, K., Stergiopoulos, S. *et al.* (2004) Safety and efficacy of analgesia-based sedation with remifentanil versus standard hypnotic-based regimens in intensive care unit patients with brain injuries: a randomised, controlled trial [ISRCTN50308308]. *Critical Care*, **8 (4)**, R268–R280.

18 Robinson, B.R., Mueller, E.W., Henson, K., Branson, R.D., Barsoum, S. & Tsuei, B.J. (2008) An analgesia-delirium-sedation protocol for critically ill trauma patients reduces ventilator days and hospital length of stay. *The Journal of Trauma* **65 (3)**, 517–526.

19 Skrobik, Y., Ahern, S., Leblanc, M., Marquis, F., Awissi, D.K. & Kavanagh, B.P. (2010) Protocolized intensive care unit management of analgesia, sedation, and delirium improves analgesia and subsyndromal delirium rates. *Anesthesia and Analgesia* **111 (2)**, 451–463.

20 Holbrook, T.L., Galarneau, M.R., Dye, J.L., Quinn, K. & Dougherty, A.L. (2010) Morphine use after combat injury in Iraq and post-traumatic stress disorder. *The New England Journal of Medicine*, **362**, 110–117.

21 Hsiang, J., Chestnut, R., Crisp, C., Klauber, M.R., Blunt, B.A., & Marshall, L.F. (1994) Early routine paralysis for intracranial pressure control in severe head injury: is it necessary? *Critical Care Medicine*, **22**, 1471–1476.

22 Bernard, S.A., Gray, T.W., Buist, M.D. *et al.* (2002) Treatment of comatose survivors of out-of-hospital cardiac arrest with induced hypothermia. *The New England Journal of Medicine*, **346**, 557–563.

23 The Hypothermia After Cardiac Arrest Study Group. (2002) Mild therapeutic hypothermia to improve the neurologic outcome after cardiac arrest. *The New England Journal of Medicine*, **346**, 549–556.

24 Clifton, G.L., Miller, E.R., Choi, S.C. *et al.* (2001) Lack of effect of induction of hypothermia after acute brain injury. *The New England Journal of Medicine*, **344**, 556–563.

25 Clifton, G.L., Valadka, A., Zygun, D. *et al.* (2011) Very early hypothermia induction in patients with severe brain injury (the National Acute Brain Injury Study: Hypothermia II): a randomised trial. *The Lancet Neurology*, **10 (2)**, 131–139.

26 Polderman, K.H., Tjong Tjin Joe, R., Peerdeman, S.M., Vandertop, W.P. & Girbes, A.R. (2002) Effects of therapeutic hypothermia on intracranial pressure and outcome in patients with severe head injury. *Intensive Care Medicine*, **28 (11)**, 1563–1573.

27 Tokutomi, T., Miyagi, T., Takeuchi, Y., Karukaya, T., Katsuki, H. & Shigemori, M. (2009) Effect of 35 degrees C hypothermia on intracranial pressure and clinical outcome in patients with severe traumatic brain injury. *The Journal of Trauma*, **66 (1)**, 166–173.

28 Lee, H.C., Chuang, H.C., Cho, D.Y., Cheng, K.F., Lin, P.H. & Chen, C.C. (2010) Applying cerebral hypothermia and brain oxygen monitoring in treating severe traumatic brain injury. *World Neurosurgery*, **74 (6)**, 654–660.

29 Thompson, H.J., Tkacs, N.C., Saatman, K.E., Raghupathi, R. & McIntosh, T.K. (2003) Hyperthermia following traumatic brain injury: a critical evaluation. *Neurobiology of Disease*, **12**, 163–173.

30 Thompson, H.J., Pinto-Martin, J. & Bullock, M.R. (2003) Neurogenic fever after traumatic brain injury: an epidemiological study *Journal of Neurology, Neurosurgery and Psychiatry*, **74 (5)**, 614–619.

31 Hinz, J., Rosmus, M., Popov, A., Moerer, O., Frerichs, I. & Quintel, M. (2007) Effectiveness of an intravascular cooling method compared with a conventional cooling technique in neurologic patients. *Journal of Neurosurgical Anesthesiology*, **19 (2)**, 130–135.

32 Diringer, M.N.; Neurocritical Care Fever Reduction Trial Group. (2004) Treatment of fever in the neurologic intensive care unit with a catheter-based heat exchange system. *Critical Care Medicine*, **32 (2)**, 559–564.

33 Fischer, M., Lackner, P., Beer, R. *et al.* (2011) Keep the brain cool—endovascular cooling in patients with severe traumatic brain injury: a case series study. *Neurosurgery*, **68 (4)**, 867–873.

34 Puccio, A.M., Fischer, M.R., Jankowitz, B.T., Yonas, H., Darby, J.M., & Okonkwo, D.O. (2009) Induced normothermia attenuates intracranial hypertension and reduces fever burden after severe traumatic brain injury. *Neurocritical Care*, **11 (1)**, 82–87.

35 Zygun, D.A., Kortbeek, J.B., Fick, G.H., Laupland, K.B. & Doig, C.J. (2005) Non-neurologic organ dysfunction in severe traumatic brain injury. *Critical Care Medicine*, **33**, 654–660.

36 Burchiel, K.J., Steege, T.D. & Wyler, A.R. (1981) Intracranial pressure changes in brain-injured patients requiring positive end-expiratory pressure ventilation. *Neurosurgery*, **8 (4)**, 443–449.

37 Huynh, T., Messer, M., Sing, R.F., Miles, W., Jacobs, D.G. & Thomason, M.H. (2002) Positive end-expiratory pressure alters intracranial and cerebral perfusion pressure in severe traumatic brain injury. *The Journal of Trauma*, **53 (3)**, 488–492; discussion 492–493.

38 Videtta, W., Villarejo, F., Cohen, M. *et al.* (2002) Effects of positive end-expiratory pressure on intracranial pressure and cerebral perfusion pressure. *Acta Neurochirurgica Supplement*, **81**, 93–97.

39 Caricato, A., Conti, G., Della Corte, F. *et al.* (2005) Effects of PEEP on the intracranial system of patients with head injury and subarachnoid hemorrhage: the role of respiratory system compliance. *The Journal of Trauma*, **58 (3)**, 571–576.

40 Koutsoukou, A., Perraki, H., Raftopoulou, A.. *et al.* (2006) Respiratory mechanics in brain-damaged patients. *Intensive Care Medicine*, **32**, 1947–1954.

41 Abbushi, W., Herkt, G., Speckner, E. & Birk, M. (1980) Intracranial pressure—variations in brain-injured patients caused by PEEP ventilation and lifted position of the upper part of the body. *Anaesthesist*, **29 (10)**, 521–524.

42 Clarke, J.P. (1997) The effects of inverse ratio ventilation on intracranial pressure: a preliminary report. *Intensive Care Medicine*, **23 (1)**, 106–109.

43 Salim, A., Miller, K., Dangleben, D., Cipolle, M. & Pasquale, M. (2004) High-frequency percussive ventilation: an alternative mode of ventilation for head-injured patients with adult respiratory distress syndrome. *The Journal of Trauma*, **57 (3)**, 542–546.

44 Fuke, N., Murakami, Y., Tsutsumi, H. *et al.* (1984) The effect of high frequency jet ventilation on intracranial pressure in the patients with severe head injury. *No Shinkei Geka*, **12 (3 Suppl)**, 297–302.

45 Hurst, J.M., Saul, T.G., DeHaven, C.B., Jr. & Branson, R. (1984) Use of high frequency jet ventilation during mechanical hyperventilation to reduce intracranial pressure in patients with multiple organ system injury. *Neurosurgery* **15 (4)**, 530–534.

46 Papadimos, T.J., Medhkour, A. & Yermal, S. (2009) Successful use of inhaled nitric oxide to decrease intracranial pressure in a patient with severe traumatic brain injury complicated by acute respiratory distress syndrome: a role for an anti-inflammatory mechanism? *Scandinavian Journal of Trauma, Resuscitation and Emergency Medicine*, **17**, 5.

47 Jaskulka, R., Weinstabl, C. & Schedl, R. (1993) The course of intracranial pressure during respiratory weaning after severe craniocerebral trauma. *Unfallchirurgie*, **96 (3)**, 138–141.

48 Holland. M.C., Mackersie, R.C., Morabito, D. *et al.* (2003) The development of acute lung injury is associated with worse neurologic outcome in patients with severe traumatic brain injury. *The Journal of Trauma*, **55**, 106–111.

49 Bronchard, R., Albaladejo, P., Brezac, G. *et al.* (2004) Early onset pneumonia. *Risk factors and consequences in head trauma patients. Anesthesiology* **100**, 234–239.

50 Ibrahim, E.H., Tracy, L., Hill, C., Fraser, V.J. & Kollef, M.H. (2001) The occurrence of ventilator-associated pneumonia in a community hospital: risk factors and clinical outcomes. *Chest*, **120**, 555–561.

51 George, D.L., Falk, P.S., Wunderink, R.G. *et al.* (1998) Epidemiology of ventilator-acquired pneumonia based on protected bronchoscopic sampling. *American Journal of Respiratory and Critical Care Medicine*, **158**, 1839–1847.

52 Chastre, J. & Fagon, J.Y. (2002) Ventilator-associated pneumonia. *American Journal of Respiratory and Critical Care Medicine*, **165**, 867–903.

53 Heyland, D.K., Cook, D.J., Griffith, L., Keenan, S.P., & Brun-Buisson, C. (1999) The attributable morbidity and mortality of ventilator-associated pneumonia in the critically ill patient. The Canadian Critical Trials Group. *American Journal of Respiratory and Critical Care Medicine*, **159**, 1249–1256.

54 Kerwin, A.J., Croce, M.A., Timmons, S.D., Maxwell, R.A., Malhotra, A.K., & Fabian, T.C. (2000) Effects of fiberoptic bronchoscopy on intracranial pressure in patients with brain injury: a prospective clinical study. *The Journal of Trauma*, **48 (5)**, 878–882; discussion 882–883. doi: 10.1097/00005373-200005000-00011.

55 Chastre, J., Wolff, M., Fagon, J.Y. *et al.* (2003) Comparison of 8 vs 15 days of antibiotic therapy for ventilator-associated pneumonia in adults: a randomized trial. *Journal of American Medical Association*, **290**, 2588–2598.

56 Zygun, D.A., Zuege, D.J., Boiteau, P.J. *et al.* (2006) Ventilator-associated pneumonia in severe traumatic brain injury. *Neurocritical Care*, **5**, 108–114.

57 Drakulovic, M.B., Torres, A., Bauer, T.T., Nicolas, J.M., Nogué, S. & Ferrer, M. (1999) Supine body position as a risk factor for nosocomial pneumonia in mechanically ventilated patients: a randomised trial. *Lancet*, **354**, 1851–1858.

58 Cook, D.J., Reeve, B.K., Guyatt, G.H. *et al.* (1996) Stress ulcer prophylaxis in critically ill patients. Resolving discordant meta-analyses. *Journal of American Medical Association,* **275,** 308–314.

59 Cocanour, C.S., Peninger, M., Domonoske, B.D. *et al.* (2006) Decreasing ventilator-associated pneumonia in a trauma ICU. *The Journal of Trauma,* **61,** 122–129.

60 Gurkin, S.A., Parikshak, M., Kralovich, K.A., Horst, H.M., Agarwal, V. & Payne, N. (2002) Indicators for tracheostomy in patients with traumatic brain injury. *American Surgery* **68,** 324–328.

61 Ahmed, N. & Kuo, Y.H. (2007) Early versus late tracheostomy in patients with severe traumatic head injury. *Surgical Infections,* **8,** 343–347.

62 Pittet, D., Tarara, D. & Wenzel, R.P. (1994) Nosocomial bloodstream infection in critically ill patients. Excess length of stay, extra costs, and attributable mortality. *Journal of American Medical Association,* **271,** 1598–1601.

63 Reed, C.R., Sessler, C.N., Glauser, F.L. & Phelan, B.A. (1995) Central venous catheter infections: concepts and controversies. *Intensive Care Medicine,* **21,** 177–183.

64 Merrer, J., De Jonghe, B., Golliot, F. *et al.* (2001) Complications of femoral and subclavian venous catheterization in critically ill patients: a randomized controlled trial. *Journal of American Medical Association,* **286,** 700–707.

65 McGee, D.C. & Gould, M.K. (2003) Preventing complications of central venous catheterizations. *The New England Journal of Medicine,* **348,** 1123–1133.

66 Maki, D.G., Stolz, S.M., Wheeler, S. & Mermel, L.A. (1997) Prevention of central venous catheter-related bloodstream infection by use of an antiseptic-impregnated catheter. A randomized, controlled trial. *Annals of Internal Medicine,* **127,** 257–266.

67 Darouiche, R.O., Raad, I.I., Heard, S.O. *et al.* (1999) A comparison of two antimicrobial-impregnated central venous catheters. *Catheter Study Group. The New England Journal of Medicine,* **340,** 1–8.

68 Veenstra, D.L., Saint, S. & Sullivan, S.D. (1999) Cost-effectiveness of antiseptic-impregnated central venous catheters for the prevention of catheter-related bloodstream infection. *Journal of American Medical Association,* **282,** 554–560.

69 Raad, I.I., Hohn, D.C., Gilbreath, B.J. *et al.* (1994) Prevention of central venous catheter-related infections by using maximal sterile barrier precautions during insertion. *Infection Control and Hospital Epidemiology,* **15,** 231–238.

70 Maki, D.G., Ringer, M. & Alvarado, C.J. (1991) Prospective randomised trial of povidone-iodine, alcohol, and chlorhexidine for prevention of infection associated with central venous and arterial catheters. *Lancet,* **338,** 339–343.

71 DesJardin, J.A., Falagas, M.E., Ruthazer, R. *et al.* (1991) Clinical utility of blood cultures drawn from indwelling central venous catheters in hospitalized patients with cancer. *Annals of Internal Medicine,* **131,** 641–647.

72 Ekeh, A.P., Dominguez, K.M., Markert, R.J. & McCarthy, M.C. (2010) Incidence and risk factors for deep venous thrombosis after moderate and severe brain injury. *The Journal of Trauma,* **68 (4),** 912–915.

73 Buller, H.R., Agnelli, G., Hull RD, Hyers, T.M., Prins, M.H. & Raskob, G.E. (2004) Antithrombotic therapy for venous thromboembolic disease: the Seventh ACCP Conference on Antithrombotic and Thrombolytic Therapy. *Chest,* **126,** 401S–428S.

74 Page, R.B., Spott, M.A., Krishnamurthy, S., Taleghani, C. & Chinchilli, V.M. (2004) Head injury and pulmonary embolism: a retrospective report based on the Pennsylvania Trauma Outcomes study. *Neurosurgery,* **54,** 143–148.

75 Koehler, D.M., Shipman, J., Davidson, M.A. & Guillamondegui, O. (2011) Is early venous thromboembolism prophylaxis safe in trauma patients with intracranial hemorrhage. *The Journal of Trauma,* **70 (2),** 324–329.

76 Black, P.M, Baker, M.F., & Snook, C.P. (1986) Experience with external pneumatic calf compression in neurology and neurosurgery. *Neurosurgery,* **18**, 440–444.

77 Kim, J., Gearhart, M.M., Zurick, A., Zuccarello, M., James, L., & Luchette, F.A. (2002) Preliminary report on the safety of heparin for deep venous thrombosis prophylaxis after severe head injury. *The Journal of Trauma,* **53**, 38–42.

78 www.braintrauma.org [accessed on July 16, 2007].

79 McIntyre, L.A., Fergusson, D.A., Hutchison, J.S. *et al.* (2006) Effect of a liberal versus restrictive transfusion strategy on mortality in patients with moderate to severe head injury. *Neurocritical Care,* **5**, 4–9.

80 Taylor, R.W., Manganaro, L., O'Brien, J., Trottier, S.J., Parkar, N. & Veremakis, C. (2002) Impact of allogenic packed red blood cell transfusion on nosocomial infection rates in the critically ill patient. *Critical Care Medicine,* **30**, 2249–2254.

81 Toy, P. & Lowell, C. (2007) TRALI—definition, mechanisms, incidence and clinical relevance. *Best Practice and Research Clinical Anaesthesiology,* **21**, 183–193.

82 Warner, M.A., O'Keeffe, T., Bhavsar, P. *et al.* (2010) Transfusions and long-term functional outcomes in traumatic brain injury. *Journal of Neurosurgery,* **113 (3)**, 539–546.

83 Smith, M.J., Stiefel, M.F., Magge, S. *et al.* (2005) Packed red blood cell transfusion increases local cerebral oxygenation. *Critical Care Medicine,* **33 (5)**, 1104–1108.

84 Leal-Noval, S.R., Rincón-Ferrari, M.D., Marin-Niebla, A. *et al.* (2006) Transfusion of erythrocyte concentrates produces a variable increment on cerebral oxygenation in patients with severe traumatic brain injury: a preliminary study. *Intensive Care Medicine,* **32 (11)**, 1733–1740.

85 Zygun, D.A., Nortje, J., Hutchinson, P.J., Timofeev, I., Menon, D.K. & Gupta, A.K. (2009) The effect of red blood cell transfusion on cerebral oxygenation and metabolism after severe traumatic brain injury. *Critical Care Medicine,* **37 (3)**, 1074–1078.

86 Piek, J., Chestnut, R.M., Marshall, L.F. *et al.* (1992) Extracranial complications of severe head injury. *Journal of Neurosurgery,* **77**, 901–907.

87 Clifton, G.L., Miller, E.R., Choi, S.C. & Levin, H.S. (2002) Fluid thresholds and outcome from severe brain injury. *Critical Care Medicine,* **30 (4)**, 739–745.

88 Härtl, R., Gerber, L.M., Ni, Q. & Ghajar, J. (2008) Effect of early nutrition on deaths due to severe traumatic brain injury. *Journal of Neurosurgery,* **109 (1)**, 50–56.

89 Acosta-Escribano, J., Fernández-Vivas, M., Grau Carmona, T. *et al.* (2010) Gastric versus transpyloric feeding in severe traumatic brain injury: a prospective, randomized trial. *Intensive Care Medicine,* **36 (9)**, 1532–1539.

90 Garcia-de-Lorenzo, A., Ortiz-Leyba, M., Planas, J.C. *et al.* (1997) Parenteral administration of different amounts of branch-chain amino acids in septic patients: clinical and metabolic aspects. *Critical Care Medicine,* **25**, 418–424.

91 Lam, A.M., Winn, H.R., Cullen, B.F. & Sundling, N. (1991) Hyperglycemia and neurological outcome in patients with head injury. *Journal of Neurosurgery,* **75**, 545–551.

92 Jeremitsky, E., Omert, L.A., Dunham, C.L., Wilberger, J. & Rodriguez, A. (2005) The impact of hyperglycemia on patients with severe brain injury. *The Journal of Trauma,* **58**, 47–50.

93 Griesdale, D.E., Tremblay, M.H., McEwen, J. & Chittock, D.R. (2009) Glucose control and mortality in patients with severe traumatic brain injury. *Neurocritical Care,* **11 (3)**, 311–316.

94 Graffagnino, C., Gurram, A.R., Kolls, B. & Olson, D.M. (2010) Intensive insulin therapy in the neurocritical care setting is associated with poor clinical outcomes. *Neurocritical Care,* **13 (3)**, 307–312.

95 Young, B., Ott, L., Dempsey, R., Haack, D. & Tibbs, P. (1989) Relationship between admission hyperglycemia and neurologic outcome of severely brain-injured patients. *Annals of Surgery,* **210**, 466–472.

96 Van Beek, J.G., Mushkudiani, N.A., Steyerberg, E.W. *et al.* (2007) Prognostic value of admission laboratory parameters in traumatic brain injury: results from the IMPACT study. *Journal of Neurotrauma*, **24 (2)**, 315–328.

97 Van den Berghe, G., Schoonheydt, K., Becx, P., Bruyninckx, F., & Wouters, P.J. (2005) Insulin therapy protects the central and peripheral nervous system of intensive care patients. *Neurology*, **64**, 1348–1353.

98 Yang, M., Guo, Q., Zhang, X. *et al.* (2009) Intensive insulin therapy on infection rate, days in NICU, in-hospital mortality and neurological outcome in severe traumatic brain injury patients: a randomized controlled trial. *International Journal of Nursing Studies*, **46 (6)**, 753–758.

99 Coester, A., Neumann, C.R. & Schmidt, M.I. (2010) Intensive insulin therapy in severe traumatic brain injury: a randomized trial. *The Journal of Trauma*, **68 (4)**, 904–911.

100 Bilotta, F., Caramia, R., Cernak, I. *et al.* (2008) Intensive insulin therapy after severe traumatic brain injury: a randomized clinical trial. *Neurocritical Care*, **9 (2)**, 159–166.

101 Meier, R., Béchir, M., Ludwig, S. *et al.* (2008) Differential temporal profile of lowered blood glucose levels (3.5 to 6.5 mmol/l versus 5 to 8 mmol/l) in patients with severe traumatic brain injury. *Critical Care*, **12 (4)**, R98.

102 Vespa, P., Boonyaputthikul, R., McArthur, D.L. *et al.* (2006) Intensive insulin therapy reduces microdialysis glucose values without altering glucose utilization or improving the lactate/pyruvate ratio after traumatic brain injury. *Critical Care Medicine*, **34 (3)**, 850–856.

103 Oddo, M., Schmidt, J.M., Carrera, E. *et al.* (2008) Impact of tight glycemic control on cerebral glucose metabolism after severe brain injury: a microdialysis study. *Critical Care Medicine*, **36 (12)**, 3233–3238.

104 Annegers, J.F., Hauser, W.A., Coan, S.P. & Rocca, W.A. (1998) A population-based study of seizures after traumatic brain injuries. *The New England Journal of Medicine*, **338**, 20–24.

105 Hauser, W.A. (1990) Prevention of post-traumatic epilepsy. *The New England Journal of Medicine*, **323**, 540–542.

106 Dauch, W.A., Schutze, M., Guttinger, M. & Bauer, B.L. (1996) Post-traumatic seizure prevention—results of a survey of 127 neurosurgery clinics. *Zentralblatt fur Neurochirurgie*, **57**, 190–195.

107 Temkin, N.R., Dikmen, S.S., Wilensky, A.J., Keihm, J., Chabal, S. & Winn, H.R. (1990) A randomized, double-blind study of phenytoin for the prevention of post-traumatic seizures. *The New England Journal of Medicine*, **323**, 497–502.

108 Jones, K.E, Puccio, A.M., Harshman, K.J. *et al.* (2008) Levetiracetam versus phenytoin for seizure prophylaxis in severe traumatic brain injury. *Neurosurgical Focus*, **25 (4)**, E3.

109 Szaflarski, J.P., Sangha, K.S., Lindsell, C.J. & Shutter, L.A. (2010) Prospective, randomized, single-blinded comparative trial of intravenous levetiracetam versus phenytoin for seizure prophylaxis. *Neurocritical Care*, **12 (2)**, 165–172.

110 Claassen, J., Mayer, S.A., Kowalski, R.G., Emerson, R.G. & Hirsch, L.J. (2004) Detection of electrographic seizures with continuous EEG monitoring in critically ill patients. *Neurology*, **62 (10)**, 1743–1748.

111 Vespa, P.M., Nuwer, M.R., Nenov, V. *et al.* (1999) Increased incidence and impact of nonconvulsive and convulsive seizures after traumatic brain injury as detected by continuous electroencephalographic monitoring. *Journal of Neurosurgery*, **91**, 750–760.

112 Vespa, P.M., Miller, C., McArthur, D. *et al.* (2007) Nonconvulsive electrographic seizures after traumatic brain injury result in a delayed, prolonged increase in intracranial pressure and metabolic crisis. *Critical Care Medicine*, **35 (12)**, 2830–2836.

113 Vespa, P.M., McArthur, D.L. & Xu, Y. (2010). Nonconvulsive seizures after traumatic brain injury are associated with hippocampal atrophy. *Neurology*, **75 (9)**, 792–798.

114 Bacic, A., Gluncic, I., & Gluncic, V. (1999) Disturbances in plasma sodium in patients with war head injuries. *Military Medicine* **164**, 214–217.

115 Vingerhoets, F. & de Tribolet, N. (1988) Hyponatremia hypo-osmolarity in neurosurgical patients. "Appropriate secretion of ADH" and "cerebral salt wasting syndrome". *Acta Neurochirurgica (Wien)* **91**, 50–54.

116 Doczi, T., Tarjanyi, J., Huszka, E. & Kiss, J. (1982) Syndrome of inappropriate secretion of antidiuretic hormone (SIADH) after head injury. *Neurosurgery,* **10 (6 Pt 1)**, 685–688.

117 www.clinicaltrials.gov [accessed on 27 September 2007].

118 Dhar, R. & Murphy-Human, T. (2011) A bolus of conivaptan lowers intracranial pressure in a patient with hyponatremia after traumatic brain injury. *Neurocritical Care,* **14 (1)**, 97–102.

119 Sandel, M. & Mysiw, W. (1996) The agitated brain injured patient. Part 1: Definitions, differential diagnosis, and assessment. *Archives of Physical Medicine and Rehabilitation,* **77**, 617–623.

120 Brooke, M., Questad, K., Patterson, D. & Bashak, K. (1992) Agitation and restlessness after closed head injury: a prospective study of 100 consecutive admissions. *Archives of Physical Medicine and Rehabilitation* **73**, 320–323.

121 Reyes, R. & Bhattacharyya, A. (1981) Traumatic brain injury: restlessness and agitation as prognosticators of physical and psychologic improvement in patients. *Archives of Physical Medicine and Rehabilitation,* **62**, 20–23.

122 Levin, H. & Grossman, R. (1978) Behavioral sequelae of closed head injury. A quantitative study. *Archives of Neurology,* **35**, 720–727.

123 Corrigan, J. & Mysiw, W. (1988) Agitation following traumatic head injury: Equivocal evidence for a discrete stage of cognitive recovery. *Archives of Physical Medicine and Rehabilitation,* **69**, 487–492.

124 Goldstein, L. (1993) Basic and clinical studies of pharmacologic effects on recovery from brain injury. *Journal of Neural Transplantation and Plasticity,* **4**, 175–192.

125 Goldstein, L. (1995) Prescribing of potentially harmful drugs to patients admitted to hospital after head injury. *Journal of Neurology, Neurosurgery and Psychiatry,* **58**, 753–755.

126 Ely, E.W., Truman, B., Shintani, A. *et al.* (2003) Monitoring sedation status over time in ICU patients: reliability and validity of the Richmond Agitation-Sedation Scale (RASS). *Journal of American Medical Association,* **289 (22)**, 2983–2991.

127 Sessler, C.N., Gosnell, M.S., Grap, M.J. *et al.* (2002) The Richmond Agitation-Sedation Scale: validity and reliability in adult intensive care unit patients. *American Journal of Respiratory and Critical Care Medicine,* **166 (10)**, 1338–1344.

128 Ely, E.W., Inouye, S.K., Bernard, G.R. *et al.* (2001) Delirium in mechanically ventilated patients: validity and reliability of the confusion assessment method for the intensive care unit (CAM-ICU). *Journal of American Medical Association,* **286 (21)**, 2703–2710.

129 Ely, E.W., Margolin, R., Francis, J. *et al.* (2001) Evaluation of delirium in critically ill patients: validation of the Confusion Assessment Method for the Intensive Care Unit (CAM-ICU). *Critical Care Medicine,* **29 (7)**, 1370–1379.

130 Pandharipande, P., Cotton, B.A., Shintani, A. *et al.* (2007) Motoric subtypes of delirium in mechanically ventilated surgical and trauma intensive care unit patients. *Intensive Care Medicine,* **33 (10)**, 1726–1731. [Epub 2007 Jun 5.]

131 Nakase-Thompson, R., Sherer, M., Yablon, S.A., Nick, T.G. & Trzepacz, P.T. (2004) Acute confusion following traumatic brain injury. *Brain Injury,* **18 (2)**, 131–142.

132 Pandharipande, P., Cotton, B.A., Shintani, A. *et al.* (2008) Prevalence and risk factors for development of delirium in surgical and trauma intensive care unit patients. *The Journal of Trauma,* **65 (1)**, 34–41.

133 Vasilevskis, E.E., Pandharipande, P.P., Girard, T.D. & Ely, E.W. (2010) A screening, prevention, and restoration model for saving the injured brain in intensive care unit survivors. *Critical Care Medicine*, **38 (10 Suppl)**, S683–S691.

134 Lescot, T., Pereira, A.R., Abdennour, L. *et al.* (2007) Effect of loxapine on electrical brain activity, intracranial pressure, and middle cerebral artery flow velocity in traumatic brain-injured patients. *Neurocritical Care*, **7 (2)**, 124–127.

135 Baguley, I.J., Heriseanu, R.E., Cameron, I.D., Nott, M.T. & Slewa-Younan, S. (2008) A critical review of the pathophysiology of dysautonomia following traumatic brain injury. *Neurocritical Care*, **8(2)**, 293–300.

136 Baguley, I.J. (2008) Autonomic complications following central nervous system injury. *Seminars in Neurology* **28 (5)**, 716–725.

137 Perkes, I., Baguley, I.J., Nott, M.T. & Menon, D.K. (2010) A review of paroxysmal sympathetic hyperactivity after acquired brain injury. *Annals of Neurology* **68 (2)**, 126–135.

138 Meythaler, J.M. & Stinson, A.M. III. (1994) Fever of central origin in traumatic brain injury controlled with propranolol. *Archives of Physical Medicine and Rehabilitation*, **75**, 816–818.

139 Baguley, I.J., Cameron, I.D., Green, A.M., Slewa-Younan, S., Marosszeky, J.E. & Gurka, J.A. (2004) Pharmacological management of Dysautonomia following traumatic brain injury. *Brain Injury* **18**, 409–417.

140 Baguley, I.J., Heriseanu, R.E., Gurka, J.A., Nordenbo, A. & Cameron, I.D. (2007) Gabapentin in the management of dysautonomia following severe traumatic brain injury: a case series. *Journal of Neurology, Neurosurgery and Psychiatry*, **78**, 539–541.

141 Lacomis, D., Petrella, J.T. & Giuliani, M.J. (1998) Causes of neuromuscular weakness in the intensive care unit: a study of ninety-two patients. *Muscle and Nerve*, **21**, 610–617.

142 De Jonghe, B., Sharshar, T., Lefaucheur, J.P. *et al.* (2002) Paresis acquired in the intensive care unit: a prospective multicenter study. *Journal of American Medical Association*, **288**, 2859–2867.

143 Coakley, J.H., Nagendran, K., Honavar, M., & Hinds, C.J. (1993) Preliminary observations on the neuromuscular abnormalities in patients with organ failure and sepsis. *Intensive Care Medicine*, **19**, 323–328.

144 Hund, E., Genzwurker, H., Bohrer, H., Jakob, H., Thiele, R. & Hacke, W. (1997) Predominant involvement of motor fibres in patients with critical illness polyneuropathy. *British Journal of Anaesthesia*, **78**, 274–278.

PART IV
Rehabilitation

CHAPTER 9

Rehabilitation of cognitive deficits after traumatic brain injury

Philippe Azouvi[1,2,3] and Claire Vallat-Azouvi[3,4]

[1] *AP-HP, Department of Physical Medicine and Rehabilitation, Raymond Poincaré Hospital, Garches, France*
[2] *EA HANDIREsP, Université de Versailles, Saint Quentin, France*
[3] *ER 6, Université Pierre et Marie Curie, Paris, France*
[4] *Antenne UEROS and SAMSAH 92, UGECAM Ile-de-France, France*

Severe traumatic brain injury (TBI) is associated with a wide range of cognitive impairments, which may compromise social and vocational reintegration. The field of cognitive rehabilitation has experienced significant progress these last 30 years, and several recent reviews and meta-analyses have reached the conclusion that there is substantial evidence to support cognitive interventions for people with TBI [1–3]. In this chapter, we will first present a brief overview of cognitive deficits after severe TBI. Then, we will review in more detail the rehabilitation of each of the main different cognitive deficits that may occur after TBI and the level of evidence for neuropsychological rehabilitation.

Cognitive deficits, behavioral changes, and outcome after severe TBI

Survivors of a severe TBI frequently may suffer from deficits of long-term episodic memory, slowed information processing, and deficits of attention, working memory, and executive functions [4]. For example, Masson *et al.* [5] showed that 5 years after a severe TBI, 44.4% of survivors had a Moderate Disability, and 14.4% a Severe Disability, mainly due to cognitive impairments. Cognitive impairments are frequently associated with behavioral and personality changes [6], poor self-awareness [7] and mental fatigue [8, 9]. Brooks and colleagues [10] reported that, 1 year after the accident, 60% of relatives answered that the patient was "not the same as before," and this proportion increased up to 74% at 5 years.

Traumatic Brain Injury, First Edition. Edited by Pieter E. Vos and Ramon Diaz-Arrastia.

Long-term memory

After emerging from coma and the vegetative state, TBI patients usually pass through a phase of global cognitive disturbance, termed posttraumatic amnesia (PTA), characterized by confusion, disorientation for time and place, inability to store and retrieve new information, and some degree of retrograde amnesia [11]. The consistent return to continuous memory indicates clearing of PTA, but memory problems frequently persist. Indeed, memory deficit is one of the most frequent complaints from patients and their relatives after a severe TBI [12]. Brooks *et al.* [10] found that memory problems were reported by 67% of relatives 1 and 5 years after a severe TBI. Memory failures were the second most frequent relatives' complaints 5 years postinjury, just after behavioral modifications.

Many studies have shown that patients with TBI suffer from a deficit in the ability to acquire new information (for a recent review see Vakil [13]). Patients perform poorer than controls on all types of memory tasks, whatever the task demand or the nature of the material to be remembered (verbal or visual) [14]. The underlying cognitive mechanisms are still debated [13]. Experimental studies suggest that TBI is associated with a slower, inconsistent, and disorganized learning rate [15, 16], an accelerated forgetting rate [17, 18], a higher number of intrusions in free recall, and a reduced ability to spontaneously use active or effortful semantic encoding or mental imagery to improve learning efficiency [19]. In many aspects, memory impairments after TBI seem closely related to attentional and executive impairments, and resemble the kind of memory disorders found after frontal lobe lesion.

In addition, a high prevalence of retrograde memory deficits has been reported after TBI, encompassing both the domains of autobiographical and public events memories and also early acquired basic and cultural knowledge [20, 21].

Working memory

Working memory is a system for both storage and manipulation of information, hence playing a central role in complex cognitive abilities [22]. It is assumed to be divided into three subsystems [22]. The central executive is an attentional control system, while the phonological loop and the visuospatial sketchpad are two modality-specific slave systems, responsible for storage and rehearsal of verbal and visuospatial information, respectively. Although the two modality-specific slave systems are relatively well preserved after TBI, central executive aspects of working memory (particularly the ability to simultaneously store and process complex information or to monitor and update information) seem to be impaired [23].

Attention and speed of processing

One of the most popular models [24] assumes that attention can be subdivided into two broad domains, intensity (the ability to modulate the level of attention on a given task) and selectivity (the ability to select relevant stimuli in the environment). Each of these two domains can be again divided in two components. Within the intensity domain, phasic alterness refers to the ability to respond faster when a stimulus is preceded by a warning signal, while sustained attention refers to the ability to maintain a stable level of performance during a monotonous long-duration task. Within the selectivity domain, focused attention refers to the ability to focus on a relevant stimulus, and hence to discard irrelevant, distracting stimuli, while divided attention refers to the concurrent performance of two competing tasks at the same time.

Mental slowness is one of the most robust findings after severe TBI and may compromise all aspects of attentional functioning. Whether attentional functions are additionally impaired remains debated. Experimental studies suggested that there is little if any specific impairment of phasic alterness, sustained attention, and focused attention beyond slowed processing [25]. However, several studies found a specific impairment of divided attention that depends on the nature and complexity of the task [26–29]. As suggested in a meta-analysis, TBI patients did not differ from controls when the divided attention tasks could be performed relatively automatically, while they were impaired relative to controls on tasks including substantial working memory load [30].

Mental fatigue is a frequent complaint after TBI, and seems closely related to attention deficits. According to Van Zomeren *et al.* [31], fatigue could be due to the constant compensatory effort required to reach an adequate level of performance in everyday life, despite cognitive deficits and slowed processing. This is known as the *coping hypothesis,* which has received support from recent experimental studies [9, 32, 33].

Deficits of executive functions

Executive functions are the cognitive abilities involved in programming, regulation, and verification of novel and/or goal-directed behavior [34]. Survivors from a traumatic coma frequently show dramatic personality and behavioral changes. These changes may be related to lack of control (disinhibition, impulsivity, irritability, hyperactivity, aggressiveness) or lack of drive (apathy, reduced initiative, poor motivation) [6]. These modifications are frequently associated with lack of awareness (anosognosia) [7].

From a cognitive perspective, impairments in planning, conceptualization, set shifting, mental flexibility, generation of new information, and inhibition have been documented, although objective assessment of these functions is difficult, due to a lack of sensitivity of most commonly used neuropsychological tasks. Several studies outlined the necessity to use ecologically valid assessment measures of executive functions [35–37].

Global intellectual efficiency

Measures of global intellectual functioning are frequently used in the neuropsychological assessment of patients with TBI [38]. The most widely used instrument is the Wechsler Adult Intelligence Scale, which has the advantage of extensive normative data, permitting statistical comparisons. Patients with severe TBI usually show a pattern of global intellectual decline. However, some measures and indexes are more sensitive to TBI. A discrepancy between verbal and performance IQ has been repeatedly reported, the lower performance IQ being related to slowed visuomotor processing. Similarly, processing speed or working memory indexes are particularly sensitive to TBI, while other subtests, such as verbal comprehension or perceptual organization, appear more resistant to brain injury [39].

Rehabilitation of executive functions

Problem-solving training

Following the pioneer work from Luria and Tsvetkova [40], several studies were conducted to assess the effectiveness of problem-solving training (PST) and of learning metacognitive strategies to improve executive functioning after brain injury. Most of these programs relied on increasing awareness, reducing the problem complexity by breaking it down into easier subtasks, and learning a systematic controlled stepwise processing. Cicerone and Wood [41] reported a single-case study of PST in a chronic frontally injured patient, 4 years postinjury. The patient was trained to use self-instructions to solve a task. An improvement was found, but generalization to everyday life situations only occurred after the use of more ecologically based training tasks.

Von Cramon and colleagues, in Germany, devised a comprehensive rehabilitation program, named PST, that was used in a randomized controlled study [42]. Twenty patients receiving PST were compared to 17 patients receiving memory training as a control treatment. Patients in the PST group showed more improvement than the control group in measures of general intelligence and problem solving and in behavioral ratings of awareness, goal-directed ideas, problem solving, and action style. The same group reported the effectiveness of problem-solving training in a professional context in a single-case study of a patient with a severe chronic dysexecutive syndrome [43]. This patient, a pathologist, was trained specifically on professional tasks during 30 weeks. However, although his diagnosis accuracy improved, no generalization was found in other everyday life tasks, even though these latter tasks required similar cognitive processes.

Rath *et al.* [44] conducted a randomized controlled study in a chronic patient group (4 years postinjury on average) with apparent good recovery but persisting socioprofessional difficulties. Experimental training consisted of two successive phases: problem orientation, based on emotional regulation to control for impulsive reactions, and problem solving, based on role-play in ecological situations. Patients receiving this experimental rehabilitation during 24 weeks ($n = 27$) improved more on cognitive testing, everyday life functioning, and self-awareness than a control group ($n = 19$) who was given conventional cognitive training.

Levine *et al.* [45] evaluated the effectiveness of another problem-solving intervention, goal management training (GMT), in a randomized controlled study. GMT relied on the goal neglect model as proposed by Duncan [46]. According to this model, dysexecutive patients tend to neglect the ultimate goal and the intermediate subgoals necessary to complete a task. Patients learned a systematic strategy to generate goals and subgoals to solve a problem. Participants ($n = 15$) received only 1 h of GMT, compared to 1 h of motor skill training in the control group. The experimental group showed an improved accuracy on a set of paper and pencil tests that were assumed to simulate everyday activities. However, the generalization to actual everyday situations remains to be demonstrated. GMT was also used by the same authors in a more ecologically oriented approach in a single-case study [45]. A postencephalitic patient received two sessions of GMT training focusing on cooking tasks. After training, the number of errors during cooking sessions decreased, and the effect remained stable 6 months after the end of the therapy.

Spikman *et al.* [47] recently reported a large ($n = 75$) multicenter randomized controlled study of a new multifaceted treatment program for executive dysfunction. This program relied heavily on GMT and PST described earlier, but a special care was given to assess the effect on executive functions in daily life. Rehabilitation was administered step-by-step during 3 months in three stages: information and awareness, goal setting and planning, and initiation, execution, and regulation. The experimental group improved significantly more than controls in the primary outcome measure, named the Role Resumption List, which is a questionnaire addressing the amount and quality of activities in different domains (vocational functioning, social interactions, leisure activities, and mobility). A significant improvement was also found on an ecological executive task, simulating a job situation, and in patients' ability to set realistic goals. Improvement lasted at least 6 months posttreatment.

Other strategies

Environmental modifications can also be used to help patients to deal more effectively with complex tasks. External cueing, by periodic auditory alerts has been used by Manly *et al.* [48]. Within the goal neglect model, randomly occurring auditory cues were intended to serve as external reminders of the goal and subgoals of the task at hand. Ten patients (mainly post-TBI) were included in this study and compared to a control group. With periodic auditory alerts, they were able to reach a nearly normal performance on an ecological multitask: they improved in their ability to deal with more tasks within a given time limit.

Compensatory strategies can also be used. Fasotti *et al.* [49] developed the time pressure management, aimed at helping patients compensate for slow information processing. This technique was based on teaching self-instructions. Patients were trained to anticipate and adapt their plans to their actual level of performance and speed, in order to reduce time pressure at the operational level.

This strategy was found effective in a randomized group study, but the generalization to everyday life remains to be demonstrated [49].

Behavioral management techniques have been less studied. A few individual case studies have been reported, suggesting that negative reinforcement techniques such as *time-out* or *response cost* could reduce aggressiveness or inappropriate repetitive behaviors [50, 51]. Medd and Tate [52] conducted on 16 patients a randomized controlled study of a cognitive–behavioral program of anger management that involved self-awareness and self-instructional training. Results showed a significant decrease of anger outbursts, without change in patients' awareness of anger problems. Onsworth *et al.* [53] conducted a study aimed at improving awareness in a group of 21 chronic patients (mainly TBI) with severe cognitive impairments and anosognosia. Treatment included problem-solving training, role-playing and compensatory strategies during 16 weeks. Self-awareness improved after the therapy and 6 months later.

Rehabilitation of attention

Studies on rehabilitation of attention after TBI have been reported, with mixed results [54]. Sohlberg and Mateer [55] reported positive results in four patients (three with TBI). A rehabilitation program of focused, sustained, and divided attention, of distractibility and of flexibility was compared to visual function training. Attentional performance only improved after attentional training, while visual function only improved after visual training. On the opposite, Ponsford and Kinsella [56], in a well-designed multiple single-case design, found that attention training was not more effective than spontaneous recovery. In a meta-analysis, Park and Ingles [57] concluded that studies that used an adequate control condition produced only small and statistically nonsignificant improvements in performance of cognitive functions and specific measures of attention. They found however that specific skills training significantly improved performance of trained tasks requiring attention.

However, there is some evidence suggesting that more specific approaches, using a training program focusing on one specific attentional process may be more effective. Indeed, attention is not a unitary construct, and it is assumed to include several dissociable cognitive processes, as described earlier in this chapter. Severe TBI is associated with slowed processing, but also with impaired ability to deal with complex multiple tasks (divided attention deficit) [58]. Only few studies assessed the effectiveness of training programs addressing specifically one or several impaired attentional subcomponents. Sturm and colleagues conducted two randomized studies in patients with brain injuries of various origins (stroke or TBI) and showed that specific attention deficits need specific training [59, 60]. They found highly specific training effects, especially for intensity aspects of attention performance (vigilance and alertness) but also for divided attention. They concluded that it is very important to start an attention therapy by comprehensive diagnostics to work out the specific attention deficits the patient suffers from. However, they did not look for improvements of daily life activities related to attentional functions.

A preliminary randomized controlled trial of dual-tasking training has been recently reported [61]. Ten patients with dual-tasking difficulties after stroke or TBI practiced exercises that involved walking being combined with cognitive tasks. An improvement was found on a task similar to the trained tasks, but without generalization to other dual-task situations. In a recent group randomized crossover study, Couillet *et al.* [62] proposed a training program of divided attention to 12 severe TBI patients. A significant improvement was found on measures of dual-task processing and, to a lesser degree, on measures of executive functioning, while no change occurred on nontarget measures, such as long-term memory and speed of processing. In addition, an improvement was found on a questionnaire addressing dual tasking in everyday life. These results suggest that rehabilitation of attention might be effective if training specifically addresses the impaired attentional subcomponents.

Rehabilitation of working memory

There has been to date little research on rehabilitation of working memory after TBI. Training of working memory has been found useful in a few other conditions, such as children with ADHD [63], stroke patients [64, 65], or a patient with a brain tumor in the left temporal lobe [66]. Significant training-induced changes in brain activity have been found in a functional imaging study in healthy individuals [67]. To our knowledge, only three studies on rehabilitation of working memory after TBI have been reported [68–70]. The first study included eight patients with mild TBI in a randomized study. Compared to controls, rehabilitation of working memory (one session per week during 11–27 weeks) resulted in a greater improvement of tests of attention and of working memory, and of complaints in daily life, while speed of processing was not modified [68]. Serino *et al.* [69] reported a group study of rehabilitation of central executive deficits in nine patients with TBI of various degrees of severity. After 4 weeks training, patients improved significantly in all cognitive functions dependent on the central executive, but not in those functions not thought to tap this system. A significant improvement was also found on psychosocial outcome measures. Vallat-Azouvi *et al.* [70] reported two single-case studies of chronic TBI patients (respectively 30 and 36 months postinjury) suffering from relatively isolated deficits of the central executive of working memory. Both patients improved significantly, both on psychometric measures and on everyday life functioning, after 6 or 8 months of a comprehensive program of rehabilitation addressing the different subcomponents of working memory [65].

Rehabilitation of long-term memory

Although direct memory training by strategies such as *learning by heart* are of very limited effect, different strategies might be helpful in brain-injured patients with memory deficits. Wilson [71] identified four major approaches within memory rehabilitation: (1) environmental adaptations, (2) new technology, (3) new learning, and (4) holistic approaches.

Environmental adaptations can be used in patients with very severe memory deficits. The principle is to change or adapt the environment to reduce the load on the patient's memory (e.g., with signposts, labels, diaries, notebooks). The ability to use such compensatory strategies depends on patient's awareness of his or her deficits and on the preservation of other cognitive abilities.

External aids and new technology such as electronic organizers or computers may be useful. The system that has been studied most extensively is the Neuropage®, which uses a computer linked by modem or telephone to a paging company. The paging system transmits automatically the reminder information that has been entered into the computer to the paging company, who transmits the message at the appropriate day and time to the patient. This system has been found to be beneficial in a randomized study of patients with moderate-to-severe memory impairments [72].

Several methods have been proposed to improve learning strategies in brain-injured individuals. Such methods include various mnemonic techniques, such as visual imagery, notebook training, using a diary with self-instructional training [73, 74]. Spaced retrieval is based on the finding that a more efficient learning is obtained if learning trials are spaced or distributed, rather than presented in one chunk [71]. Errorless learning is based on the finding that amnesic patients learn better when they are prevented from making mistakes during the learning process. The basic assumption is that patients with severe memory problems cannot remember their mistakes so fail to correct them. Errorless learning has been found useful mainly in patients with severe memory deficits [75, 76].

Holistic rehabilitation

Holistic rehabilitation relies on an integrated treatment approach, addressing cognitive, social, and emotional sequelae of TBI, as well as awareness, motivation, and interpersonal skills [77, 78]. Group and individual therapy are often combined, either on an inpatient or an outpatient basis. The main objective is to optimize adjustment through realistic goals and compensatory strategies to improve activity, participation, and quality of life, rather than restoring underlying cognitive deficits. There are unfortunately very few controlled studies of holistic rehabilitation, with contradictory results. A randomized trial in a large group of patients ($n = 120$) at an early stage after TBI (38 days on average) failed to find any significant difference at 1 year between patients who were given an intensive inpatient cognitive rehabilitation during 8 weeks and a control group receiving a less intensive treatment at home [79]. However, as noted by Cicerone *et al.* [1], the ability to generalize from the results of this study is limited due to the limited course of treatment (8 weeks), and to the very good outcomes of the participants in each group (more than 90% returned to work). Other studies reported favorable outcomes. Powell *et al.* [80] reported a randomized study of community-based rehabilitation. Treatment included multidisciplinary rehabilitation and social support twice a week during 27.3 weeks on average. Patients improved more than a control group in terms of independence, organization, and well-being.

Reviews and meta-analyses

Several recent reviews, consensus conferences, or meta-analyses addressed the issue of the effectiveness of cognitive rehabilitation, after TBI or other brain injuries, such as stroke. An NIH conference consensus on rehabilitation of persons with TBI, in 1999, concluded that data were still limited, due to heterogeneity of patients, intervention modalities, and assessment measures [81]. More recently, Cicerone and colleagues conducted three systematic reviews of evidence-based cognitive rehabilitation [1–3]. Their reviews were not limited to, but included a number of studies with TBI patients. A summary of these three reviews is presented in Table 9.1. They identified, up to 2008, 42 studies of rehabilitation of executive functions. Six of these studies were rated as class I (randomized controlled study). The authors concluded that there was enough evidence to recommend problem-solving training in clinical practice. Cicerone *et al.* [1–3] identified 71 studies (up to 2008) on memory rehabilitation, among which 10 were rated as class I; 24 studies on rehabilitation of attention, among which 10 were rated class I, and 36 studies based on holistic rehabilitation, among which only four were rated as class I (with opposite results).

Table 9.1 Evidence-based cognitive rehabilitation.

Domain	Total number	Class I studies
Visuospatial	66	18
Language	122	16
Memory	71	10
Attention	24	6
Executive functions	42	6
Holistic	36	4

Data from Cicerone *et al.*, 2000, 2005, 2011 [1–3]. It presents the total number of studies included across these three reviews for each cognitive domain and the number of class I studies.

Rohling *et al.* [82] reexamined the first two Cicerone *et al.* [1, 2] reviews in a quantitative meta-analysis. The overall effect of cognitive rehabilitation, across all functions and after adjustment for improvement in nontreated control patients, was moderate but significantly different from zero (mean effect size, 0.30; 95% CI, 0.22–0.37). These authors identified 14 studies on rehabilitation of executive functions and attention, with a mean effect size of 0.61 (95% CI, 0.37–0.95). However, they also reported that control patients also significantly improved (mean effect size, 0.39). This stresses the importance of controlling for confounding effects such as placebo effect, the nonspecific effect of global cognitive training, or spontaneous recovery. Nevertheless, after control of these confounding effects, the mean effect size of the difference between experimental rehabilitation and control training was modest but significantly different from zero (mean ES = 0.27; CI 95%, 0.04–0.50), thus suggesting the effectiveness of rehabilitation of executive functions. Regarding memory rehabilitation, Rohling *et al.* [82] included 14 studies associated with an effect size of 0.61 (95% CI, 0.37–0.85). However, the effect of holistic rehabilitation (24 studies) was not significant (effect size, 0.03; 95% CI, −0.13 to 0.19). This analysis also showed that treatment effects were moderated by time since injury (larger effects at the early stage, although the effect is still significant more than 1 year after injury).

Kennedy *et al.* [83] conducted a meta-analysis of rehabilitation of executive functions. They identified 15 studies, including 5 rated as class I, which used metacognitive strategy instructions [42, 44, 45, 49, 84]. Effect sizes were computed on these 5 latter studies. Results showed that effect sizes from immediate impairment outcomes did not significantly differ from control intervention. However, effect-sizes from activity/participation outcomes (mean = 0.57; 95% CI, 0.48–0.67) were significantly larger than effect sizes from control intervention (mean = 0.38; 95% CI, 0.27–0.50), suggesting that rehabilitation resulted in better functioning in daily life.

Conclusion

There is now a growing consensus on the efficacy of cognitive rehabilitation in patients with severe TBI, despite the relatively small number of randomized controlled trials. However, effect sizes remain in the small-to-moderate range. The efficacy of cognitive rehabilitation clearly depends on the intensity and duration of therapy. However, other factors that may influence outcome should be taken into consideration, related either to staff (providing good interdisciplinary teamwork, focusing therapy on functional goals relevant to the injured person) or to the patient and his or her family (awareness, motivation, active involvement in the therapy process). The use of novel technologies such as computer-based cognitive rehabilitation, while still in its infancy, shows promise for expanding the availability of this therapy.

References

1 Cicerone, K.D., Dahlberg, C., Malec, J.F. *et al.* (2005) Evidence-based cognitive rehabilitation: updated review of the literature from 1998 through 2002. *Archives of Physical Medicine and Rehabilitation,* **86**, 1681–1692.

2 Cicerone, K.D., Dahlberg, C., Kalmar, K., *et al.* (2000) Evidence-based cognitive rehabilitation: recommendations for clinical practice. *Archives of Physical Medicine and Rehabilitation,* **81**, 1596–1615.

3 Cicerone, K.D., Langenbahn, D.M., Braden, C., *et al.* (2011) Evidence-based cognitive rehabilitation: updated review of literature from 2003 through 2008. *Archives of Physical Medecine of Rehabilitation,* **92**, 519–530.

4 Azouvi, P., Vallat-Azouvi, C., & Belmont, A. (2009). Cognitive deficits after traumatic coma. *Progress in Brain Research,* **177**, 89–110.

5 Masson, F., Maurette, P., Salmi, L.R. *et al.* (1996) Prevalence of impairments 5 years after a head injury, and relationship with disabilities and outcome. *Brain Injury,* **10**, 487–497.

6 Brooks, D.N., & McKinlay, W.W. (1983) Personality and behavioural change after severe blunt head injury: a relative's view. *Journal of Neurology, Neurosurgery and Psychiatry,* **46**, 336–344.

7 Prigatano, G.P., & Altman, I.M. (1990) Impaired awareness of behavioral limitations after traumatic brain injury. *Archives of Physical Medicine and Rehabilitation,* **71**, 1058–1064.

8 Ziino, C., & Ponsford, J. (2005) Measurement and prediction of subjective fatigue following traumatic brain injury. *Journal of the International Neuropsychological Society,* **11**, 416–425.

9 Belmont, A., Agar, N., & Azouvi, P. (2009) Subjective fatigue, mental effort, and attention deficits after severe traumatic brain injury. *Neurorehabilitation and Neural Repair,* **23**, 939–944.

10 Brooks, D.N., Campsie, L., Symington, C., Beattie, A., & MacKinlay W. (1986) The five year outcome of severe blunt head injury: a relative's view. *Journal of Neurology, Neurosurgery and Psychiatry,* **49**, 764–770.

11 Russel, W.R., & Smith, A. (1961) Post traumatic amnesia in closed head injury. *Archives of Neurology,* **5**, 16–29.

12 van Zomeren, A.H., & van den Burg, W. (1985) Residual complaints of patients two years after severe head injury. *Journal of Neurology, Neurosurgery, and Psychiatry,* **48**, 21–28.

13 Vakil, E. (2005) The effect of moderate to severe traumatic brain injury (TBI) on different aspects of memory: a selective review. *Journal of Clinical and Experimental Neuropsychology,* **27**, 977–1021.

14 Brooks, D.N. (1976) Wechsler Memory Scale performance and its relationship to brain damage after severe closed head injury. *Journal of Neurology, Neurosurgery and Psychiatry,* **39**, 593–601.

15 Zec, R.F., Zellers, D., Belman, J. *et al.* (2001) Long-term consequences of severe closed head injury on episodic memory. *Journal of Clinical and Experimental Neuropsychology,* **23**, 671–691.

16 Levin, H.S., Grossman, R.G., Rose, J.E., & Teasdale, G. (1979) Long-term neuropsychological outcome of closed head injury. *Journal of Neurosurgery,* **50**, 412–422.

17 Vanderploeg, R.D., Crowell, T.A., & Curtiss, G. (2001) Verbal learning and memory deficits in traumatic brain injury: encoding, consolidation, and retrieval. *Journal of Clinical and Experimental Neuropsychology,* **23**, 185–195.

18 Crosson, B., Novack, T.A., Trenerry, M.R., & Craig, P.L. (1988) California Verbal Learning Test (CVLT) performance in severely head-injured and neurologically normal adult males. *Journal of Clinical and Experimental Neuropsychology,* **10**, 754–768.

19 Levin, H.S. (1989) Memory deficit after closed head injury. *Journal of Clinical and Experimental Neuropsychology.* **12**, 129–153.

20 Levin, H.S., High, W.M., Meyers, C.A., Von Laufen, A., Hayden, M.E., & Eisenberg, H.M. (1985) Impairment of remote memory after closed head injury. *Journal of Neurology, Neurosurgery and Psychiatry*, **48**, 556–563.

21 Piolino, P., Desgranges, B., Manning, L., North, P., Jokic, C., & Eustache, F. (2007) Autobiographical memory, the sense of recollection and executive functions after severe traumatic brain injury. *Cortex*, **43**, 176–195.

22 Baddeley, A.D. (1986) *Working Memory*. Oxford University Press, New York.

23 Vallat-Azouvi, C., Weber, T., Legrand, L., & Azouvi, P. (2007) Working memory after severe traumatic brain injury. *Journal of the International Neuropsychological Society*, **13**, 770–780.

24 van Zomeren, A.H., & Brouwer, W.H. (1994) *Clinical Neuropsychology of Attention*. Oxford University Press, New York.

25 Ponsford, J., & Kinsella, G. (1992) Attentional deficits following severe closed head injury. *Journal of Clinical and Experimental Neuropsychology*, **14**, 822–838.

26 Azouvi, P., Couillet, J., Leclercq, M., Martin, Y., Asloun, S., & Rousseaux, M. (2004) Divided attention and mental effort after severe traumatic brain injury. *Neuropsychologia*, **42**, 1260–1268.

27 Azouvi, P., Jokic, C., Van der Linden, M., Marlier, N., & Bussel, B. (1996) Working memory and supervisory control after severe closed head injury. A study of dual task performance and random generation. *Journal of Clinical and Experimental Neuropsychology*, **18**, 317–337.

28 Leclercq, M., Couillet, J., & Azouvi, P., *et al.* (2000) Dual task performance after severe diffuse traumatic brain injury or vascular prefrontal damage. *Journal of Clinical and Experimental Neuropsychology*, **22**, 339–350.

29 McDowell, S., Whyte, J., & D'Esposito, M. (1997) Working memory impairments in traumatic brain injury: evidence from a dual-task paradigm. *Neuropsychologia*, **35**, 1341–1353.

30 Park, N.W., Moscovitch, M., Robertson, I.H. (1999) Divided attention impairments after traumatic brain injury. *Neuropsychologia*, **37**, 1119–1133.

31 Van Zomeren, A.H., Brouwer, W.H., & Deelman, B.G. (1984) Attentional deficits: the riddles of selectivity, speed, and alertness. In: D. Brooks (ed). *Closed Head Injury: Psychological, Social and Family Consequences*, pp. 74–107. Oxford University Press, Oxford.

32 Ziino, C., & Ponsford, J. (2006) Vigilance and fatigue following traumatic brain injury. *Journal of the International Neuropsychological Society*, **12**, 100–110.

33 Ziino, C., & Ponsford, J. (2006) Selective attention deficits and subjective fatigue following traumatic brain injury. *Neuropsychology*, **20**, 383–390.

34 Shallice, T. (1988) *From Neuropsychology to Mental Structure*. Cambridge University Press, Cambridge.

35 Burgess, P.W., Alderman, N., Evans, J., Emslie, H., & Wilson, B. (1998) The ecological validity of tests of executive function. *Journal of the International Neuropsychological Society*, **4**, 547–558.

36 Wood, R.L., & Liossi, C. (2006) The ecological validity of executive tests in a severely brain injured sample. *Archives of Clinical Neuropsychology*, **21**, 429–437.

37 Chevignard, M., Pillon, B., Pradat-Diehl, P., *et al.* (2000) An ecological approach to planning dysfunction: script execution. *Cortex*, **36**, 649–669.

38 Mandleberg, I.A., & Brooks, D.N. (1975) Cognitive recovery after severe head injury. 1. Serial testing on the Wechsler Adult Intelligence Scale. *Journal of Neurology, Neurosurgery and Psychiatry*, **38**, 1121–1126.

39 Axelrod, B.N., Fichtenberg, N.L., Liethen, P.C., Czarnota, M.A., & Stucky, K. (2001) Performance characteristics of postacute traumatic brain injury patients on the WAIS-III and WMS-III. *Clinical Neuropsychology*, **15**, 516–520.

40 Luria, A.R., & Tsvetkova, L.S. (1967) *Les troubles de la résolution de problèmes*. Gauthier Villars, Paris.

41 Cicerone, K.D., & Wood, J.C. (1987) Planning disorder after closed head injury: a case study. *Archives of Physical Medicine and Rehabilitation*, **68**, 111–115.

42 Von Cramon, D.Y., Matthes-Von Cramon, G., & Mai, N. (1991) Problem-solving deficits in brain-injured patients: a therapeutic approach. *Neuropsychological Rehabilitation*, **1**, 45–64.

43 Von Cramon, D.Y., & Matthes-Von Cramon, G. (1994) Back to work with a chronic dysexecutive syndrome? (a case report). *Neuropsychological Rehabilitation*, **14**, 399–417.

44 Rath, J.F., Simon, D., Langenbahn, D.M., Sherr, R.L., & Diller, L. (2003) Group treatment of problem solving deficits in outpatients with traumatic brain injury: a randomised outcome study. *Neuropsychological Rehabilitation*, **13**, 461–488.

45 Levine, B., Robertson, I.H., Clare, L. *et al.* (2000) Rehabilitation of executive functioning: an experimental-clinical validation of goal management training. *Journal of the International Neuropsychological Society*, **6**, 299–312.

46 Duncan, J. (1986) Disorganization of behaviour after frontal lobe damage. *Cognitive Neuropsychology*, **37**, 271–290.

47 Spikman, J.M., Boelen, D.H., Lamberts, K.F., Brouwer, W.H., & Fasotti, L. (2010) Effects of a multifaceted treatment program for executive dysfunction after acquired brain injury on indications of executive functioning in daily life. *Journal of the International Neuropsychological Society*, **16**, 118–129.

48 Manly, T., Hawkins, K., Evans, J., Woldt. K., & Robertson, I.H. (2002) Rehabilitation of executive function: facilitation of effective goal management on complex tasks using periodic auditory alerts. *Neuropsychologia*, **40**, 271–281.

49 Fasotti, L., Kovacs, F., Eling, P.A.T.M., & Brouwer, W.H. (2000) Time pressure management as a compensatory strategy training after closed head injury. *Neuropsychological Rehabilitation*, **10**, 47–65.

50 Alderman, N., Fry, R.K., & Youngson, H.A. (1995) Improvement of self-monitoring skills, reduction of behavior disturbance and the dysexecutive syndrome. *Neuropsychological Rehabilitation*, **5**, 193–222.

51 Alderman, N., & Ward, A. (1991) Behavioural treatment of the dysexecutive syndrome: reduction of repetitive speech using response cost and cognitive overlearning. *Neuropsychological Rehabilitation*, **1**, 65–80.

52 Medd, J., & Tate, R.L. (2000) Evaluation of an anger management therapy programme following ABI: a preliminary study. *Neuropsychological Rehabilitation*, **10**, 185–201.

53 Ownsworth, T.L., McFarland, K., & Young, R.M. (2000) Self-awareness and psychosocial functioning following acquired brain injury: An evaluation of a group support programme. *Neuropsychological Rehabilitation*, **10**, 465–484.

54 Ponsford, J. (2008) Rehabilitation of attention following traumatic brain injury. In: D.T. Stuss, G. Winocur, I.H. Robertson (eds), *Cognitive Neuro-rehabilitation, Second Edition Evidence and Application*, pp. 507–521. Cambridge University Press, Cambridge.

55 Sohlberg, M.M., & Mateer, C.A. (1987) Effectiveness of an attention training program. *Journal of Clinical and Experimental Neuropsychology*, **9**, 117–130.

56 Ponsford, J.L., & Kinsella, G. (1988) Evaluation of a remedial programme for attentional deficits following closed-head injury. *Journal of Clinical and Experimental Neuropsychology*, **10**, 693–708.

57 Park, N.W., & Ingles, J.L. (2001) Effectiveness of attention rehabilitation after an acquired brain injury: a meta-analysis. *Neuropsychology*, **15**, 199–210.

58 Leclercq M, Azouvi P. (2002) Attention after traumatic brain injury. In: M. Leclercq, & P. Zimmermann (eds). *Applied Neuropsychology of Attention*, pp. 251–73. Psychology Press, Hove.

59 Sturm, W., Willmes, K., Orgass, B., & Hartje, W. (1997) Do specific attention deficits need specific training ? *Neuropsychological Rehabilitation*, **7**, 81–103.

60 Sturm, W., Fimm, B., Cantagallo, A. *et al.* (2002) Computerized training of specific attention deficits in stroke and traumatic brain-injured patients: a multicentric efficacy study. In: M. Leclercq, & P. Zimmermann (eds), *Applied Neuropsychology of Attention*, pp. 365–380. Psychology Press, London.

61 Evans, J.J., Greenfield, E., Wilson, B.A., & Bateman, A. (2009) Walking and talking therapy: improving cognitive-motor dual-tasking in neurological illness. *Journal of the International Neuropsychological Society*, **15**, 112–120.

62 Couillet, J., Soury, S., Lebornec, G. *et al.* (2010) Rehabilitation of divided attention after severe traumatic brain injury: a randomised trial. *Neuropsychological Rehabilitation*, **20**, 321–339.

63 Klingberg, T., Fernell, E., Olesen, P.J. *et al.* (2005) Computerized training of working memory in children with ADHD—a randomized, controlled trial. *Journal of the American Academy of Child and Adolescent Psychiatry*, **44**, 177–186.

64 Westerberg, H., Jacobaeus, H. Hirvikoski, T. *et al.* (2007) Computerized working memory training after stroke—a pilot study. *Brain Injury*, **21**, 21–29.

65 Vallat, C., Azouvi, P., Hardisson, H., Meffert, R., Tessier, C., & Pradat-Diehl, P. (2005) Rehabilitation of verbal working memory after left hemisphere stroke. *Brain Injury*, **19**, 1157–1164.

66 Duval, J., Coyette, F., & Seron, X. (2008) Rehabilitation of the central executive component of working memory: a re-organisation approach applied to a single case. *Neuropsychological Rehabilitation*, **1**, 430–460.

67 Olesen, P.J., Westerberg, H., & Klingberg, T. (2004) Increased prefrontal and parietal activity after training of working memory. *Nature Neuroscience*, **7**, 75–79.

68 Cicerone, K. (2002) Remediation of "working attention" in mild traumatic brain injury. *Brain Injury*, **16**, 185–195.

69 Serino, A., Ciaramelli, E., Santantonio, A.D., Malagu, S., Servadei, F., & Ladavas, E. (2007) A pilot study for rehabilitation of central executive deficits after traumatic brain injury. *Brain Injury*, **21**, 11–19.

70 Vallat-Azouvi, C., Pradat-Diehl, P., & Azouvi, P. (2009) Rehabilitation of the central executive of working memory after severe traumatic brain injury: two single-case studies. *Brain Injury*, **23**, 585–594.

71 Wilson, B.A. (2003) Rehabilitation of memory deficits. In: B.A. Wilson (ed). *Neuropsychological Rehabilitation: Theory and Practice*, pp. 71–87. Psychology Press, Hove.

72 Wilson, B.A., Emslie, H.C., Quirk, K., & Evans, J.J. (2001) Reducing everyday memory and planning problems by means of a paging system: a randomised control crossover study. *Journal of Neurology, Neurosurgery and Psychiatry*, **70**, 477–482.

73 Kaschel, R., Della Salla, S., Cantagallo, A., Fahlbock, A., Laaksonen, R., & Kazen, M. (2002) Imagery mnemonics for the rehabilitation of memory: a randomised group controlled trial. *Neuropsychological Rehabilitation*, **12**, 127–153.

74 Ownsworth, T.L., & McFarland, K. (1999) Memory remediation in long-term acquired brain injury: two approaches in diary training. *Brain Injury*, **13**, 605–626.

75 Baddeley, A., & Wilson, B.A. (1994) When implicit learning fails: amnesia and the problem of error elimination. *Neuropsychologia*, **32**, 53–68.

76 Wilson, B.A., Baddeley, A., Evans, J.J., & Shiel, A. (1994) Errorless learning in the rehabilitation of memory impaired people. *Neuropsychological Rehabilitation*, **4**, 307–326.

77 Ben-Yishay, Y., & Gold, J. (1990) Therapeutic milieu approach to neuropsychological rehabilitation. In: R.L. Wood (ed). *Neurobehavioural Sequelae of Traumatic Brain Injury*, pp. 194–215. Taylor, & Francis, New York.

78 Prigatano, G.P., Fordyce, D.J., Zeiner, H.K., Roueche, J.R., Pepping, M., & Wood, B.C. (1984) Neuropsychological rehabilitation after closed head injury in young adults. *Journal of Neurology, Neurosurgery and Psychiatry*, **47**, 505–513.

79 Salazar, A.M., Warden, D.L., Schwab, K. *et al.* (2000) Cognitive rehabilitation for traumatic brain injury: a randomized trial. Defense and Veterans Head Injury Program (DVHIP) Study Group. *Journal of American Medical Association*, **283**, 3075–3081.

80 Powell, J., Heslin, J., & Greenwood, R. (2002) Community based rehabilitation after severe traumatic brain injury: a randomised controlled trial. *Journal of Neurology, Neurosurgery, and Psychiatry*, **72**, 193–202.

81 NIH. (1999) Consensus conference: rehabilitation of persons with traumatic brain injury. *Journal of American Medical Association,*. **282**, 974–983.

82 Rohling, M.L., Faust, M.E., Beverly, B., & Demakis, G. (2009) Effectiveness of cognitive rehabilitation following acquired brain injury: a meta-analytic re-examination of Cicerone *et al.'s* (2000, 2005) systematic reviews. *Neuropsychology*, **23**, 20–39.

83 Kennedy, M.R., Coelho, C., Turkstra, L. *et al.* (2008) Intervention for executive functions after traumatic brain injury: a systematic review, meta-analysis and clinical recommendations. *Neuropsychological Rehabilitation*, **18**, 257–299.

84 Webb, P.M., & Gluecauf, R.L. (1994) The effects of direct involvement in goal setting on rehabilitation outcome for persons with traumatic brain injuries. *Rehabilitation Psychology*, **39**, 179–188.

PART V

Postacute care and community in reintegration

CHAPTER 10

Epidemiology of traumatic brain injury

Ramon Diaz-Arrastia and Kimbra Kenney

Center for Neuroscience and Regenerative Medicine, Uniformed Services University of the Health Sciences, Bethesda, MD, USA

Traumatic brain injury (TBI) is among the oldest and most common medical afflictions affecting humankind. Injuries to the cranium are commonly found in skeletal remains of prehistoric humans. While some of these injuries occurred in the perimortem period, the majority are healed skull fractures, a consequence of nonlethal head injuries from which the victims survived for many months and years. Between 10 and 50% of skulls of prehistoric humans show evidence of cranial trauma [1, 2], with the higher number corresponding to times of climactic stress and political instability. Since most cranial trauma does not result in skull fractures, this number represents an underestimate of the true prevalence of TBI in our ancestors. It is likely that most of these injuries were a consequence of warfare, as high levels of interpersonal violence were a universal feature of early human civilizations. However, it is also likely that many of these TBIs were accidental and occurred during hunting or otherwise interacting with a harsh environment. TBI remains a common and frequently disabling feature of modern life in industrialized as well-industrializing societies. This chapter discusses the existing data on incidence of TBI, most of which comes from industrialized nations, but evolving evidence from developing countries is also included. Recent trends related to a decline in traffic-related injuries and an increase in fall-related injuries in the elderly are highlighted. Additionally, more recent information on lifetime prevalence of TBI is reviewed, as it is becoming apparent that consequences of brain trauma manifest over many years [3]. As elsewhere in this book, this information is presented with a focus on information relevant to practicing clinicians encountering patients with TBI in different medical settings.

Traumatic Brain Injury, First Edition. Edited by Pieter E. Vos and Ramon Diaz-Arrastia.

Incidence of TBI

In the USA, the Centers for Disease Control and Prevention have carried out surveillance studies of TBI incidence using standardized case definitions and methods of data collection for the past two decades [4, 5]. The most readily ascertained data are collected from the National Ambulatory Medical Care Survey (NAMCS), the National Hospital Discharge Survey (NHDS), and the National Vital Statistics System and focus on emergency department (ED) visits, hospitalizations, and deaths. The most recent data indicate that each year 1.37 million Americans are treated and released from an ED, 275 000 are hospitalized and discharged alive, and 52 000 die as a consequence of TBI [5]. It is further estimated that TBI is a contributing factor in a third (30.5%) of all injury-related deaths in the USA. It is more difficult to estimate how many individuals are seen in outpatient departments and office-based clinical settings, but recent estimates using National Hospital Ambulatory Medical Care survey and NAMCS data indicate that an additional 84 000 patients with TBI are seen annually in hospital outpatient departments and 1 080 000 are seen by office-based physicians and in community health clinics. Thus, the total number of TBIs for which individuals seek medical attention in the USA annually approaches 3.5 million [6].

Data from other developed countries are comparable to US data. Age-adjusted incidence rates in the USA (per 100 000 population) are 468 for ED visits, 93.6 for hospitalizations, and 17.4 for deaths. A systematic review of European data [7] identified rates (per 100 000) of 235 for ED visits and 15 for TBI-related mortality. Similar rates are reported from Australia [8] and Sweden [9]. Differences in rates are likely due in part to differences between countries in case ascertainment procedures and definitions. However, part of the difference is also likely due to differences in socioeconomic status, transportation and safety regulation, and the delivery of emergency medical services. Within the USA, there are wide differences among states in reported rates of hospital discharges for TBI, with a high of 99 per 100 000 in Maryland to a low of 52 per 100 000 in Rhode Island [10]. This variation is mostly accounted for by discordant rates of TBI among different American ethnic groups [11].

Epidemiologic data from low- and middle-income countries are incomplete. Many nations, particularly developing countries, do not have systematic hospital registration and reporting systems. Trauma registries and surveillance programs are in their infancy in most of the developing world. However, reviews of available data [12] indicate that TBIs due to motor vehicle accidents are significantly higher in Latin America and sub-Saharan Africa, primarily due to underdeveloped road and transportation systems.

The vast majority of these injuries are classified as *mild*, although it is recognized that the traditional definitions of mild, moderate, and severe TBI leave much to be desired and are not well suited for epidemiologic studies. It is also clear that the term *mild* does not mean inconsequential and that some mild TBIs result in significant and disabling long-term deficits. The magnitude of deficits resulting from mild TBI remains to be determined in carefully conducted, population-based studies.

Trends in incidence

One of the more gratifying trends of modern life has been a striking reduction in mortality from TBI resulting from motor vehicle accidents over the past four decades, at least in developed countries [13]. The experience of Australia is typical. Between 1970 and 1995 there was a reduction in fatalities from traffic accidents of 47%, despite a 40% increase in population and a 140% increase in the number of motor vehicles. Fatalities per registered vehicle fell over fourfold during that period, from 8.05 to 1.84% [14], and the fatality rate per billion kilometers traveled fell by 90% from 1960 to 2010 [15]. This primarily reflects increased use of safety devices (seat belts, airbags, motorcycle and bicycle helmets, child safety seats) and other improvements in road and automotive engineering, as well as improved enforcement of traffic laws, particularly those against driving while intoxicated [16]. It is also likely that improvements in medical care, both pre- and in-hospital, played a role. A retrospective review of neurosurgical databases in the USA found that mortality from severe TBI declined from 39 to 27% from 1984 to 1996 [17].

However, as the population ages throughout the world, particularly in developed countries, fatalities from TBI in individuals aged greater than 75 years have largely counterbalanced the recent decrease in deaths from road traffic accidents [18]. In the elderly, most TBIs result primarily from falls, and while these injuries are usually classified as mild, they often result in significant disability and even death.

Figure 10.1 represents CDC data [5] for TBI-related ED visits, hospitalizations, and death, by cause and age. In early life (before age 10), falls are the predominant cause of TBI requiring medical attention, and most of these are mild injuries that do not require hospitalization and rarely result in death. In adolescence and young adulthood, motor vehicle accidents predominate, and these are frequently severe injuries that often require hospitalization and are associated with high death rates. Finally, in late life (>65 years), falls are again the predominant mechanism, but in the elderly, hospitalization and death rates are high.

Prevalence of TBI

While high-quality and generally consistent data are available to estimate TBI incidence rates, at least in industrialized countries, much less is known about lifetime history or lifetime occurrence of TBI [11]. This is particularly important given the recent recognition of long-term and often delayed effects of neurotrauma [19, 20], as well as the appreciation that multiple brain injuries have an additive effect.

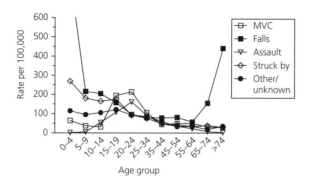

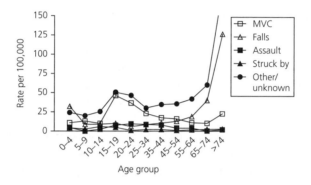

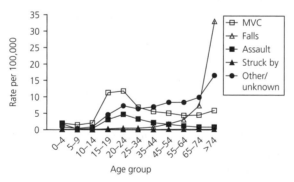

Figure 10.1 TBI-related ED visits (a), hospitalization (b), and deaths (c) by cause and age. Adapted from Ref. 5.

The Christchurch Health and Development Study (CHDS) is perhaps the best prospective, population-based study of the prevalence of TBI [21]. The CHDS enrolled 1265 children born in the municipality of Christchurch (New Zealand) in mid-1977. This number represents 97% of all births in Christchurch during the recruitment period. Participants were studied at birth, 4 months, 1 year, and annually until age 16 and then again at ages 18, 21, and 25. By age 25, the cohort consisted of 1003 participants (a loss to follow-up rate of only 21.7%). Data were gathered using multiple sources of information, including parental interview, subject self-report, teacher questionnaire, psychometric assessments, medical and hospital records, and other official records. Information about TBI was obtained at each visit through self-report and parental report, and all inpatient or outpatient hospital admissions were verified against hospital records. A total of 458 TBI events were identified from birth to 25 years in this cohort, of which 33% resulted in admission to the hospital for observation or inpatient care. The overall prevalence of TBI from birth to age 25 years was 32%, and the prevalence of injuries sufficiently severe to warrant an inpatient stay of at least one night was 12%.

A second birth cohort study that analyzed TBI prevalence was carried out in Northern Finland [22]. The Northern Finland Birth Cohort studied 12 058 residents of Oulu and Lapland provinces born in 1966. Diagnostic codes were extracted from the Finnish Hospital Discharge Registry and the Registry of Causes of Death. Outpatient visits and ED visits shorter than 24 h were not included. In this study, 3.8% of the cohort had experienced at least one hospitalization for TBI. Differences between the Finnish and the New Zealand study are likely a result of the less rigorous case ascertainment procedures used in Finland.

A retrospective but population-based study of TBI prevalence was recently carried out in the state of Colorado in the USA [23]; 2701 residents of that state participated in a random-digit-dialed computer-assisted telephone interview, which adapted the Ohio State University TBI Identification Method (OSU TBI-ID) [24]. The OSU TBI-ID is a structured questionnaire that has been validated in multiple populations as a tool for identifying lifetime TBI exposures. In this study, 24% of the sample reported one or more TBIs with loss of consciousness, and an additional 14% reported one of more TBIs without loss of consciousness. Of the 38% reporting one or more TBIs, 24% report having been hospitalized, yielding a hospitalization rate of 9%, which is comparable to the Christchurch results despite substantially different methodology.

Prevalence of disability after TBI

A second critical area in which the epidemiology is still evolving is the prevalence of long-term disability after TBI. Such estimates are of fundamental importance to policymakers and service providers to ensure adequate resources for lifelong needs of people living with TBI-related disabilities. An initial estimate based on a CDC working paper (Guerrero *et al.*, unpublished) indicated that 5.3 million Americans in 1996 were living with long-term disabilities after TBI. More recent estimates using improved methodology have revised that estimate [25]. This study used a logistic regression model developed using a population-based sample of persons with TBI from the South Carolina Traumatic Brain Injury Follow-up Registry [26] hospitalization data to estimate TBI-related long-term disability incidence by year, gender, and age for the period from 1979 to 2004. The model incorporated several potential predictors such as injury severity, mechanism, age, gender, and preexisting comorbidities, with empirically observed disability. The equation coefficients were applied to NHDS data from 1979 to 2004, and prevalence rates adjusted for life expectancy. This study concluded that 3.17 million people (95% confidence interval (CI) 3.02–3.32 million), approximately 1.1% of the US civilian population, were living with long-term disabilities resulting from TBI.

While this estimate is useful in planning for the provision of rehabilitation services and caregiving, it likely underrepresents the true prevalence of TBI-associated disability, since many of the long-term consequences of brain injury manifest years after the trauma and may not be ascribed to the TBI. For example, in the CHDS study described earlier, hospitalization for TBI during the preschool years was associated with increased risk of psychiatric symptoms manifesting during adolescence (age 14–16 years) [27]. The odds ratio (OR) for symptoms of attention-deficit/hyperactivity disorder was 4.2, for substance abuse disorder was 3.6, for mood disorder 3.1, and for conduct disorder/oppositional defiant disorder 6.2.

Late-life dementia is another recognized consequence of early or midlife TBI [28]. Plassman *et al.* [29] identified 548 US Navy and Marine veterans hospitalized for TBI in the Pacific theater during World War II. Controls were 1228 veterans hospitalized for non-TBI injuries at the same time period. Study subjects were evaluated by telephone interviews and clinical assessments 50 years after the injury. The veterans who had sustained a severe TBI (defined as loss of consciousness or posttraumatic amnesia lasting longer than 24 h) were more than four times as likely to have dementia compared to controls (hazard ratio [HR] 4.41 (95% CI 2.09–9.63), while those who had sustained a moderate TBI (defined as loss of consciousness or posttraumatic amnesia lasting longer than 30 min but <24 h) were at more than doubled risk (HR, 2.39; 95% CI, 1.24–4.58). In this study, no increased risk was evident for the veterans who suffered a mild TBI (loss of consciousness or posttraumatic amnesia fewer than 30 min), but such an association has been found in other similar studies. In the MIRAGE study [30], information on head injury was collected by interview of multiple informants and review of medical records; the OR for dementia was 4.0 (95% CI 2.9–5.5) for head injury with loss of consciousness and 2.0 (95% CI 1.5–2.7) for head injury without loss of consciousness. Available data allow a rough calculation of how much of the population's burden of dementia is attributable to TBI. Assuming that the cumulative lifetime incidence of TBI requiring hospitalization is 10%, a reasonable estimate based on the CHDS [21] and the Colorado population-based telephone survey [23], and given that the relative risk of dementia in individuals who suffered a TBI of sufficient severity as to require hospitalization ranges from

1.5-fold to threefold [29–31], the attributable risk of dementia due to TBI is in the range of 5–15% [32]. Given the high prevalence of dementia in aging industrialized societies, measures aimed at preventing TBI or at preventing the long-term consequences of brain injury are one of the most promising strategies for reducing the social burden of late-life dementia.

Conclusions and future directions

TBI is a defining feature of humankind and a common feature of modern life. Despite recent very gratifying reductions in TBIs related to motor vehicle accidents and interpersonal violence, trauma remains an important cause of morbidity and mortality, particularly in persons under the age of 45. Further, rapidly aging populations throughout the world present a special challenge, given the high and increasing rates of TBI in the elderly. Surveillance methods are in place in industrialized countries but remain to be established in low- and middle-income countries. However, even in wealthy countries, there is insufficient information regarding long-term outcomes and delayed chronic effects of TBI. Two issues are of particular importance. First is the need to better understand the relationship between childhood TBI and psychiatric and behavior disorders in adolescence and early adulthood. In the USA, the National Children's Study of environmental effects on child health and development represents an important opportunity to attain this goal. Second is the need to better understand the interaction between residual deficits after brain trauma and age-related neurodegeneration, an issue of particular importance as life expectancy increases throughout the world. Long-term cohort studies, utilizing platforms such as the TBI Model System of Care and the US Veterans Administration, will be needed to provide such information. This information is of fundamental importance to planners and policymakers, but it will also represent an opportunity for clinical investigations aimed at developing therapies designed to alter the natural history of outcome after TBI.

References

1 Tung, T.A. (2007) Trauma and violence in the Wari empire of the Peruvian Andes: warfare, raids, and ritual fights. *American Journal of Physical Anthropology*, **133**, 941–956.

2 Torres-Rouff, C. & Costa Junqueira, M.A. (2006) Interpersonal violence in prehistoric San Pedro de Atacama, Chile: behavioral implications of environmental stress. *American Journal of Physical Anthropology*, **130**, 60–70.

3 Masel, B.E. & Dewitt, D.S. (2010) Traumatic brain injury: a disease process, not an event. *Journal of Neurotrauma*, **27**, 1529–1540.

4 Adekoya, N., Thurman, D.J., White, D.D., & Webb, K.W. (2002) Surveillance for traumatic brain injury deaths—United States, 1989–1998. *MMWR Surveillance Summaries*, **51**, 1–14.

5 Faul, M., Xu, L., Wald, M.W., & Coronado, V.G. *Traumatic Brain Injury in the United States: Emergency Department Visits, Hospitalizations, and Deaths 2002–2006*, pp. 1–71, Centers for Disease Control and Prevention, National Center for Injury Prevention and Control, Atlanta, GA.

6 Coronado, V.G., McGuire, L.C., Sarmiento, K. *et al.* (2012) Trends in Traumatic Brain Injury in the U.S. and the public health response: 1995–2009. *Journal of Safety Research*, **43**, 299–307.

7 Tagliaferri, F., Compagnone, C., Korsic, M., Servadei, F., & Kraus, J. (2006) A systematic review of brain injury epidemiology in Europe. *Acta Neurochirurgica (Wien)*, **148**, 255–268.

8 Hillier, S.L., Hiller, J.E., & Metzer, J. (1997) Epidemiology of traumatic brain injury in South Australia. *Brain Injury*, **11**, 649–659.

9 Andersson, E.H., Bjorklund, R., Emanuelson, I., & Stalhammar, D. (2003) Epidemiology of traumatic brain injury: a population based study in western Sweden. *Acta Neurologica Scandinavica*, **107**, 256–259.

10 Langlois, J.A., Kegler, S.R., Butler, J.A., *et al.* (2003) Traumatic brain injury-related hospital discharges. Results from a 14-state surveillance system, 1997. *MMWR Surveillance Summary*, **52**, 1–20.

11 Corrigan, J.D., Selassie, A.W., & Orman, J.A. (2010) The epidemiology of traumatic brain injury. *The Journal of Head Trauma Rehabilitation*, **25**, 72–80.

12 Hyder, A.A., Wunderlich, C.A., Puvanachandra, P., Gururaj, G., & Kobusingye, O.C. (2007). The impact of traumatic brain injuries: a global perspective. *NeuroRehabilitation*, **22**, 341–353.

13 Peden, M., Scurfield, R., Sleet, D., *et al.* (2004) *World Report on Road Traffic Injury Prevention*. World Health Organization, Geneva, pp. 1–224.

14 Atkinson, L. & Merry, G. (2001) Advances in neurotrauma in Australia 1970–2000. *World Journal of Surgery*, **25**, 1224–1229.

15 Bureau of Infrastructure, Transport and Regional Economics (2010) Effectiveness of Measures to Reduce Road Fatality Rates. Australian Government. http://www.bitre.gov.au/publications/2010/files/is_039.pdf [accessed on November 1, 2014].

16 Reilly, P.L. (2012) Current evaluation of TBI epidemiology in an aging society with improved preventive measures. In: M.C. Morganti-Kossmann, R. Raghupathi, & A. Maas (eds), *Traumatic Brain and Spinal Cord Injury*, pp. 1–16. Cambridge University Press, New York.

17 Lu, J., Marmarou, A., Choi, S., Maas, A., Murray, G., & Steyerberg, E.W. (2005) Mortality from traumatic brain injury. *Acta Neurochirurgica Supplement*, **95**, 281–285.

18 Coronado, V.G., Xu, L., Basavaraju, S.V. *et al.* (2011) Surveillance for traumatic brain injury-related deaths—United States, 1997–2007. *MMWR Surveillance Summary*, **60**, 1–32.

19 Institute of Medicine Committee on Gulf War and Health (2009) Neurologic Outcomes. In: Institute of Medicine (ed), *Gulf War and Health. Volume 7. Long-Term Consequences of Traumatic Brain Injury*, pp. 197–264. National Academies Press, Washington, DC.

20 Institute of Medicine Committee on Gulf War and Health (2009) Psychiatric outcomes. In: Institute of Medicine (ed), *Gulf War and Health. Volume 7. Long-Term Consequences of Traumatic Brain Injury*, pp. 256–300. National Academies Press, Washington, DC.

21 McKinlay, A., Grace, R.C., Horwood, L.J., Fergusson, D.M., Ridder, E.M., & MacFarlane, M.R. (2008) Prevalence of traumatic brain injury among children, adolescents, and young adults: prospective evidence from a birth cohort. *Brain Injury*, **22**, 175–181.

22 Winqvist, S., Lehtilahti, M., Jokelainen, J., Luukinen, H., & Hillbom, M. (2007) Traumatic brain injuries in children and young adults: a birth cohort study from northern Finland. *Neuroepidemiology*, **29**, 136–142.

23 Whiteneck, G., Cuthbert, J., & Corrigan, J. D. (2012) *Lifetime history of traumatic brain injury in the general population and its relationship to outcomes. International Brain Injury Association 9th World Congress, Edinburgh*, March 21–25, 2012, Scotland.

24 Bogner, J. & Corrigan, J.D. (2009) Reliability and predictive validity of the Ohio State University TBI identification method with prisoners. *Journal of Head Trauma Rehabilitation*, **24**, 279–291.

25 Zaloshnja, E., Miller, T., Langlois, J.A., & Selassie, A.W. (2008) Prevalence of long-term disability from traumatic brain injury in the civilian population of the United States, 2005. *Journal of Head Trauma Rehabilitation*, **23**, 394–400.

26 Selassie, A.W., Zaloshnja, E., Langlois, J.A., Miller, T., Jones, P., & Steiner, C. (2008) Incidence of long-term disability following traumatic brain injury hospitalization, United States, 2003. *Journal of Head Trauma Rehabilitation*, **23**, 123–131.

27 McKinlay, A., Grace, R., Horwood, J., Fergusson, D., & MacFarlane, M. (2009) Adolescent psychiatric symptoms following preschool childhood mild traumatic brain injury: evidence from a birth cohort. *Journal of Head Trauma Rehabilitation*, **24**, 221–227.

28 Shively, S., Scher, A.I., Perl, D.P., & Diaz-Arrastia, R. (2012) Dementia resulting from traumatic brain injury: what is the pathology? *Archives of Neurology*, **69**(10), 1245–1251.

29 Plassman, B.L., Havlik, R.J., Steffens, D.C. *et al.* (2000) Documented head injury in early adulthood and risk of Alzheimer's disease and other dementias. *Neurology*, **55**, 1158–1166.

30 Guo, Z., Cupples, L.A., Kurz, A. *et al.* (2000) Head injury and risk of AD in the MIRAGE study. *Neurology*, **54**, 1316–1323.

31 Fleminger, S., Oliver, D.L., Lovestone, S., Rabe-Hesketh, S., & Giora, A. (2003) Head injury as a risk factor for Alzheimer's disease: the evidence 10 years on; a partial replication. *Journal of Neurology, Neurosurgery and Psychiatry*, **74**, 857–862.

32 Kahn, H.A. & Sempos, C.T. (1989) Attributable risk. In: *Statistical Methods in Epidemiology*, pp. 72–84. Oxford University Press, New York.

CHAPTER 11

Neuropsychiatric and behavioral sequelae

Kathleen F. Pagulayan[1,2] and Jesse R. Fann[2,3,4]

[1] VA Puget Sound Health Care System, University of Washington, Seattle, WA, USA
[2] Departments of Psychiatry and Behavioral Sciences, University of Washington, Seattle, WA, USA
[3] Departments of Rehabilitation Medicine, University of Washington, Seattle, WA, USA
[4] Departments of Epidemiology, University of Washington, Seattle, WA, USA

Neuropsychiatric symptoms and behavioral changes are significant contributors to disability following traumatic brain injury (TBI) [1]. The risk for developing a neuropsychiatric disorder increases after TBI, especially in the first year postinjury [2–4]. Due to the negative impact that these symptoms can have on rehabilitation and functional outcome [5], early diagnosis and treatment of these conditions is critical.

Assessment of psychiatric disorders following TBI: A biopsychosocial approach

Many factors contribute to the development and maintenance of postinjury psychiatric symptoms, including both preinjury characteristics (e.g., education, vocational history, psychiatric disorders) and postinjury functioning (e.g., injury-related disabilities, awareness of deficits) [6]. Comorbid conditions, preexisting psychiatric symptoms, and TBI-related cognitive impairment can complicate the clinical picture. Additional subthreshold psychiatric symptoms that detrimentally affect functioning may be present and should be monitored and potentially treated. The complexity and multifaceted nature of potential contributors to the clinical picture support the use of a biopsychosocial framework for assessment. This approach integrates injury-related factors with relevant psychiatric history, postinjury psychological adjustment, and the social impact of the injury (e.g., change in family, occupational/educational, or social functioning). Some critical elements of a post-TBI psychiatric evaluation are listed below.

Traumatic Brain Injury, First Edition. Edited by Pieter E. Vos and Ramon Diaz-Arrastia.

Relevant premorbid factors

Neurobehavioral and psychiatric symptoms after TBI likely represent the inter-action between premorbid conditions, personality characteristics, TBI-related changes in brain function, and reactions to postinjury functional changes. Race and ethnicity, age at time of injury, and preinjury alcohol use are important predictors of postinjury psychiatric symptoms [7]. In addition, preinjury educational and vocational attainment, social support, and involvement with the legal system provide a context for understanding current symptoms and their functional impact.

Emotional and behavioral functioning

Common behavioral sequelae include personality change, impulsivity, disinhibi-tion, reduced frustration tolerance, decreased motivation, and sleep disturbance. Current symptom levels and change from baseline should be evaluated. Common emotional changes include mood dysregulation, depression, irritability, anxiety, and apathy [8]. Restricted affect or expressive dysprosody can also occur and may result in an incongruence between verbally expressed emotion and affect [9]. In these cases, it is recommended that the provider focus on the content of the information being expressed. Many psychiatric symptoms overlap with TBI sequelae (e.g., sleep disturbances, concentration difficulties, psychomotor agita-tion/retardation), and this should be considered in the diagnostic process. In addition, rates of suicidal ideation, suicide attempts, and completed suicide are increased relative to the general population following TBI [10–13]. Finally, eval-uation of familial relationships and support systems, current psychosocial stressors, and coping mechanisms can be important for treatment planning.

Injury-related factors

Injury severity, brain regions affected, pain, and comorbid medical conditions (e.g., motor dysfunction, headaches, chronic pain from physical injuries, visual/sensory disturbances, hypothyroidism, seizures) can all contribute to the clinical picture.

Awareness of deficits/cognitive impairment

Reduced awareness of deficits is common after TBI, especially as injury severity increases [14]. This, as well as injury-related cognitive impairment, may limit the accuracy of self-reported psychiatric symptoms. In cases where this is a con-cern, collateral information can be used to evaluate current symptoms.

Risk factors

Premorbid psychiatric and substance abuse histories are strong risk factors for postinjury psychiatric symptoms, although individuals with no psychiatric his-tory are still at increased risk for developing symptoms [15]. Younger age, female gender, lower education, unstable preinjury employment, poorer functioning, and shorter time since injury have also been reported as risk factors, particularly for depression [6, 16–19], although these associations have not been present across all studies. Injury severity has not consistently been correlated with development of a psychiatric disorder [7, 16, 20].

Epidemiology, clinical presentation, and treatment

The most frequently occurring neuropsychiatric and behavioral conditions are presented in the following and summarized in Table 11.1. *Diagnostic and Statistical Manual of Mental Disorders*, Fourth Edition, (DSM-IV) criteria were used in the majority of the research summarized [22]. Of note, individuals with TBI often experience symptoms in more than one of these categories during the first year after their injury [7].

Depression

Major depression is the most common psychiatric disorder after TBI [23], with approximately 50% of hospitalized patients developing major depression within the first year postinjury [16]. Preinjury psychiatric illness significantly increases risk for postinjury depression [15]. Depression is associated with numerous negative outcomes, including reduced participation in rehabilitation, reduced overall functioning, and increased aggression and anxiety [5, 16, 24]. TBI is also associated with an increased risk for suicide attempt [10], especially when a psychiatric disorder and substance abuse are both present [25]. The presence of repeated TBIs may increase the risk for suicidal thoughts and behaviors as well [26]. Researchers have observed that major depressive disorder (MDD) may be more biologically determined soon after TBI [4]. Conversely, psychosocial factors, such as poor social support, family discord, and an unstable job situation, can be stronger determinants of MDD as time since injury increases [27]. In theory, pharmacotherapy, psychotherapy, and alternative approaches might be combined and balanced for individual circumstances, risk factors, and time postinjury.

Clinically, it is important to differentiate between the rapid mood fluctuations and emotional lability that can occur following TBI and a more prolonged, sustained depressed mood that would be suggestive of major depression [9]. DSM-IV diagnostic criteria for depression are applicable [28], but in patients with TBI, symptoms such as feeling hopeless and worthless, frustration, aggression, and difficulty enjoying activities may be the most useful in differentiating depressed and nondepressed individuals [29]. Assessment of suicide risk and protective factors can help identify individuals who may have increased risk for

Table 11.1 Core features, correlates and treatment of post-TBI psychiatric problems.

Psychiatric problems	Core features	Correlates	First-(and second)-line medication management
Major depression	Episodes of sadness, loss of pleasure, feelings of hopelessness or worthlessness, and suicidal thoughts, with or without psychosis	Lesions to left dorsolateral frontal and/or basal ganglia regions	Selective serotonin reuptake inhibitors (SSRIs)
		Poor pre-TBI psychosocial functioning	Tricyclic antidepressants (TCAs)
Mania	Episodes of irritability and/or elated mood, increased energy, impulsivity with or without psychosis	Lesions to temporal lobe and right orbitofrontal cortex	Valproate (lithium)
Psychosis	Loss of touch with reality, disorganized thought process, and presence of hallucinations and/or delusions	TBI prior to adolescence	Atypical antipsychotics (typical antipsychotics)
		Congenital neurological disorder	
		Frontal and temporal lesions	
Anxiety	Feeling of apprehension, panic or dread, with or without autonomic signs/symptoms	Lesions to the right hemisphere in anxious depression	SSRIs (short-term benzodiazepines)
	PTSD symptoms include reexperiencing the trauma, avoidant behavior, emotional numbing, and hypervigilance	PTSD more common with mild TBI	
Apathy	Lack of motivation and initiative in the absence of dysphoria	Damage to the mesial frontal lobe and its subcortical structures	Psychostimulants, dopamine agonists
Insomnia	Problems falling or staying asleep or early morning awakenings	Mild TBI, depression, anxiety, and pain	Sleep hygiene prior to initiation of medications
			Trazodone, mirtazapine (short-term sedative/hypnotic)
Anger/aggression	Verbal outbursts, physical assaults, property destruction	Preinjury substance abuse and aggressive behavior, frontal lobe injuries	Beta-blockers
			Valproate, SSRIs (antipsychotics in acute setting)

Source: Adapted with permission from Vaishnavi *et al.* [21]. © Elsevier.

self-harm and allow for the development of appropriate treatment to mitigate this risk [30]. Finally, apathy and fatigue are often associated with CNS impairment. These symptoms can occur concomitantly with or independently of depression [8, 31] and are often mistaken for primary depression [32]. Risk for depression remains elevated through the first year of recovery and possibly longer [16]. The average duration of depression in two studies was 4–5 months, although there was significant individual variability [4, 16]. Self-report measures such as the Patient Health Questionnaire-9 (PHQ-9) [33] and the Neurobehavioral Functioning Inventory—Depression Scale (NFI-D) [34] have been shown to be valid in TBI populations and may complement the clinical interview or serve as screening instruments.

Treatments

Empirical evidence for treatment of post-TBI depression is limited [35, 36]. The pharmacotherapy data do not provide definitive evidence of efficacy for any specific class of medications. The literature does suggest that we cannot assume that standard antidepressant medications will have the same efficacy and tolerability in persons with TBI as in persons without neurologic insult. However, few adverse effects were reported in studies of antidepressants, especially selective serotonin reuptake inhibitors (SSRIs), with the most severe adverse effects (e.g., seizures) and the most dropouts occurring with tricyclic antidepressants (TCAs). Some data suggest that antidepressants, especially TCAs and bupropion, are associated with an increased risk of seizures [37], a particular concern following severe TBI [38]; however, if the drugs are titrated cautiously, most patients will not experience increased seizures, particularly if they are taking an anticonvulsant [39]. Because of the potentially problematic adverse effects of TCAs and monoamine oxidase inhibitors (MAOIs) (e.g., sedation, hypotension, and anticholinergic effects) in patients with CNS impairment and their narrow therapeutic index (which can lead to inadvertent overdose in patients with cognitive impairment), these medications should be used with extreme caution in TBI patients.

Among the 27 studies meeting criteria for inclusion in a recent systematic review [35] there were only two evidence class I studies. The class I pharmacotherapy study [40] showed trends toward superiority of sertraline (25–200 mg/d) over placebo in a demographically heterogeneous sample that was temporally far removed from their TBI. Other SSRIs, such as citalopram, and serotonin–norepinephrine receptor inhibitors (SNRIs), such as venlafaxine, may also be effective, but more data are needed.

For apathy and fatigue, medications that augment dopaminergic activity appear to be the most useful [41]. Methylphenidate and dextroamphetamine are generally safe at standard dosages [42] (e.g., methylphenidate 10–30 mg/d in divided doses) and have been used successfully to enhance participation in rehabilitation. Therapeutic use of these oral psychostimulants in the medically ill rarely leads to abuse in patients without a personal or family history of substance abuse.

Modafinil has been efficacious in treating excessive daytime sleepiness in patients with TBI [43, 44]. Bupropion [41] and dopamine agonists, such as amantadine [45], bromocriptine [46], and levodopa/carbidopa [47], have been used for apathy states, fatigue, and cognitive impairment. Stimulants and dopamine agonists can increase the risk for delirium and psychosis and thus should be used with caution in more vulnerable patients. Amantadine has been associated with an increased risk of seizures [48], but methylphenidate, dextroamphetamine, and bromocriptine do not appear to lower seizure threshold at typical doses.

Preliminary evidence supports the use of cognitive behavioral therapy (CBT) for depression following TBI [49, 50]. Problem-solving and behavioral activation approaches delivered via regular phone interventions in the first year postinjury may also be effective in reducing depressive symptoms [51]. Patients may prefer physical exercise as a therapeutic intervention [52] and there is some evidence that higher levels of exercise may be associated with improvements in mood, sleep, and overall quality of life [53, 54]. There are also limited data supporting the efficacy and tolerability of electroconvulsive therapy (ECT), low-intensity magnetic field exposure, biofeedback, and acupuncture for treating depression after TBI [35]. However, the narrowly selected and small samples and divergent TBI severity and proximity characteristics make these results highly preliminary.

Mania

Overall, TBI does not appear to significantly increase the risk of mania [55], except for possibly in the first year postinjury. One study closely tracked individuals after their injury and found that 9% of their sample met diagnostic criteria for mania within 12 months of the injury but that symptoms lasted 2 months on average and resolved over time [56]. Lower estimates, ranging from 0% to 2%, have been found in studies evaluating the presence of psychiatric disorders multiple years postinjury (e.g., 2–30 years) [10, 23, 24, 57].

Treatment

The best evidence for treatment of manic symptoms in TBI consists of case series, with positive results for lithium (at 900 mg/d) [58], valproate (up to 750–1000 mg/d) [59], clonidine (150–600 µg/d) [60], ECT [61], and thioridazine (50 mg/d) with amitriptyline (100 mg/d) [61]. A reasonable approach is to use valproate as a first-line agent due to the evidence for efficacy and relatively low side effect risks. Lithium should be a second-line agent because it can lower the seizure threshold and TBI patients are more prone to seizures already [21]. Additionally, lithium has a narrow therapeutic index, and TBI patients may be particularly prone to neurotoxic effects due to lack of self-care (such as not hydrating properly) and difficulty with dose adherence.

Anxiety disorders, obsessive–compulsive disorder, and trauma- and stressor-related disorders

Anxiety frequently presents along with depression [16] and can range from mild mood changes to disabling symptoms such as severe panic and agoraphobia [62]. Symptoms can occur at any point postinjury but may increase at critical time points such as hospital discharge, return to school or work, anniversary of injury, or changes in rehabilitation (e.g., introduction of new skill or alteration of routine). Clinical differentiation between brief symptoms that present in response to specific triggers and the more persistent debilitating symptoms is important.

Acute stress disorder/posttraumatic stress disorder

Acute stress disorder (ASD) and posttraumatic stress disorder (PTSD) are disorders that develop in response to a traumatic event. In the DSM-IV, these were considered anxiety disorders. However, in the recently released DSM-5, ASD and PTSD are classified as trauma- and stressor-related disorders, and the diagnostic criteria have been modified. At present, there is minimal research in TBI on the updated DSM-5 criteria, so the information presented in the following summarizes the literature regarding ASD and PTSD according to DSM-IV criteria. Both disorders involve exposure to a traumatic event followed by the presence of reexperiencing, avoidance, and hyperarousal symptoms. ASD also involves dissociative symptoms. In ASD, the symptoms are present for 2 days to 4 weeks, while in PTSD the symptoms are present for at least 1 month. ASD occurs in approximately 4.5–13% of individuals with mild TBI (mTBI) [63, 64]; in this population, high endorsement of postconcussive symptoms that overlap with ASD is common (e.g., sleep disturbance, irritability, and poor concentration) [64]. Prevalence of ASD in more severely injured individuals is not well documented. ASD after mTBI is a significant predictor of later PTSD [65], and early treatment can reduce or prevent the development of PTSD [66].

PTSD can occur after TBI of all severities, with prevalence estimates ranging from 12 to 27% in the first year postinjury [67, 68]. Posttraumatic amnesia (PTA) and loss of consciousness (LOC) may have a protective role against the development of PTSD [69]. Risk factors for PTSD include postinjury ASD, recall of the traumatic event, assault-related injury, intoxication at time of injury, and history of psychiatric illness [69, 70]. Similar to ASD, the symptom overlap between some TBI and PTSD symptoms can cause diagnostic challenges. Avoidance and hyperarousal symptoms may be prominent, while reexperiencing symptoms are less common among those with PTA [69]. If present, the reexperiencing symptoms may relate to events surrounding the injury, such as being rescued or the postinjury hospitalization, as opposed to the injury itself [71]. Self-report measures such as the PTSD checklist can be useful but may overestimate the prevalence of PTSD due to the overlap between some PTSD and TBI symptoms [72].

Generalized anxiety disorder

Generalized anxiety disorder (GAD) involves at least 6 months of excessive anxiety and worry that interferes with daily functioning and is associated with symptoms such as fatigue, difficulty concentrating, irritability, muscle tension, restlessness or psychomotor agitation, and impaired sleep. Many of these symptoms overlap with TBI-related sequelae, so examination of their association with anxiety symptoms is needed for accurate diagnosis. The prevalence of GAD in TBI samples is around 10–15% [2, 73, 74]. High rates of GAD have been documented up to 15 years postinjury [23, 75]. The GAD-7 [76] and Brief Symptom Inventory [77] may be useful for assessing anxiety symptoms.

Panic disorder

Panic disorder has been documented following TBI of all severities, with estimates ranging from approximately 7 to 15% [23, 78]. Clinically, it may present as a sudden onset of increased anxiety accompanied by autonomic response (e.g., agitation, sweating, shaking, shortness of breath, chest pain). Many individuals with postinjury panic disorder did not have a prior history of that condition [79]. Although panic disorder has been documented soon after the injury, one study found a latency period of over 10 years in most cases where panic disorder developed after TBI [57].

Obsessive–compulsive disorder

Obsessive–compulsive disorder (OCD) involves the presence of recurrent disabling obsessions and/or compulsions. OCD has been documented following TBI of all severities [80, 81], but prevalence rates at 1 year postinjury are low, ranging from less than 1 to 4% [74, 78]. Comorbid mood and anxiety disorders are common [81]. Diagnosis can be challenging in individuals with TBI because differentiating between obsessive–compulsive behaviors and neurologically driven perseveration or repetition due to poor memory may be difficult [82]. Checking and repetitive behaviors that require a significant amount of time and interfere with daily functioning should raise concern about the possibility of OCD [82].

Treatment of anxiety disorders, OCD, and trauma-and stressor-related disorders

Benzodiazepines are not recommended for long-term use because TBI patients may be more susceptible to potential adverse reactions and they may actually cause a paradoxical agitation in these patients [83]. However, benzodiazepines may be effective for short-term treatment for acute anxiety, particularly in the first few weeks after injury. They should be initiated at lower doses because they may exacerbate or cause cognitive impairment and sedation. Sedating medications are of particular concern in TBI because they may impair mobility and cognition and interfere with rehabilitation, particularly if the patient is taking multiple central nervous system (CNS) depressants, such as anticonvulsants, muscle relaxants, and analgesics. In the case of severe anxiety, however, benzo-diazepines can improve focus by decreasing anxiety or panic.

The high prevalence of substance abuse in patients with TBI adds to the risk of benzodiazepine use in some patients. When possible, it is preferable to start with a scheduled dose of a shorter-acting agent such as lorazepam or promptly transition dosing from as-needed to scheduled dosing once an optimum daily total dose is determined. Assistance with dosage monitoring from a family member or caregiver can help prevent inadvertent overusage and monitoring for side effects or disinhibition.

SSRIs, SNRIs, and TCAs may have efficacy for anxiety in TBI. Although few studies exist in TBI patients, antidepressants appear to be effective for anxiety, particularly in the context of depression. SSRIs also have been found to be effective in decreasing mood lability after brain injury [84]. Because the initial activating effects of serotonergic agents may be particularly problematic for anxious individuals, these medications should be started at 50% or 25%, the usual starting dose. However, as with treatment for depression, the higher range of doses may be needed to eventually achieve maximum therapeutic effect. Potential side effects that may be more pronounced after TBI, such as sedation, apathy, agitation, and sexual dysfunction should be monitored closely.

Valproic acid, gabapentin, and pregabalin may be of benefit for anxiety, especially in patients with concomitant mood lability or seizures [85]. Buspirone is another option for generalized anxiety symptoms; however, it has rarely been associated with seizures and movement disorders [86]. These agents may also be helpful for patients with anger and aggression. Again, slow titration is indicated. There exists good evidence for the use of beta-blockers for agitation and aggression after TBI [87], but they have also been used for anticipatory anxiety in non-TBI populations. Caution should be exercised when using beta-blockers in patients with ongoing dizziness or light-headedness. Pindolol is less likely to cause bradycardia.

A combination of CBT with treatment of cognitive deficits appears to be effective for generalized anxiety and OCD [49, 88]. CBT is also effective in reducing frequency of PTSD in individuals with mTBI and ASD [89]. Cognitive processing therapy and prolonged exposure are empirically validated PTSD treatments, and there is limited evidence that these treatments are effective for comorbid mTBI and PTSD [90–92].

Psychotic symptoms

There may be a slightly elevated risk of psychosis after moderate or severe TBI [55]. However, attribution of the psychotic symptoms to the TBI is complicated by several factors, including that the symptoms frequently occurs years postinjury [93, 94] and that individuals with premorbid symptoms of psychosis and those with increased genetic risk for schizophrenia may have a greater likelihood of sustaining a brain injury [15, 95]. Post-TBI psychosis may be associated with posttraumatic epilepsy or severe mood disorder or occur as a chronic condition that is similar to schizophrenia [96]. Common clinical characteristics include delusions and hallucinations, without negative symptoms such as flat affect, avolition, and alogia [93].

Treatment

The empirical research regarding treatment of post-TBI psychosis is limited. Identifying and treating underlying conditions (e.g., epilepsy, delirium, or severe depression) are critical [96]. When the psychotic symptoms are not due to an underlying condition, case studies support the use of olanzapine [97], an atypical antipsychotic medication, at 5–20 mg/d for the treatment of delusions and auditory hallucinations in this population [98, 99]. Other atypical antipsychotics at low doses may also be beneficial (e.g., risperidone starting at 0.25–0.5 mg/d, quetiapine starting at 25 mg bid, ziprasidone starting at 5 mg/d, and aripiprazole starting at 5 mg/d [83]. Quetiapine and olanzapine may be the most sedating and, therefore, potentially most useful for comorbid sleep and anxiety problems. Sedation, weight gain, and QTc prolongation should be monitored closely. Typical antipsychotics such as haloperidol may not be as beneficial in the TBI population because of data that indicate poorer outcomes in rehabilitation [83] and poorer neuronal recovery in animal models [100]; TBI patients may also be more prone to developing extrapyramidal side effects and tardive dyskinesia [83].

Substance abuse

Substance use disorders are common among individuals with TBI. One study found that 30% of individuals reported moderate-to-heavy alcohol consumption at 1 year postinjury and 48% reported binge drinking once a month or more [101]. Marijuana is the most commonly used illicit drug in this population [102]. Preinjury substance abuse is an excellent predictor of postinjury substance abuse [103]. Substance use may decrease immediately postinjury but tends to increase with time since injury and functional independence [104]. Assessment of patterns of substance use, symptoms of dependence, and functional impact of substance use is beneficial for determining treatment needs. Screening measures such as the CAGE questionnaire [105], Alcohol Use Disorders Identification Test (AUDIT-C) [106], and Short Michigan Alcohol Screening Test (SMAST) [107] may be useful in identifying problematic substance abuse.

Treatment

Substance use screening is recommended soon after the injury. Brief educational sessions that include information regarding normative patterns of use, consequences of continued use, and treatment options have been shown to help reduce alcohol intake for patients admitted to trauma centers [108]. Motivational interviewing [109] or coping and social skills training [110, 111] may also be effective post-TBI treatments for substance abuse.

Agitation, anger, and aggression

Reduced impulse control, behavioral and cognitive disinhibition, difficulty modulating emotional reactions, increased aggression, and irritability are all common following TBI, especially as injury severity increases [8, 112]. Agitation among patients emerging from a coma, characterized by restlessness, confusion, and disorientation, may be a sign of delirium [113]. Persisting anger and aggression may reflect injury-related personality change or exacerbation of premorbid personality characteristics [114]; individuals are often unable to inhibit or control the behavior postinjury. Comorbid medical illness, substance use, depression, and executive dysfunction may increase the risk for aggression.

Treatment

Treatment can be divided into acute treatment, in which the goal is timely management of behavior to prevent injury to self or others, and chronic treatment, in which the goal is long-term management and prevention [115]. Many agents take from 2 to 8 weeks to gain full effectiveness. Medications that worsen cognition or sedation can actually worsen confusion and may, therefore, worsen agitation during the confusional state of PTA after TBI. Because the effects of medications on the patient with TBI can be unpredictable, and their side effects actually may potentiate the behavior problem (e.g., akathisia from antipsychotics), systematically eliminating certain medications can prove beneficial. A rationale for such an approach is the clinical observation that some patients have a natural course of recovery and that some medication efficacy may decrease over time.

The best evidence for the treatment of aggression in TBI is for beta-blockers (propranolol, with a maximum of 160–320 mg/d or pindolol, with a maximum of 40–100 mg/d) [87, 97]. Other options include SSRIs, valproate (750–2250 mg/d), lithium (titrated to a serum level of 0.4–1.4 mEq/L), TCAs, buspirone (10–60 mg/d), and methylphenidate [97]. For acute aggression, antipsychotics and benzodiazepines are most often used. For chronic aggression, one should treat the maximum number of comorbid symptoms with the fewest medications as possible. For example, one may use SSRIs or valproate/carbamazepine, depending on the presence of comorbid depression or mania/irritability, respectively.

Beta-blockers are a reasonable choice for isolated chronic aggression in the absence of significant mood changes [21].

Behavioral interventions and environmental modifications are often essential, including identification of factors that precede aggressive behavior. Common precipitating factors include overstimulation, frustration related to new functional limitations and/or inability to effectively communicate, cognitive deficits, and poor social support [116]. Environmental modifications might include reducing sources of overstimulation (e.g., limiting number of visitors, turning off TV/radio), increasing consistency in rehabilitation staff, and identifying cognitive strengths and weaknesses and incorporating this into the rehabilitation plan. Aggressive behaviors resulting from frustration may decrease as cognition and communication improves and functional impairments decrease.

Sleep disturbance

Approximately 30–70% of individuals report post-TBI sleep disturbance [117], and a recent meta-analysis found that approximately one-quarter of individuals have a diagnosed sleep disorder following TBI [118]. Sleep disorders including insomnia, hypersomnia, obstructive sleep apnea, periodic limb movement, and narcolepsy all occur at rates higher than the general public [118]. Finally, this meta-analysis found that individuals with a TBI were two to four times more likely to have sleep disturbance, including reduced sleep maintenance and efficiency, nightmares, sleep walking, and somnolence. Contributors to sleep disruption include the brain injury itself, physical injuries and pain, and psychiatric disturbances [119].

Treatment

Few specific data exist on treating insomnia or other sleep disorders in TBI, but trazodone is widely used in these patients for middle or late insomnia, and hypnotics are used in as many as 20% of TBI patients [120]. Trazodone-associated orthostatic hypotension may be particularly problematic in the rehabilitation setting, however. The sedating antidepressant, mirtazapine, may be another viable choice. Antihistamines such as diphenhydramine should be avoided because of their anticholinergic properties, as cognitive problems can occur with TBI patients· For the same reason, most nonprescription drugs and nortriptyline/ amitriptyline may not be the first choice.

Psychological interventions including relaxation training, sleep restriction, sleep hygiene education, stimulus control, and cognitive therapy are helpful for treating insomnia in the general population [121]. Limited research has investigated this among individuals with TBI, but a case study reported that CBT for insomnia reduced sleep-onset latencies and nocturnal awakenings and increased sleep efficiency in an individual with TBI [122].

Conclusions

Neuropsychiatric and behavioral sequelae of TBI are common, occurring in both the acute and chronic phases of recovery and distressing both patients and their families. Comprehensive evaluation of symptoms should include an integration of preinjury characteristics with injury-related features and current psychosocial and environmental factors. Although the neuropsychiatric and behavioral symptoms following TBI may present differently from psychiatric symptoms in non-TBI populations, they should be carefully monitored and treated if they are significantly impacting function [21].

Acknowledgments

Work on this chapter was supported in part by the US Department of Veterans Affairs, Office of Research and Development Clinical R&D Career Development Award Program (IK2 CX00516); the National Institutes of Health (R21HD053736); and the National Institute on Disability and Rehabilitation Research (H133G070016).

References

1 NIH Consensus Panel on Rehabilitation of Persons with Traumatic Brain Injury (1999) Rehabilitation of persons with traumatic brain injury. *Journal of American Medical Association*, **282 (10)**, 974–983.

2 van Reekum, R., Cohen, T., & Wong, J. (2000) Can traumatic brain injury cause psychiatric disorders? *The Journal of Neuropsychiatry and Clinical Neuroscience*, **12 (3)**, 316–327.

3 Ashman, T.A., Spielman, L.A., Hibbard, M.R., Silver, J.M., Chandna, T., & Gordon, W.A. (2004) Psychiatric challenges in the first 6 years after traumatic brain injury: cross-sequential analyses of Axis I disorders. *Archives of Physical Medicine and Rehabilitation*, **85 (4 Suppl 2)**, S36–S42.

4 Jorge, R., Robinsons, R., Arndt, S., Starkstein, S.E., Forrester, A.W., & Geisler, F. (1993) Depression following traumatic brain injury: a 1 year longitudinal study. *Journal of Affective Disorders*, **27 (4)**, 233–243.

5 Rapoport, M.J., McCullagh, S., Streiner, D., & Feinstein, A. (2003) The clinical significance of major depression following mild traumatic brain injury. *Psychosomatics*, **44 (1)**, 31–37.

6 Dikmen, S.S., Bombardier, C.H., Machamer, J.E., Fann, J.R., & Temkin, N.R. (2004) Natural history of depression in traumatic brain injury. *Archives of Physical Medicine and Rehabilitation*, **85 (9)**, 1457–1464.

7 Hart, T., Benn, E.K., & Bagiella, E. *et al.* (2014) Early trajectory of psychiatric symptoms after traumatic brain injury: relationship to patient and injury characteristics. *Journal of Neurotrauma*, **31 (7)**, 610–617.

8 Ciurli, P., Formisano, R., Bivona, U., Cantagallo, A., & Angelelli, P. (2011) Neuropsychiatric disorders in persons with severe traumatic brain injury: prevalence, phenomenology, and relationship with demographic, clinical, and functional features. *The Journal of Trauma Rehabilitation*, **26 (2)**, 116–126.

9 McAllister, T. (2007) Neuropsychiatric aspects of TBI. In: N. Zasler, D. Katz, & R. Zafonte (eds). *Brain Injury Medicine*, pp. 835–864. Demos Medical Publishing, New York.

10 Silver, J.M., Kramer, R., Greenwald, S., & Weissman, M. (2001) The association between head injuries and psychiatric disorders: findings from the New Haven NIMH Epidemiologic Catchment Area Study. *Brain Injury*, **15 (11)**, 935–945.

11 Simpson, G. & Tate, R. (2007) Suicidality in people surviving a traumatic brain injury: prevalence, risk factors and implications for clinical management. *Brain Injury*, **21 (13/14)**, 1335–1351.

12 Teasdale, T. & Engberg, A. (2001). Suicide after traumatic brain injury: a population study. *Journal of Neurology, Neurosurgery and Psychiatry*, **71 (4)**, 436–440.

13 Brenner, L.A., Ignacio, R.V., & Blow, F.C. (2011) Suicide and traumatic brain injury among individuals seeking Veterans Health Administration Services. *Journal of Head Trauma Rehabilitation*, **26 (4)**, 257–264.

14 Hart, T., Seignourel, P., & Sherer, M. (2009) A longitudinal study of awareness of deficit after moderate to severe traumatic brain injury. *Neuropsychological Rehabilitation*, **19 (2)**, 161–176.

15 Fann, J.R., Burington, B., Leonetti, A., Jaffe, K., Katon, W.J., & Thompson, R.S. (2004) Psychiatric illness following traumatic brain injury in an adult health maintenance organization population. *Archives of General Psychiatry*, **61 (1)**, 53–61.

16 Bombardier, C.H., Fann, J.R., Temkin, N.R., Esselman, P.C., Barber, J., & Dikmen, S.S. (2010) Rates of major depressive disorder and clinical outcomes following traumatic brain injury. *Journal of American Medical Association*, **303**, 1938–1945.

17 Rapoport, M.J., McCullagh, S., Streiner, D., & Feinstein, A. (2003) Age and major depression after mild traumatic brain injury. *The American Journal of Geriatric Psychiatry*, **11**, 365–369.

18 Whelan-Goodinson, R., Ponsford, J.L., Schonberger, M., & Johnston, L. (2010) Predictors of psychiatric disorders following traumatic brain injury. *The Journal of Trauma Rehabilitation*, **25**, 320–329.

19 Hart, T., Hoffman, J.M., Pretz, C., Kennedy, R., Clark, A.N., & Brenner, L.A. (2012) A longitudinal study of major and minor depression following traumatic brain injury. *Archives of Physical Medicine and Rehabilitation*, **93**, 1343–1349.

20 Holsinger, T., Steffens, D., Phillips, C. *et al.* (2002) Head injury in early adulthood and the lifetime risk of depression. *Archives of General Psychiatry*, **59 (1)**, 17–22.

21 Vaishnavi, S., Rao, V., & Fann, J.R. (2009) Neuropsychiatric problems after traumatic brain injury: unraveling the silent epidemic. *Psychosomatics*, **50 (3)**, 198–205.

22 American Psychiatric Association (1994) *Diagnostic and Statistical Manual of Mental Disorders*. 4th ed. American Psychiatric Association, Washington, DC.

23 Hibbard, M.R., Uysal, S., Kepler, K., Bogdany, J., & Silver, J. (1998) Axis I psychopathology in individuals with traumatic brain injury. *The Journal of Head Trauma Rehabilitation*, **13 (4)**, 24–39.

24 Fann, J.R., Katon, W.J., Uomoto, J.M., & Esselman, P.C. (1995) Psychiatric disorders and functional disability in outpatients with traumatic brain injuries. *American Journal of Psychiatry*, **152 (10)**, 1493–1499.

25 Simpson, G. & Tate, R. (2005) Clinical features of suicide attempts after traumatic brain injury. *The Journal of Nervous and Mental Disease*, **193 (10)**, 680–685.

26 Bryan, C.J. & Clemans, T.A. (2013) Repetitive traumatic brain injury, psychological symptoms, and suicide risk in a clinical sample of deployed military personnel. *JAMA Psychiatry*, **70 (7)**, 686–691.

27 Gomez-Hernandez, R., Max, J.E., Kosier, T., Paradiso, S., & Robinson, R.G. (1997) Social impairment and depression after traumatic brain injury. *Archives of Physical Medicine and Rehabilitation*, **78 (12)**, 1321–1326.

28 Seel, R.T., Macciocchi, S., & Kreutzer, J.S. (2010) Clinical considerations for the diagnosis of major depression after moderate to severe TBI. *The Journal of Trauma Rehabilitation*, **25 (2)**, 99–112.

29 Seel, R.T., Kreutzer, J.S., Rosenthal, M., Hammond, F.M., Corrigan, J.D., & Black, K. (2003) Depression after traumatic brain injury: a National Institute on Disability and Rehabilitation Research Model Systems multicenter investigation. *Archives of Physical Medicine and Rehabilitation*, **84 (2)**, 177–184.

30 Dennis J.P., Ghahramanlou-Holloway, M., Cox, D.W., & Brown, G.K.A. (2011) A guide for the assessment and treatment of suicidal patients with traumatic brain injuries. *Journal of Head Trauma Rehabilitation*, **26 (4)**, 244–256.

31 Andersson, S., Gundersen, P.M., & Finset, A. (1999) Emotional activation during therapeutic interaction in traumatic brain injury: effect of apathy, self-awareness and implications for rehabilitation. *Brain Injury*, **13**, 393–404.

32 Marin, R.S. (1991) Apathy: a neuropsychiatric syndrome. *The Journal of Neuropsychiatry and Clinical Neurosciences*, **3 (3)**, 243–254.

33 Fann, J.R., Bombardier, C.H., Dikmen, S. *et al.* (2005) Validity of the Patient Health Questionnaire-9 in assessing depression following traumatic brain injury. *The Journal of Head Trauma Rehabilitation*, **20 (6)**, 501–511.

34 Seel, R.T. & Kreutzer, J.S. (2003) Depression assessment after traumatic brain injury: an empirically based classification method. *Archives of Physical Medicine and Rehabilitation*, **84 (11)**, 1621–1628.

35 Fann, J.R., Hart, T., & Schomer, K.G. (2009) Treatment for depression after traumatic brain injury: a systematic review. *Journal of Neurotrauma*, **26 (12)**, 2383–2402.

36 Rapoport, M. (2012) Depression following traumatic brain injury. *Epidemiology*, risk factors, and management. *CNS Drugs*, **26 (2)**, 111–121

37 Davidson, J. (1989) Seizures and bupropion: a review. *Journal of Clinical Psychiatry*, **50 (7)**, 256–261.

38 Wroblewski, B.A., McColgan, K., Smith, K., Whyte, J., & Singer, W.D. (1990) The incidence of seizures during tricyclic antidepressant drug treatment in a brain-injured population. *Journal of Clinical Psychopharmacology*, **10 (2)**, 124–128.

39 Ojemann, L.M., Baugh-Bookman, C. & Dudley, D.L. Effect of psychotropic medications on seizure control in patients with epilepsy. *Neurology*, **37 (9)**, 1525–1527.

40 Ashman, T.A., Cantor, J.B., Gordon, W.A. *et al.* (2009) A randomized controlled trial of sertraline for the treatment of depression in persons with traumatic brain injury. *Archives of Physical Medicine and Rehabilitation*, **90 (5)**, 733–740.

41 Marin, R.S., Fogel, B.S., Hawkins, J., Duffy, J., & Krupp, B. (1995) Apathy: a treatable syndrome. *The Journal of Neuropsychiatry and Clinical Neurosciences*, **7 (1)**, 23–30.

42 Alban, J.P., Hopson, M.M., Ly, V., & Whyte, J. (2004) Effect of methylphenidate on vital signs and adverse effects in adults with traumatic brain injury. *American Journal of Physical Medicine and Rehabilitation*, **83 (2)**, 131–137.

43 Teitelman, E. (2001) Off-label uses of modafinil. *American Journal of Psychiatry*, **158 (8)**, 1341.

44 Sheng, P., Hou, L., Wang, X., *et al.* (2013) Efficacy of modafinil on fatigue and excessive daytime sleepiness associated with neurological disorders: a systematic review and meta-analysis. *PLoS one* **8 (12)**, e81802. doi:10.1371/journal.pone.0081802

45 Sawyer, E., Mauro, L.S., & Ohlinger, M.J. (2008) Amantadine enhancement of arousal and cognition after traumatic brain injury. *Annals of Pharmacotherapy*, **42 (2)**, 247–252.

46 McDowell, S., Whyte, J., & D'Esposito, M. (1998) Differential effect of a dopaminergic agonist on prefrontal function in traumatic brain injury patients. *Brain*, **121 (Pt 6)**, 1155–1164.

47 Lal, S., Merbtiz, C.P., & Grip, J.C. (1988) Modification of function in head-injured patients with Sinemet. *Brain Injury*, **2 (3)**, 225–233.

48 Gualtieri, T., Chandler, M., Coons, T.B., & Brown, L.T. (1989) Amantadine: a new clinical profile for traumatic brain injury. *Clinical Neuropharmacology*, **12 (4)**, 258–270.

49 Tiersky, L.A., Anselmi, V., Johnston, M.V. *et al.* (2005) A trial of neuropsychologic rehabilitation in mild-spectrum traumatic brain injury. *Archives of Physical Medicine and Rehabilitation,* **86 (8)**, 1565–1574.

50 Gurr, B. & Coetzer, B.R. (2005) The effectiveness of cognitive-behavioural therapy for post-traumatic headaches. *Brain Injury,* **19 (7)**, 481–491.

51 Bombardier, C.H., Bell, K.R., Temkin, N.R., Fann, J.R., Hoffman, J., & Dikmen, S. (2009) The efficacy of a scheduled telephone intervention for ameliorating depressive symptoms during the first year after traumatic brain injury. *The Journal of Trauma Rehabilitation,* **24 (4)**, 230–238.

52 Fann, J.R., Jones, A.L., Dikmen, S.S., Temkin, N.R., Esselman, P.C., & Bombardier, C.H. (2009) Depression treatment preferences after traumatic brain injury. *The Journal of Trauma Rehabilitation,* **24 (4)**, 272–278.

53 Hoffman, J.M., Bell, K.R., Powell, J.M. *et al.* (2010) A randomized controlled trial of exercise to improve mood after traumatic brain injury. *Physical Medicine and Rehabilitation,* **2 (10)**, 911–919.

54 Wise, E.K., Hoffman, J.M., Powell, J.M., Bombardier, C.H., & Bell, K.R. (2012). Benefits of exercise maintenance after TBI. *Archives of Physical Medicine and Rehabilitation,* **93 (8)**, 1319–1323.

55 Hesdorffer, D.C., Rauch, S.L., & Tamminga, C.A. (2009) Long-term psychiatric outcomes following traumatic brain injury: a review of the literature. *The Journal of Trauma Rehabilitation,* **24 (6)**, 452–459.

56 Jorge, R., Robinson, R., Starkstein, S., Arndt, S., Forrester, A., & Geisler, F. (1993) Secondary mania following traumatic brain injury. *American Journal of Psychiatry,* **150 (6)**, 916–921.

57 Koponen, S., Taiminen, T., Portin, R. *et al.* (2002) Axis I and II psychiatric disorders after traumatic brain injury: a 30-year follow-up study. *American Journal of Psychiatry,* **159 (8)**, 1315–1321.

58 Hale, M.S. & Donaldson, J.O. (1982) Lithium carbonate in the treatment of organic brain syndrome. *The Journal of Nervous and Mental Disease,* **170 (6)**, 362–365.

59 Pope, H.G., Jr., McElroy, S.L., Satlin, A., Hudson, J.I., Keck, P.E., Jr., & Kalish, R. (1988) Head injury, bipolar disorder, and response to valproate. *Comprehensive Psychiatry,* **29 (1)**, 34–38.

60 Bakchine, S., Lacomblez, L., Benoit, N., Parisot, D., Chain, F., & Lhermitte, F. (1989) Manic-like state after bilateral orbitofrontal and right temporoparietal injury: efficacy of clonidine. *Neurology,* **39 (6)**, 777–781.

61 Clark, A.F. & Davison, K. (1987) Mania following head injury. A report of two cases and a review of the literature. *British Journal of Psychiatry,* **150**, 841–844.

62 Fann, J.R. & Jakupcak, M. (2013) Anxiety disorders. In: D. Arciniegas, N. Zasler, R. Vanderploeg, & M. Jaffee (eds), *Management of Adults with Traumatic Brain Injury.* American Psychiatric Publishing, Inc., Washington, DC.

63 Bryant, R. & Harvey, A. (1998) Relationship between acute stress disorder and posttraumatic stress disorder following mild traumatic brain injury. *American Journal of Psychiatry,* **155 (5)**, 625–629.

64 Broomhall, L.G., Clark, C.R., McFarlane, A.C. *et al.* (2009) Early stage assessment and course of acute stress disorder after mild traumatic brain injury. *The Journal of Nervous and Mental Disease,* **197 (3)**, 178–181.

65 Harvey, A. & Bryant, R. (2000) Two-year prospective evaluation of the relationship between acute stress disorder and posttraumatic stress disorder following mild traumatic brain injury. *American Journal of Psychiatry,* **157 (4)**, 626–628.

66 Bryant, R., Harvey, A., Dang, S., Sackville, T., & Basten, C. (1998) Treatment of acute stress disorder: a comparison of cognitive-behavioral therapy and supportive counseling. *Journal of Consulting and Clinical Psychology,* **66 (5)**, 862–866.

67 Bryant, R.A., Marosszeky, J.E., Crooks, J., & Gurka, J.A. (2000) Posttraumatic stress disorder after severe traumatic brain injury. *American Journal of Psychiatry,* **157 (4)**, 629–631.

68 Glaesser, J., Neuner, F., Lutgehetmann, R., Schmidt, R., & Elbert, T. (2004) Posttraumatic stress disorder in patients with traumatic brain injury. *BMC Psychiatry*, **9 (4)**, 5.

69 Gil, S., Caspi, Y., Ben-Ari, I.Z., Koren, D., & Klein, E. (2005) Does memory of a traumatic event increase the risk for posttraumatic stress disorder in patients with traumatic brain injury? A prospective study. *American Journal of Psychiatry*, **162 (5)**, 963–969.

70 Bombardier, C.H., Fann, J.R., Temkin, N. *et al.* (2006) Posttraumatic stress disorder symptoms during the first six months after traumatic brain injury. *The Journal of Neuropsychiatry and Clinical Neurosciences*, **18 (4)**, 501–508.

71 Bryant, R.A. (2001) Posttraumatic stress disorder and traumatic brain injury: can they co-exist? *Clinical Psychological Reveiw*, **21 (6)**, 931–948.

72 Sumpter, R.E. & McMillan, T.M. (2005) Misdiagnosis of post-traumatic stress disorder following severe traumatic brain injury. *British Journal of Psychiatry*, **186**, 423–426.

73 Hiott, D. & Labbate, L. (2002) Anxiety disorders associated with traumatic brain injuries. *Neurorehabilitation*, **17**, 345–355.

74 Bryant, R.A., O'Donnell, M.L., Creamer, M., McFarlane, A.C., Clark, C.R., & Silove, D. (2010) The psychiatric sequelae of traumatic injury. *American Journal of Psychiatry*, **167 (3)**, 312–320.

75 Hoofien, D., Gilboa, A., Vakil, E., & Donovick, P.J. (2001) Traumatic brain injury (TBI) 10–20 years later: a comprehensive outcome study of psychiatric symptomatology, cognitive abilities and psychosocial functioning. *Brain Injury*, **15 (3)**, 189–209.

76 Spitzer, R.L., Kroenke, K., Williams, J.B., & Lowe, B. (2006) A brief measure for assessing generalized anxiety disorder: the GAD-7. *Archives of Internal Medicine*, **166 (10)**, 1092–1097.

77 Meachen, S.J., Hanks, R.A., Millis, S.R., & Rapport, L.J. (2008) The reliability and validity of the brief symptom inventory-18 in persons with traumatic brain injury. *Archives of Physical Medicine and Rehabilitation*, **89 (5)**, 958–965.

78 Deb, S., Lyons, I., Koutzoukis, C., Ali, I., & McCarthy, G. (1999) Rate of psychiatric illness 1 year after traumatic brain injury. *American Journal of Psychiatry*, **156 (3)**, 374–378.

79 Whelan-Goodinson, R., Ponsford, J., Johnston, L., & Grant, F. (2009) Psychiatric disorders following traumatic brain injury: their nature and frequency. *The Journal of Trauma Rehabilitation*, **24 (5)**, 324–332.

80 Kant, R., Smith-Seemiller, L., & Duffy, J. (1996) Obsessive-compulsive disorder after closed head injury: review of the literature and report of four cases. *Brain Injury*, **10 (1)**, 55–63.

81 Berthier, M.L., Kulisevsky, J.J., Gironell, A., & Lopez, O.L. (2001) Obsessive-compulsive disorder and traumatic brain injury: behavioral, cognitive, and neuroimaging findings. *Neuropsychiatry, Neuropsychology and Behavioral Neurology*, **14 (1)**, 23–31.

82 Coetzer, B. & Stein, D. (2003) Obsessive compulsive disorder following traumatic brain injury: diagnostic issues. *Journal of Cognitive Rehabilitation*, **4**, 4–8.

83 Lee, H.B., Lyketsos, C.G., & Rao, V. (2003) Pharmacological management of the psychiatric aspects of traumatic brain injury. *International Review of Psychiatry*, **15 (4)**, 359–370.

84 Nahas, Z., Arlinghaus, K.A., Kotrla, K.J., Clearman, R.R., & George, M.S. (1998) Rapid response of emotional incontinence to selective serotonin reuptake inhibitors. *The Journal of Neuropsychiatry and Clinical Neurosciences*, **10 (4)**, 453–455.

85 Pande, A.C., Pollack, M.H., Crockatt, J. *et al.* (2000) Placebo-controlled study of gabapentin treatment of panic disorder. *Journal of Clinical Psychopharmacology*, **20 (4)**, 467–471.

86 Levitt, P., Henry, W., & McHale, D. (1993) Persistent movement disorder induced by buspirone. *Movement Disorder*, **8**, 331–334.

87 Fleminger, S., Greenwood, R.J., & Oliver, D.L. (2006) Pharmacological management for agitation and aggression in people with acquired brain injury. *Cochrane Database of Systematic Review*, **(4)**, CD003299.

88 Williams, W., Evans, J., & Fleminger, S. (2003) Neurorehabilitation and cognitive-behaviour therapy of anxiety disorders after brain injury: an overview and a case illustration of obsessive-compulsive disorder. *Neuropsychological Rehabilitation*, **13 (1–2)**, 133–148.

89 Bryant, R.A., Moulds, M., Guthrie, R., & Nixon, R.D. (2003) Treating acute stress disorder following mild traumatic brain injury. *American Journal of Psychiatry*, **160 (3)**, 585–587.

90 Report of (VA) Consensus Conference: Practice Recommendations for Treatment of Veterans with Comorbid TBI, Pain, and PTSD. (2010) http://www.ptsd.va.gov/professional/pages/handouts-pdf/TBI_PTSD_Pain_Practice_Recommend.pdf [accessed on July 12, 2014].

91 Davis, J.J., Walter, K.H., Chard, K.M., Parkinson, R.B., & Houston, W.S. (2013) Treatment adherence in cognitive processing therapy for combat related PTSD with history of mild TBI. *Rehabilitation Psychology*, **58 (1)**, 36–42.

92 Sripada, R.K., Rauch, S.A.M., Tuerk, P.W. *et al.* (2013) Mild traumatic brain injury and treatment response in prolonged exposure for PTSD. *Journal of Traumatic Stress*, **26 (3)**, 369–375.

93 Fujii, D. & Ahmed, I. (2002) Psychotic disorder following traumatic brain injury: a conceptual framework. *Cognitive Neuropsychiatry*, **7 (1)**, 41–62.

94 Sachdev, P., Smith, J.S., & Cathcart, S. (2001) Schizophrenia-like psychosis following traumatic brain injury: a chart-based descriptive and case-control study. *Psychological Medicine*, **31 (2)**, 231–239.

95 Malaspina, D., Goetz, R.R., Friedman, J.H. *et al.* (2001) Traumatic brain injury and schizophrenia in members of schizophrenia and bipolar disorder pedigrees. *American Journal of Psychiatry*, **158 (3)**, 440–446.

96 McAllister, T.W. & Ferrell, R.B. (2002) Evaluation and treatment of psychosis after traumatic brain injury. *NeuroRehabilitation*, **17 (4)**, 357–368.

97 Warden, D.L., Gordon, B., McAllister, T.W. *et al.* (2006) Guidelines for the pharmacologic treatment of neurobehavioral sequelae of traumatic brain injury. *Journal of Neurotrauma*, **23 (10)**, 1468–1501.

98 Umansky, R. & Geller, V. (2000) Olanzapine treatment in an organic hallucinosis patient. *International Journal of Neuropsychopharmacology*, **3 (1)**, 81–82.

99 Butler, P.V. (2000) Diurnal variation in Cotard's syndrome (copresent with Capgras delusion) following traumatic brain injury. *Australian and New Zealand Journal of Psychiatry*, **34 (4)**, 684–687.

100 Feeney, D.M., Gonzalez, A., & Law, W.A. (1982) Amphetamine, haloperidol, and experience interact to affect rate of recovery after motor cortex injury. *Science*, **217 (4562)**, 855–857.

101 Horner, M.D., Ferguson, P.L., Selassie, A.W., Labbate, L.A., Kniele, K., & Corrigan, J.D. (2005) Patterns of alcohol use 1 year after traumatic brain injury: a population-based, epidemiological study. *Journal of International Neuropsychological Society*, **11 (3)**, 322–330.

102 Taylor, L., Kreutzer, J., Demm, S., & Meade, M. (2003) Traumatic brain injury and substance abuse: a review and analysis of the literature. *Neuropsychological Rehabilitation*, **13 (1/2)**, 165–188.

103 Bombardier, C.H., Rimmele, C.T., & Zintel, H. (2002) The magnitude and correlates of alcohol and drug use before traumatic brain injury. *Archives of Physical Medicine and Rehabilitation*, **83 (12)**, 1765–1773.

104 Kreutzer, J.S., Witol, A.D., & Marwitz, J.H. (1996) Alcohol and drug use among young persons with traumatic brain injury. *Journal of Learning Disabilities*, **29 (6)**, 643–651.

105 Ewing, J.A. (1984) Detecting alcoholism. The CAGE questionnaire. *Journal of American Medical Association*, **252 (14)**, 1905–1907.

106 Bush, K., Kivlahan, D., McDonell, M., Fihn, S., & Bradley, K. (1998) The AUDIT alcohol consumption questions (AUDIT-C): an effective brief screening test for problem drinking. Ambulatory Care Quality Improvement Project (ACQUIP). Alcohol Use Disorders Identification Test. *Archives of Internal Medicine*, **158 (16)**, 1789–1795.

107 Selzer, M., Vinokur, A., & van Rooijen, L. (1975) A self-administered Short Michigan Alcoholism Screening Test (SMAST). *Journal of Studies on Alcohol*, **36**, 127–132.

108 Soderstrom, C.A., DiClemente, C.C., Dischinger, P.C., *et al.* (2007) A controlled trial of brief intervention versus brief advice for at-risk drinking trauma center patients. *The Journal of Trauma*, **62 (5)**, 1102–1111.

109 Bombardier, C. & Rimmele, C. (1999) Motivational interviewing to prevent alcohol abuse after traumatic brain injury: a case series. *Rehabilitation Psychology*, **44**, 52–67.

110 Langley, M. & Kiley, D. (1992) Prevention of substance abuse in persons with neurological disabilities. *NeuroRehabilitation*, **2**, 52–64.

111 Cox, W.M., Heinemann, A.W., Miranti, S.V., Schmidt, M., Klinger, E., & Blount, J. (2003) Outcomes of systematic motivational counseling for substance use following traumatic brain injury. *Journal of Addictive Disease*, **22 (1)**, 93–110.

112 Rao, V. & Lyketsos, C.G. (2002) Psychiatric aspects of traumatic brain injury. *Psychiatric Clinics of North America*, **25 (1)**, 43–69.

113 Sandel, M.E. & Mysiw, W.J. (1996) The agitated brain injured patient. Part 1: definitions, differential diagnosis, and assessment. *Archives of Physical Medicine and Rehabilitation*, **77 (6)**, 617–623.

114 Kim, E., Lauterbach, E.C., Reeve, A., *et al.* (2007) Neuropsychiatric complications of traumatic brain injury: a critical review of the literature. *The Journal of Neuropsychiatry and Clinical Neurosciences*, **19 (2)**, 106–127.

115 Silver, J., Hales, R., & Yudofsky, S. (2002) Neuropsychiatric aspects of traumatic brain injury. In: S. Yudofsky & R. Hales (eds). *The American Psychiatric Publishing Textbook of Neuropsychiatry and Clinical Neurosciences*, pp. 625–672. American Psychaitric Publishing, Washington, DC.

116 Corrigan, P. & Mueser, K. (2000) Behavior therapy for aggressive psychiatric patients. In: M. Crowner (ed). *Treating Violent Psychiatric Patients: Progress in Psychiatry #60*, pp. 69–85. American Psychiatric Press, Washington DC.

117 Ouellet, M., Savard, J., & Morin C. (2004) Insomnia following traumatic brain injury: a review. *Neurorehabilitation and Neural Repair*, **18 (4)**, 187–198.

118 Mathias, J.L. & Alvaro, P.K. (2012). Prevalence of sleep disturbances, disorders, and problems -following traumatic brain injury: a meta-analysis. *Sleep Medicine*, **13**, 898–905.

119 Zeitzer, J., Friedman, L., & O'Hara, R. (2009) Insomnia in the context of traumatic brain injury. *Journal of Rehabilitation Research and Development*, **46 (6)**, 827–836.

120 Worthington, A.D. & Melia, Y. (2006) Rehabilitation is compromised by arousal and sleep disorders: results of a survey of rehabilitation centres. *Brain Injury*, **20 (3)**, 327–332.

121 National Institutes of Health (2005) National Institutes of Health State of the Science Conference Statement on manifestations and management of chronic insomnia in adults. *Sleep*, **28 (9)**, 1049–1057.

122 Ouellet, M.C. & Morin, C.M. (2007) Efficacy of cognitive-behavioral therapy for insomnia associated with traumatic brain injury: a single-case experimental design. *Archives of Physical Medicine and Rehabilitation*, **88 (12)**, 1581–1592.

CHAPTER 12

Follow-up and community integration of mild traumatic brain injury

Joukje van der Naalt[1] and Joke M. Spikman[2]

[1]Department of Neurology, University Medical Center Groningen, Groningen, the Netherlands
[2]Department of Neuropsychology, University Medical Center Groningen, Groningen, the Netherlands

Traumatic brain injury (TBI) is an important cause of disability and death in young adults [1, 2]. The majority (80–90%) of patients admitted to the emergency department are classified as mild TBI [3]. The definition of mild TBI according to the Task Force on mild TBI of the WHO Collaborating Center for Neurotrauma [4] comprises the following criteria:

1 Glasgow Coma Scale on admission 13–15
2 Loss of consciousness less than 30 min
3 Posttraumatic amnesia less than 24 h

Most of these patients recover within weeks to months without specific therapy. However, a subgroup of 15–25% patients continues to experience disabling postconcussive symptoms (PCS) that interfere with their return to work or resumption of social activities [5, 6]. These symptoms cause a social economical burden, since TBI often affects young patients in their twenties and thirties with full occupational status. The financial costs associated with unemployment after TBI are substantial, given that TBI disproportionally affects young people of working age [7]. Lost work productivity after mild TBI may be the largest component of economic costs of brain trauma in the USA [8]. In the USA, costs associated with care and management of TBI are estimated to be $22 billion annually [9]. In health care, indirect costs are much higher than direct costs. Admission and radiological policies are determining factors for the level of direct costs, whereas loss of productivity is the main expense for indirect costs. As minimal data are available regarding the lost work productivity in the majority of patients who are not hospitalized, economic costs of brain injury are substantially underestimated. Given the economic consequences, it is of paramount importance to identify those patients who are prone to develop chronic postconcussive problems in order to institute early rehabilitation focusing on resumption of previous activities [10, 11].

Traumatic Brain Injury, First Edition. Edited by Pieter E. Vos and Ramon Diaz-Arrastia.
© 2015 John Wiley & Sons, Ltd. Published 2015 by John Wiley & Sons, Ltd.

Care as usual

Several protocols are applied to optimize patient care and management. According to international guidelines, a brain computed tomography (CT) scan is performed at the Emergency Department (ER) on all patients with a GCS of 15 or less and in the presence of certain risk factors (see Chapter 4) [12, 13].

Only patients with documented brain injury are admitted to the neurological or surgical ward. In general, follow-up of patients after sustaining a mild TBI is only done in patients with abnormalities on admission CT. When a CT scan reveals no abnormalities in the acute phase after injury, the patient is regarded as having sustained no relevant TBI and is not seen for follow-up. However, routine CT imaging appears rather insensitive for detecting structural brain changes which may account for persistent symptoms as 20% of the patients with a normal CT scan on admission will develop cognitive complaints. On the other hand, 22% of patients with CT abnormalities showed good outcome [14]. Especially in mild TBI, CT abnormalities are rather nonspecific, and therefore, clinical variables and age are found to be stronger predictions for outcome than CT abnormalities [15]. Only when a patient experiences residual deficits does a referral to a neurologist or rehabilitation specialist occur, and eventually, a neuropsychological examination and magnetic resonance imaging (MRI) are performed. In general, referral occurs within several months after injury due to late recognition of residual impairments and because no practice-based guidelines for a multidisciplinary approach are available [6].

Follow-up

Routine follow-up or interventions are not useful for most patients with mild TBI as the vast majority of improvement occurs between the time of injury and 3 months following the injury. For those patients admitted to the hospital, one regular follow-up either at the hospital or with the general practitioner is advised in most recent guidelines [14]. Mostly, patients are admitted to the outpatient clinic within 4–6 weeks after injury. In those patients with complaints that interfere with resumption of work, additional diagnostic procedures (MRI, neuropsychological assessment) are performed to evaluate whether these impairments are related to the injury or to concomitant anxiety or depression. With the acquired information of these diagnostic procedures, individual targeted rehabilitation therapy can be instituted (Figure 12.1).

Some studies reveal that early targeted educational intervention that includes reassuring information can reduce long-term complaints [16]. A single-session educational intervention within 3 weeks after injury was found to be as effective as a more elaborate assessment. However, many patients had returned to

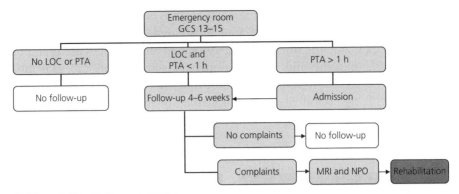

Figure 12.1 Flow diagram with follow-up scheme of mild TBI. LOC, loss of consciousness; MRI, magnetic resonance imaging; NPO, neuropsychological assessment; PTA, posttraumatic amnesia.

work before the intervention and as such the lack of treatment effect may be due to lack of persistent symptoms in the participants [17]. Early follow-up within 7 days after injury was only found to be effective in hospitalized patients with PTA durations of more than 1 h, resulting in significantly fewer difficulties with everyday activities and lower ratings of PCS at 6 months after injury [18]. In a systematic review [19], it was recommended to apply cognitive behavioral therapy (CBT) in those patients with symptoms not responding to information and education alone as this treatment may not be as beneficial as previously thought. Future research on effective treatments can probably focus more on developing early brief treatments targeted to a specific problem group than studying potentially more extensive and expensive rehabilitation models for all mild TBI survivors.

Imaging

In the acute phase after injury, CT is the standard imaging technique because of more accurate detection of intracranial blood to determine eligibility for eventual neurosurgical intervention (see Chapter 4) [20]. For mild TBI, the incidence of abnormalities is about 15% increasing to 50% when a CT scan is done only in those with neurological symptoms [21]. Conventional CT has limited ability to detect structural and functional abnormalities as suggested by the fact that 20% of patients with a normal CT scan on admission show unfavorable outcome [14]. MRI is the preferred imaging technique in the subacute phase and during follow-up of mild TBI as MRI is more sensitive in detecting diffuse axonal injury and nonhemorrhagic contusions (see Chapter 2) [22]. For years, T1- and T2-weighted spin echo and FLAIR-weighted sequences were the most commonly used MRI modalities in TBI. Nowadays, T2*-weighted gradient echo is used instead of these conventional sequences because of better detection of diffuse axonal injury, with visualization of hemosiderin deposits as a result of hemorrhage [23, 24]. The number of T2*-weighted abnormalities are found to correlate with outcome and with neuropsychological deficits [23, 25, 26]. Susceptibility-weighted imaging is the most recently developed structural MRI technique with high sensitivity for hemosiderin. The first studies are promising as they show high sensitivity but a rather inconsistent relation with outcome [27, 28] (Figure 12.2).

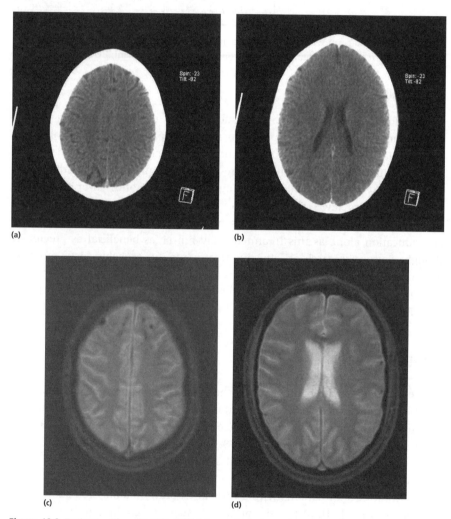

Figure 12.2 Patient with mild TBI, GCS 14 on admission, after a bicycle accident. CT on admission reveals no abnormalities (a and b). MRI performed 3 months after injury due to persisting cognitive complaints reveals microhemorrhages corresponding with diffuse axonal injury in the frontal regions bilaterally (c) and in the corpus callosum and in the cortex (d).

Outcome of mild TBI

Postconcussive symptoms

The outcome after mild TBI in general is favorable with 75–90% of patients achieving good outcome 1 year after injury [29] measured with the Glasgow Outcome Scale. Although the majority of symptoms are present in the first 3 months after injury, still, 25–50% of patients will have persistent complaints interfering with resumption of work and social activities. The most frequent complaints after mild TBI are forgetfulness, concentration problems, and increased fatigue [30–32]. In one of the first studies on outcome of mild TBI, moderate disability was found in one out of four patients [33]. For determination of outcome and return to work, timing of follow-up is important. One month after injury, physical limitations play a role in resuming work [34] with considerable improvement noted over the first 6 months postinjury, whereas some of the reported limitations in communication and emotional domains remain constant over time [35].

Cognitive impairment

Deficits in cognitive functioning are not consistently demonstrated with standard neuropsychological tests despite the often reported attention and memory complaints. Some studies report cognitive deficits in the early stage postinjury. For instance, Kwok *et al.* [36] found mild TBI patients to be impaired on tests for speed of information processing, attention, and memory at 1 month postinjury. However, at 3 months postinjury, patients were reassessed, and most test performances had returned to a normal level or were only present in those patients with CT abnormalities on admission [37]. A meta-analysis by Binder *et al.* [38] showed evidence for subtle neuropsychological deficits in mild TBI patients assessed more than 3 months postinjury, but more recent meta-analyses fail to detect significant long-term neuropsychological impairments [39–41]. Furthermore, poor test performances of mild TBI might be the consequence of poor effort [42]. More than 25% of a sample of mild TBI patients failed a symptom validity test, indicating poor effort. Strikingly, this was not related to litigation, but to lower educational levels as well as reported high levels of distress. It is also demonstrated that the mere expectation that an individual will experience cognitive symptoms influences the extent to which they are actually experienced. Studies investigating mild TBI patients under a condition of *diagnosis threat* (in which they were told that they may be experiencing cognitive problems due to the injury) versus a neutral condition found lower performances on cognitive tests as well as higher complaint ratings for the first group, even on a long term [43–45].

Return to work

The majority of patients with mild TBI will have returned to work by 3 months after injury [30, 46]. In most studies, only the first day of working is noted without defining the level of work that the patient could achieve or the percentage of the total working hours. One recent study showed that the majority of patients with mild TBI (56%) started working until 1 and 3 months after injury. Ultimately, 91% of the patients were working in a full-time job at 6 months postinjury [47]. However, this does not imply that patients resuming work are without complaints. Work-related problems were reported by up to half of employed patients. Even patients who have resumed work completely report temporary increase of postconcussive complaints in the first months after regaining full activities, suggesting that patients who are resuming activities show suboptimal performance [32]. Given the long-term consequences, lost work productivity should not only be measured by work absence but also by estimation of reduced performance on the job.

Long-term outcome and community integration

Outcome studies beyond 10 years after injury contain patients with varying severity of injury hampering the precise estimation of long-term outcome. Furthermore, the response rate is often low in mild TBI probably due to relative favorable outcome of this patient category. However, the few studies on long-term follow-up on mild TBI ultimately show good recovery varying from 50 to 88 % of patients [48, 49]. Approximately 95% of patients found their life as a whole at follow-up good or at least acceptable. An important factor influencing survival seemed to be whether relations with family and friends could be maintained at preinjury levels [50]. Up to 30% reported distressed family relations 1 year after injury. Emotional and behavioral impairments are also noted 1 year after injury [51]. Even though patients are found to live and work independently several years postinjury, they still may have difficulties in social interactions due to personality disturbances [52]. Over the years, changes in adjustment show improvement of emotional stability but increased difficulties with anger management and self-monitoring [53]. In those with milder injuries, adverse psychosocial factors are associated with deterioration [54]. At follow-up 5–7 years after injury, as many had deteriorated (12%) as had improved (13%). Those who deteriorated were more depressed and anxious and had more alcohol-related problems [55]. When comparing a mild to a moderate–severe TBI group in a cohort study beyond 10 years after injury, no substantial difference was found between injury severity groups in case of living arrangements, marital status, education, or quality of life. In addition, cognitive impairment and emotional problems were more commonly reported than physical impairment in the long term with 10–25% of patients reporting some degree of feelings of depression or anxiety [56, 57]. Approximately 1 in 10 patients was found to have lost their jobs because of persistent complaints [58]. Long-term outcome surveys in mild TBI indicate that self-reported outcomes and adaptation to impairment-related limitations improve as the time since injury increase, especially in the mild TBI group [59] (Table 12.1).

Table 12.1 Long-term outcome studies of mild TBI. Studies with 100 or more patients are selected.

Author	Severity	Follow-up	Impairments	Outcome (for mild TBI)	Return to previous work	
Engberg [50]	Register-based questionnaire survey	2–5 years n=240 mild TBI	42%, behavioral disturbances	65%, good recovery* 25%, less social contacts	42%	Response 76%
Kashluba [37]	Prospective outcome study	1 year n=102 mild TBI with abnormal CT	29%, cognitive problems	Not specified	61%	
Huang [52]	Level 1 trauma center	1–10 years n=327 75% mild TBI	Not assessed	Good recovery† 49%, 1 year 41%, 3 years	50%, 1 year 75%, 3 years	Response 33%
Brown [59]	Prospective cohort study	10–30 years n=1623 79% mild TBI	24%, depression or anxiety	75%, satisfied with quality of life	62%	Response 37%
vanderPloeg [54]	Cross-sectional cohort study	10–30 years n=254 mild TBI	14%, depression	22%, concentration	75%	
Asikainen [48]	Retrospective cohort study	n=508 TBI 115 mild TBI 5–20 years	16%, anxiety disorder	28%, memory 73%, good recovery†	68%	
Masson [49]	Prospective cohort study	n=176 TBI 114 mild TBI 5 years	Not assessed	88%‡, good recovery	77%	

TBI, traumatic brain injury.
Outcome defined by the Glasgow Outcome Scale—Extended (GOSE) with * = 8 or † = 7 and 8, ‡ = recovered from brain and initial injury.

Prediction of outcome

The factors predictive for outcome have to be defined, both in the acute and chronic phases in order to facilitate treatment strategies for TBI.

Acute injury characteristics such as mechanism of injury [60], extracranial injuries [34, 61], duration of PTA [32], and clinical findings [62] have been related to outcome. Furthermore, preinjury characteristics such as personality traits, vocational status, and education level are related to residual impairments [42, 63, 64]. Few studies have examined which symptoms in the immediate postinjury period best predict subsequent development of PCS [65–68]. Postural instability and dizziness have been related to PCS at 3 months postinjury but not with specific outcome measures. Vomiting and headache at the ER together with noise intolerance and pain assessed within days to weeks after injury have been found to be predictive for PCS [62, 69–71]. However, in the setting of acute trauma care it is not always possible to obtain information on all these variables and therefore early identification of patients who are likely to develop residual complaints is difficult.

It is estimated that 15–25% of patients having sustained mild TBI are at increased risk of developing chronic symptoms, but there is controversy on the actual rate of poor outcome as many studies focus on symptom manifestation rather than on actual level of functioning. The predictive power of most commonly reported complaints after mild TBI is poor because of nonspecificity of complaints that may be reported by those with other injuries [72, 73] and the fact that patients seem to underestimate the prevalence of their preinjury complaints compared to controls.

Furthermore, several factors are associated with the development of chronic postconcussive impairments comprising coping strategies that subjects use, premorbid anxiety, and depression levels, as well as having social support of relatives and close others [63, 67, 74–77]. Mild TBI patients with many complaints have a significantly higher risk on a negative vocational outcome than those with lesser or no complaints [40, 76]. Having postconcussion complaints is significantly related to higher levels of stress and depression which in turn can be conceived as the result of an inadequate coping style [76, 78]. Patients with inadequate coping styles showed a worse psychosocial outcome than patients with adequate coping styles [79, 80].

Treatment strategies

Postconcussive complaints

Because anxiety in the acute phase after injury has been found to be related to persistent PCS [71, 73], interventions aimed at reducing anxiety would be expected to decrease prolonged symptomatology. This is consistent with

Mittenberg's work that reported a beneficial effect of a brief, early cognitive behavioral intervention in reducing the incidence of PCS [72]. In one of the first studies on CBT in mild TBI, reduced anxiety and depression were found although no changes were noted in cognitive measures [81]. However, in this study over half of patients were involved in litigation and were seen several years after injury. One nonrandomized study suggests that the treatment of depression in patients with mild TBI may improve cognitive function [82].

Inadequate coping skills have been found to be a major factor in the development of residual impairments in TBI patients. Inadequate coping pertains to the inability to regulate emotions and adapt responses to a distressing situation and is related to frontal network dysfunction. It manifests itself as unrealistic illness perception, leading to increased feelings of anxiety or depression. This results in persisting residual complaints and impairments and eventually unfavorable outcome. Psychotherapeutic intervention by means of CBT aimed at improving coping skills in order to reduce stress- and anxiety-related responses has proven to be effective in the chronic stage [83, 84] in patients with varying severity of injury.

Whitaker [75] demonstrated that in mild TBI patients, illness perception is decisive for the eventual outcome with higher risk for those who tend to catastrophize on long-term postconcussion complaints interfering with their social and vocational reintegration. Hence, coping style and specifically early illness perception seem plausible targets for psychotherapeutic intervention. In a range of studies, the effectivity of CBT in reducing stress-, depression- and anxiety-related complaints and improving coping skills and adaptive behavior in TBI patients in the chronic stage (6 months or longer postinjury) was proved [83, 85–88].

Return to work

Return to work is another important outcome measure in rehabilitation after TBI. There is little evidence to suggest what should be considered the best approach for vocational rehabilitation [7] although Mateer and Sira [89] argue that CBT is very effective for improving coping styles in TBI patients. Three main categories of vocational rehabilitation for TBI patients are identified based on program-based vocational rehabilitation, supported employment, and case-coordinated care. A postintervention study of mild TBI patients within a rehabilitation setting showed 60% resumption of work, with two-thirds of patients being full-time employed. Age and a high symptom load were found to be negative predictors [90]. After long-term follow-up, approximately 80% of patients fully employed before the injury were found to have resumed full-time work [32]. As a clinical implication, early identification of patients with mild TBI at risk of prolonged time off work is mandatory. Available predictors such as preinjury job status are not sufficient to select suitable patients for intervention. An alternative approach to identify high-risk TBI patients would be a brief screening interview or questionnaire used during the first weeks after injury.

Summary

Most patients with mild TBI recover without specific therapy with a subgroup experiencing residual impairments that interfere with resumption of work and social activities. Routine follow-up may not be needed, but given the consequences of late referral when residual impairments interfere with return to work, it is mandatory to identify those patients at risk for developing persistent symptoms in an early stage. Such knowledge would facilitate risk stratification directly at the emergency department, to help decide which patients need specialized follow-up care focused on return to work and social activities.

References

1 Thornhill, S., Teasdale, G.M., Murray, G.D., McEwen, J., Roy, C.W., & Penny, K.I. (2000) Disability in young people and adults one year after head injury: prospective cohort study. *British Medical Journal*, **320**, 1631–1635.

2 Tagliaferri, F., Compagnone, C., Korsic, M., Servadei, F., & Kraus, J. (2006) A systematic review of brain injury epidemiology in Europe. *Acta Neurochirurgica*, **148**, 255–268.

3 Carroll, L.J., Cassidy, J.D., Holm, L., Kraus, J., & Coronado, V.G.; WHO Collaborating Centre Task Force on Mild Traumatic Brain Injury (2004) Methodological issues and research recommendations for mild traumatic brain injury: the WHO collaborating Centre Task Force on Mild Traumatic Brain Injury. *Journal of Rehabilitation Medicine*, **36 (S43)**, 113–125.

4 Holm, L., Cassidy, J.D., Carroll, L.J., & Borg, J. (2005) Summary of the WHO collaborating Centre for Neurotrauma Task force on Mild traumatic brain injury. *Journal of Rehabilitation Medicine*, **37**, 137–141.

5 Ponsford, J., Willmott, C., Rothwell, A. *et al*. (2000) Factors influencing outcome following mild traumatic brain injury in adults. *Journal of International Neuropsychological Society*, **6**, 568–579.

6 Carroll, L.J., Cassidy, J.D., Peloso, P.M. *et al*.; WHO Collaborating Centre Task Force on Mild Traumatic Brain Injury (2004) Prognosis for mild traumatic brain injury: results of the WHO collaborating centre task force on mild traumatic brain injury. *Journal of Rehabilitation Medicine*, **36 (S43)**, 84–105.

7 Fadyl, J.K. & McPherson, K.M. (2009) Approaches to vocational rehabilitation after traumatic brain injury: a review of the evidence. *The Journal of Head Trauma Rehabilitation*, **24 (3)**, 195–212.

8 Fife, D. (1987) Head injury with and without hospital admission: comparisons of incidence and short-term disability. *Journal of Public Health*, **77**, 810–812.

9 Yasuda, S., Wehman, P., Tagett, P., Cifu, D., & West, M. (2001) Return to work for persons with traumatic brain injury. *American Journal of Physical Medicine and Rehabilitation*, **80 (11)**, 852–864.

10 Ragnarsson, K.T., Moses, L.G., Clarke, W.R. *et al*. (1999) Rehabilitation of persons with traumatic brain injury. *Journal of American Medical Association*, **282**, 974–983.

11 Cassidy, J.D., Carroll, L.J., Peloso, P.M. *et al*.; WHO Collaborating Centre Task Force on Mild Traumatic Brain Injury (2004) Incidence, risk factors and prevention of mild traumatic brain injury: results of the WHO collaborating centre task force on mild traumatic brain injury. *Journal of Rehabilitation Medicine*, **36**, 28–60.

12 Vos, P.E., Battistin, L., Birmarner, G. *et al*.; European Federation of Neurological Societies (2002) EFNS guideline on mild traumatic brain injury: report of an EFNS task force. *European Journal of Neurology*, **9 (3)**, 207–219 [Review].

13 National Institute for Health and Clinical Excellence (2007) *Head Injury: Triage, Assessment, Investigation and Early Management of Head Injury in Infants, Children and Adults.* NICE, London.

14 Naalt van der, J., Hew, J.M., Zomeren van, A.H., Sluiter, W.J., & Minderhoud, J.M. (1999) Computed tomography and magnetic resonance imaging in mild to moderate head injury: early and late imaging related to outcome. *Annals of Neurolgy*, **46**, 70–78.

15 Jacobs, B., Beems, T., Stulemeijer, M. *et al.* (2010) Outcome prediction in mild traumatic brain injury: age and clinical variables are stronger predictors than CT abnormalities. *Journal of Neurotrauma*, **27**, 655–668.

16 Borg, J., Holm, L., Peloso, P.M. *et al.*; WHO Collaborating Centre Task Force on Mild Traumatic Brain Injury (2004) Non-surgical intervention and cost for mild traumatic brain injury: results of the WHO Collaborating Centre Task Force on Mild Head Injury. *Journal of Rehabilitation Medicine*, **S43**, 76–83.

17 Paniak, C., Toller-Lobe, G., Reynolds, S., Melnyk, A., & Nagy, J. (2000) A randomized trial of 2 treatments for mild traumatic brain injury: 1 year follow-up. *Brain Injury*, **14**, 219–226.

18 Wade, D.T., Crawford, S., Wendon, F.J., King, N.S., & Moss, N.E.G. (1997) Does routine follow-up after head injury help? A randomized controlled trial. *Journal of Neurology, Neurosurgery and Psychiatry*, **62**, 478–484.

19 Al Sayegh, A., Sandford, D., & Carson, A.J. Psychological approaches to treatment of post-concussion syndrome: a systematic review. *Journal of Neurology, Neurosurgery and Psychiatry*, **81**, 1128–1134.

20 Parizel, P.M., van Goethem, J.W., Ozsarlak, O., Maes, M., & Phillips, C.D. (2005) New developments in the neuroradiological diagnosis of cranial cerebral trauma. *European Radiology*, **15**, 569–581.

21 Gomez, P., Lobato, R., Ortega, J.M., & Dela Cruz, J. (1996) Mild head injury: differences in prognosis among patients with a Glasgow Coma Score of 13 to 15 associated with abnormal CT-findings. *British Journal of Neurosurgery*, **10**, 453–460.

22 Metting, Z., Rodiger, L.A., DeKeyser, J., & van der Naalt, J. (2007) Structural and functional neuroimaging in mild-to-moderate head injury. *Lancet Neurology*, **6**, 699–710.

23 Yaganawa, Y., Tsushima, T., Tokumaru, A. *et al.* (2000) A quantitative analysis of head injury using T2*-weighted gradient-echo imaging. *The Journal of Trauma*, **49**, 272–277.

24 Scheid, R., Preul, C., Gruber, O., Wiggins, C., & von Cramon, D.Y. (2003) Diffuse axonal injury associated with chronic traumatic brain injury: evidence from T2*-weighted gradient-echo imaging at 3T. *American Journal of Neuroradiology*, **24**, 1049–1054.

25 Hughes, D.G., Jackson, A., Mason, D.L., Berry, E., Hollis, S., & Yates, D.W. (2004) Abnormalities on magnetic resonance imaging seen acutely following mild traumatic brain injury: correlation with neuropsychological tests and delayed recovery. *Neuroradiology*, **46**, 550–558.

26 Kurca, E., Sivak, S., & Kucera, P. (2006) Impaired cognitive functions in mild traumatic brain injury patients with normal and pathologic magnetic resonance imaging. *Neuroradiology*, **48**, 661–669.

27 Sigmund, G.A., Tong, T.A, Nickerson, J.P., Wall, C.J., Oyoyo, U., & Ashwal, S. (2007) Multimodality comparison of neuroimaging in pediatric traumatic brain injury. *Pediatric Neurology*, **36**, 217–226.

28 Chastain, C.A., Oyoyo, U.E., Zipperman, M. *et al.* (2009) Predicting outcome of traumatic brain injury by imaging modality and injury distribution. *Journal of Neurotrauma*, **26**, 1183–1196.

29 Naalt van der, J. (2001) Prediction of outcome in mild to moderate head injury: a review. *Journal of Clinical and Experimental Neuropsychology*, **23 (6)**, 837–851.

30 Englander, J., Hall, K., Stimpson, T., & Chaffin, S. (1992) Mild traumatic brain injury in an insured population: subjective complaints and return to employment. *Brain Injury*, **6**, 161–166.

31 Stambrook, M. (1990) Effects of mild, moderate and severe closed head injury on long-term vocational status. *Brain Injury*, **4**, 183–190.

32 Naalt van der, J., Zomeren van, A.H., Sluiter, W.J., & Minderhoud, J.M. (1999) One year outcome in mild to moderate head injury: the predictive value of acute injury characteristics related to complaints and return to work. *Journal of Neurology, Neurosurgery and Psychiatry*, **66**, 207–213.

33 Rimel, R.W. (1981) Disability caused by minor head injury. *Neurosurgery*, **9**, 221–228.

34 Dacey, R., Dikmen, S., Temkin, N., McLean, A., Armsden, G., & Winn, H.R. (1991) Relative effects of brain and non-brain injuries on neuropsychological and psychosocial outcome. *The Journal of Trauma*, **31 (2)**, 217–222.

35 Pagulayan, K.F., Temkin, N.R., Mahamer, J., & Dikmen, S.S. (2006) A longitudinal study of health-related quality of life after traumatic brain injury. *Archives of Physical Medicine and Rehabilitation*, **87**, 611–618.

36 Kwok, F.Y., Lee, T.M.C., Leung, C.H.S., & Poon, W.S. (2008). Changes of cognitive functioning following mild traumatic brain injury over a 3-month period. *Brain Injury*, **22 (10)**, 740–751.

37 Kashluba, S., Hanks, R.A., Casey, J.E., & Millis, S.R. (2008) Neuropsychologic and functional outcome after complicated mild traumatic brain injury. *Archives of Physical Medicine and Rehabilitation*, **89**, 904–911.

38 Belanger, H.G., Curtiss, G., Demery, J.A., Lebowitz, B.K., & Vanderploeg, R.D. (2005) Factors moderating neuropsychological outcomes following mild traumatic brain injury: a meta-analysis. *Journal of the International Neuropsychological Society*, **11**, 215–227.

39 Binder, L.M., Rohling, M.L., & Larrabee, G.J. (1997) A review of mild head trauma. Part 1. Meta-analytic review of neuropsychological studies. *Journal of Clinical and Experimental Neuropsychology*, **19**, 421–431.

40 Frencham, K.A., Fox, A.M., & Maybery, M.T. (2005) Neuropsychological studies of mild traumatic brain injury: a meta-analytic review of research since 1995. *Journal of Clinical and Experimental Neuropsychology*, **27**, 334–351.

41 Dikmen, S.S., Corrigan, J.D., Levin, H.S., Machamer, J., Stiers, W., & Weisskopf, M.G. (2009) Cognitive outcome following traumatic brain injury. *The Journal of Head Trauma Rehabilitation*, **24**, 430–438.

42 Stulemeijer, M., Andriessen, T.M.J.C., Brauer, J.M.P., Vos, P.E., & Van Der Werf, S. (2007) Cognitive performance after mild head injury: the impact of poor effort on test results and its relation to distress, personality and litigation. *Brain Injury*, **21**, 309–318.

43 Suhr, J.A. & Gunstad, J. (2002) "Diagnosis Threat": the effect of negative expectations on cognitive performance in head injury. *Journal of Clinical and Experimental Neuropsychology*, **24**, 448–457.

44 Suhr, J.A. & Gunstad, J. (2005) Further exploration of the effect of "diagnosis threat" on cognitive performance in individuals with mild head injury. *Journal of the International Neuropsychological Society*, **11**, 23–29.

45 Ozen, L.J. & Fernandes, M.A. (2011) Effects of "Diagnosis Threat" on cognitive and affective functioning long after mild head injury. *Journal of the International Neuropsychological Society*, **17**, 219–229.

46 Dikmen, S.S., Temkin, N.R., Machamer, J.E., Holubkov, A.L., Fraser, R.T., & Winn, H.R. (1994) Employment following traumatic head injuries. *Archives of Neurology*, **51**, 177–186.

47 Boake, C., McCauley, S.R., Pedroza, C., Levin, H.S., Brown, S.A., & Brundage, S.I. (2005) Lost productive work time after mild to moderate traumatic brain injury with and without hospitalization. *Neurosurgery*, **56**, 994–1003.

48 Asikainen, I., Kaste, M., & Sarnas, S. (1998) Predicting late outcome for patients with traumatic brain injury referred to a rehabilitation programme: a study of 508 Finnish patients 5 years or more after injury. *Brain Injury*, **12 (2)**, 95–107.

49 Masson, F., Maurette, P., Salmi, L.R. *et al.* (1996) Prevalence of impairments 5 years after a head injury and their relationship with disabilities and outcome. *Brain Injury,* **10 (7)**, 487–497.

50 Engberg, A.W. & Teasdale, T.W. (2004) Psychosocial outcome following traumatic brain injury in adults: a long-term population based follow-up. *Brain Injury,* **18 (6)**, 533–545.

51 Testa, J.A., Malec, J.F., Moessner, A.M. *et al.* (2006) Predicting family functioning after TBI. Impact of neurobehavioral factors. *The Journal of Head Trauma Rehabilitation,* **3**, 236–247.

52 Huang, S.J., Ho, H.L., & Yang, C.C. (2010) Longitudinal outcomes of patients with traumatic brain injury: a preliminary study. *Brain Injury,* **24**, 1606–1615.

53 Hanks, R.A., Temkin, N., Machamer, J., & Dikmen, S.S. (1999) Emotional and behavioral adjustment after traumatic brain injury. *Archives of Physical Medicine and Rehabilitation,* **80**, 991–999.

54 Vander Ploeg, R., Curtiss, G., Luis, C.A., & Salazar, A.M. (2007) Long-term morbidities following self-reported mild traumatic brain injury. *Journal of Clinical and Experimental Neuropsychology,* **29 (6)**, 585–598.

55 Whitnall, L., McMillan, T.M., Murray, G.D., & Teasdale, G.M. (2006) Disability in young people and adults after head injury: 5–7 year follow up of a prospective cohort study. *Journal of Neurology, Neurosurgery and Psychiatry,* **77**, 640–645.

56 Konrad, C., Geburek, A.J., Rist, F. *et al.* (2011) Long-term cognitive and emotional consequences of mild traumatic brain injury. *Psychological Medicine,* **41**(6), 1197–1202.

57 Hessen, E., Nestvold, K., & Anderson, V. (2007) neuropsychological function 23 years after mild traumatic brain injury: a comparison of outcome after paediatric and adult head injuries. *Brain Injury,* **21**, 963–979.

58 Zumstein, M.A., Moser, M., Mottini, M. *et al.* (2011) Long-term outcome in patients with mild traumatic brain injury: a prospective observational study. *The Journal of Trauma,* **71**(1):120–127.

59 Brown, A.W., Moessner, A.M., Mandrekr, J., Diehl, N.N., Leibson, C.L., & Malec, J.F. (2011) A survey of very-long-term outcomes after traumatic brain injury among members of a population-based incident cohort. *Journal of Neurotrauma,* **28**, 167–176.

60 Hanlon, R.E., Dermery, J.A., Martinovich, Z., & Kelly, J.P. (1999) Effects of acute injury characteristics on neuropsychological status and vocational outcome following mild traumatic brain injury. *Brain Injury,* **13 (11)**, 873–878.

61 Stulemeijer, M., van der Werff, S.P., Jacobs, B. *et al.* (2006) Impact of additional extracranial injuries on outcome after mild traumatic brain injury. *Journal of Neurotrauma,* **23**, 1561–1569.

62 Fabbri, A., Servadei, F., Marchesini, G. *et al.* (2004) Prospective validation of a proposal for diagnosis and management of patients attending the emergency department for mild head injury. *Journal of Neurology, Neurosurgery and Psychiatry,* **75**, 410–416.

63 Dawson, D.R., Schwartz, M.L., & Winocur, G. (2007) Return to productivity following traumatic brain injury: cognitive, psychological, physical, spiritual and environmental correlates. *Disability and Rehabilitation,* **29 (4)**, 301–313.

64 Dikmen, S., Machamer, J., & Temkin, N. (2001) Mild head injury: facts and artifacts. *Journal of Clinical Experimental Neuropsychology,* **23 (6)**, 729–738.

65 De Kruijk, J.R., Menheere, P.P.C.A., Meerhoff, S., Meerhoff, S., Rutten, J., & Twijnstra, A. (2002) Prediction of post-traumatic complaints after mild traumatic brain injury: early symptoms and biochemical markers. *Journal of Neurology, Neurosurgery and Psychiatry,* **73**, 727–732.

66 Savola, O. & Hilbom, M. (2003) Early predictors of post-concussion symptoms in patients with mild head injury. *European Journal of Neurology,* **10**, 175–181.

67 Lundin, A., de Boussard, C., Edman, G., & Borg, J. (2006) Symptoms and disability until 3 months after mild TBI. *Brain Injury,* **20 (8)**, 799–806.

68 Sheedy, J., Harvey, E., Faux, S., Geffen, G., & Shores, E.A. (2009) Emergency department assessment of mild traumatic brain injury and the prediction of postconcussive symptoms: a 3-month prospective study. *The Journal of Head Trauma Rehabilitation,* **24 (5)**, 333–343.

69 Bohnen, N., Twijstra, A., Wijnen, G., & Jolles, J. (1991) Tolerance for light and sound of patients with persistent post-concussional symptoms 6 months after mild head injury. *Journal of Neurology*, **238**, 443–446.

70 Stulemeijer, M., van der Werff, S., Borm, G.F., & Vos, P.E. (2008) Early prediction of favorable recovery after mild traumatic brain injury. *Journal of Neurology, Neurosurgery and Psychiatry*, **79**, 936–942.

71 Dischinger, P.C., Ryb, G.E., Kufera, J.A., & Auman, K.M. (2009) Early predictors of postconcussive syndrome in a population of trauma patients with mild traumatic brain injury. *The Journal of Trauma*, **66**, 289–297.

72 Mittenberg, W., DiGuilio, D.V., Perin, S., & Bass, A.E. (1992) Symptoms following mild head injury: expectation as etiology. *Journal of Neurology, Neurosurgery and Psychiatry*, **55**, 200–204.

73 Meares, S., Shores, E.A., Taylor, A.J. *et al.* (2008) Mild traumatic brain injury does not predict acute postconcussion syndrome. *Journal of Neurology, Neurosurgery and Psychiatry*, **79**, 300–306.

74 Bernstein, D.M. (1999) Recovery from mild head injury. *Brain Injury*, **13**, 151–172.

75 Whittaker, R., Kemp, S., & House, A. (2007) Illness perceptions and outcome in mild head injury: a longitudinal study. *Journal of Neurology, Neurosurgery and Psychiatry*, **78**, 644–646.

76 King, N.S. (1996) Emotional, neuropsychological, and organic postconcussion factors: their use in the prediction of persisting postconcussion symptoms after moderate and mild head injuries. *Journal of Neurology, Neurosurgery and Psychiatry*, **61**, 75–81.

77 Malec, J.F., Testa, J.A., Rush, B.K., Brown, A.W., & Moessner, A.M. (2007) Self-assessment of impairment, impaired self-awareness and depression after traumatic brain injury. *The Journal of Head Trauma Rehabilitation*, **22 (3)**, 156–166.

78 Mateer, C.A. & Sira, C.S. (2006) Cognitive and emotional consequences of TBI: intervention strategies for vocational rehabilitation. *Neurorehabilitation*, **21**, 315–326.

79 Guerin, F., Kennepohl, S., Leveille, G., Dominique, A., & McKerral, M. (2006) Vocational outcome indicators in atypically recovering mild TBI: a post-intervention study. *Neurorehabilitation*, **21**, 295–303.

80 Machulda, M.M., Bergquist, T.F., Ito, V., & Chew, S. (1998) Relationship between stress, coping and postconcussion symptoms in a healthy adult population. *Archives of Clinical Neuropscyhology* **13 (5)**, 415–424.

81 Malia, K., Powell, G., & Torode, S. (1995) Coping and psychosocial function after brain injury. *Brain Injury*, **9**, 607–618.

82 Moore, A.D. & Stambrook, M. (1995) Cognitive moderators of outcome following traumatic brain injury: a conceptual model and implications for rehabilitation. *Brain Injury*, **9**, 109–130.

83 Tiersky, L.A., Anselmi, V., Johnston, M.V. *et al.* (2005) A trial of neuropsychological rehabilitation in mild-spectrum traumatic brain injury. *Archives of Physical Medicine and Rehabilitation*, **86 (8)**, 1565–1574.

84 Fann, J.R., Uomoto, J.M., & Katon, W.J. (2001) Cognitive improvement of depression following mild traumatic brain injury. *Psychosomatics*, **42**, 48–54.

85 Pastore, V., Colombo, K., Liscio, M. *et al.* (2011) Efficacy of cognitive behavioural therapy for children and adolescents with traumatic brain injury. *Disability and Rehabilitation* , **33**(8):675–683.

86 Wolters, G., Stapert, S., Brands, I., & van Heugten, C. (2010) Coping styles in relation to cognitive rehabilitation and quality of life after brain injury. *Neuropsychological Rehabilitation*, **20 (4)**, 587–600.

87 Huckans, M., Pavawalla, S., Demadura, T. *et al.* (2010) A pilot study examining effects of group-based Cognitive Strategy Training treatment on self-reported cognitive problems, psychiatric symptoms, functioning and compensatory strategy use in OIF/OEF combat veterans with persistent cognitive disorder and history of traumatic brain injury. *Journal of Rehabilitation Research Development*, **47**, 43–60.

88 Soo, C. & Tate, R. (2007) Psychological treatment for anxiety in people with traumatic brain injury. *Cochrane Database of Systematic Review*, **18**, CD005239.

89 Williams, W.H., Evans, J.J., & Wilson, B.A. (2003) Neurorehabilitation for two cases of post-traumatic stress disorder following traumatic brain injury. *Cognitive Neuropsychiatry*, **8**, 1–18.

90 Anson, K. & Ponsford, J. (2006) Coping and emotional adjustment following traumatic brain injury. *The Journal of Head Trauma Rehabilitation*, **21 (3)**, 248–259.

Index

Traumatic Brain Injury, First Edition. Edited by Pieter E. Vos and Ramon Diaz-Arrastia.
© 2015 John Wiley & Sons, Ltd. Published 2015 by John Wiley & Sons, Ltd.